Current Practices in Ophthalmology

Current Practices in Ophthalmology

Editor: Ray George

AMERICAN
MEDICAL PUBLISHERS
www.americanmedicalpublishers.com

AMERICAN
MEDICAL PUBLISHERS
www.americanmedicalpublishers.com

Cataloging-in-publication Data

Current practices in ophthalmology / edited by Ray George.
p. cm.
Includes bibliographical references and index.
ISBN 979-8-88740-032-7
1. Ophthalmology. 2. Eye--Diseases. I. George, Ray.
RE46 .C87 2023
617.7--dc23

American Medical Publishers,
41 Flatbush Avenue,
1st Floor, New York,
NY 11217, USA

ISBN 979-8-88740-032-7 (Hardback)

Contents

Preface

Ophthalmology is a branch of medicine that studies eye physiology, eye disorders, and different types of treatments. Techniques used within this field can help diagnose a wide range of eye diseases and ailments. Some of the major diseases studied within this area of medicine are cataract, thyroid eye disease, dry eye syndrome, refractive errors and macular degeneration. There are numerous subspecialties within ophthalmology such as neuro-ophthalmology, refractive surgery, plastic and reconstructive surgery and ocular oncology. Neuro-ophthalmology focuses on the eye issues related to the nervous system. Refractive surgery focuses on reducing the dependency on contact lenses and prescription glasses by improving the refractive state of the eye. This book consists of contributions made by international experts and aims to shed light on some of the current practices in opthalmology. It presents some of the vital pieces of work being conducted across the world, on various topics related to this field. This book will serve as a resource guide for experts as well as students.

This book is a comprehensive compilation of works of different researchers from varied parts of the world. It includes valuable experiences of the researchers with the sole objective of providing the readers (learners) with a proper knowledge of the concerned field. This book will be beneficial in evoking inspiration and enhancing the knowledge of the interested readers.

In the end, I would like to extend my heartiest thanks to the authors who worked with great determination on their chapters. I also appreciate the publisher's support in the course of the book. I would also like to deeply acknowledge my family who stood by me as a source of inspiration during the project.

Editor

1

Imaging Devices and Glaucoma Management

Pinakin Gunvant Davey

1. Introduction

The definition of glaucoma varies depending upon the source or criteria of the randomized controlled trial evaluated. Thus the diagnosis of glaucoma can be enigmatic due to lack of universally accepted definition of glaucoma that covers all facets of glaucoma pathogenesis. The classic definition of having the triad of visual field damage, nerve head damage and elevated intraocular pressure is no longer valid. Although intraocular pressure remains arguably the most important risk factor its absolute value may be elevated or remain within the statistical limits of normality depending upon the type of glaucoma. Issues related to glaucoma management are anything but cookbook type Therefore glaucoma remains interesting for clinicians that manage patients with glaucoma and researchers that study its pathogenesis.

The patients at risk of glaucoma undergo cellular level damage that is manifests as both structural damage at posterior pole of the eye and damage to functional vision. The major goals of glaucoma management are quite clear; to halt the progressive damage of the disease and maintain functional vision with least disruption to quality of life. As we know now that structure damage (optic nerve or retinal nerve fiber layer) often precede functional damage, however this is not universal as imaging devices many not be sensitive enough to pick up subtle damages.[1] Given that scenario it is the recommendation of both and American Optometric association and American Academy of Ophthalmology to record both structure and visual function in patients at risk of glaucomatous optic neuropathy.[2 3]

Obtaining objective data on the morphology and the structure of optic nerve and nerve fiber layer is of great advantage particularly if it is repeatable and reproducible because there is great amount of intra and inter observer variability amongst clinicians. To this accord the computerized imaging technologies can obtain automated evaluation of structural damage in eyes at risk of glaucoma particularly because imaging is less influenced by disease severity and has low long term variability. [4] This article will cover: 1) the technology behind each imaging device, 2) understand parts of the output that is important parameters that have shown to be clinically useful, having diagnostic or prognostic ability. This article will also evaluate: 3) the output of imaging devices to evaluate progressive damage in individuals at risk of glaucoma. Further this article will also discuss the common imaging artifacts that can influence the outcome of the imaging tests.

Most experts in the field will agree to the fact that stereo optic disc imaging is perhaps the gold standard of all techniques of optic disc evaluation.[3 5 6] Fundus cameras can generate a stereo disc images by either displacing the camera system thus creating an offset and obtain two pictures sequentially. The disadvantage of such a technique is that the amount of displacement can differ from one visit to another that can lead to erroneous judgment. Ideally stereo optic disc pictures should be captured by simultaneously this can be achieved by having a dual camera system that captures two images simultaneously. Also until recent years automated analysis of the optic disc morphology was not readily available and investigators of various studies performed planimetry to evaluate disc morphology.[5 6] With the advances in automated analysis this technique may see a revival and increased use in clinical care.

The computerized imaging devices are fundamentally Scanning Laser Ophthalmoscope, Scanning Laser Polarimeter or Optical Coherence Tomograph. These technologies may provide similar information but there are fundamental differences between devices that makes the measurements obtained from each non-interchangeable. Furthermore there is benefit to be gained by performing multiple imaging on the same patient as it may yield additional clinical details.

2. Scanning laser ophthalmoscope

Heidelberg Engineering manufactures Heidelberg Retina Tomograph III (HRT which is the current generation scanning laser ophthalmoscope that provides topographical data of the optic nerve and peri-papillary retina. Using high speed raster scanning technique and diode laser for illumination HRT obtains two-dimensional images of retina and optic nerve. The depth of focal plane is automatically adjusted to obtain multiple two-dimensional images. The HRT III acquires 16 to 64 2-dimentional images to a maximum depth of 4 mm that starts at vitreo-retinal interface to beyond the bottom of the optic disc cupping. The number of optic section varies in different eyes. The eye with deep cupping has an increase in number of sections (two-dimensional images). The optic sections are combined to produce a three-dimensional topography of the optic disc surface. This is repeated up to six time and the best three are selected and averaged to obtain the final output.

2.1. Interpretation of a HRT III output

There are various reports with different level of information that is produced by the device. The author believes that the OU report (Figure 1) is an excellent output of various parameters that are clinically useful in making judgment and patient education. The quality of the scan is judged on the value of standard deviation; the lower the value of standard deviation the better is the quality of the scan (see section A Figure 1). The HRT III provides useful information on optic disc size. The device software classifies the optic disc, average or large once the user has outlined the optic disc margin (see section A Figure 1). Overall HRT's optic disc analysis provides details of cup information, neuro-retinal rim information and retinal nerve fiber layer (RNFL) information. The right eye of the patient is compared to the left eye and the between eyes asymmetry is also provided. All parameters provided are also compared to the normative database to evaluate if parameters are within statistical limits of normality, borderline or outside normal limits.

A color coded figure provides the cupping information (section B Figure 1). The cupping is represented by the red color where as the neuro retinal rim is represented by blue and green with blue being sloping rim and the green the stable rim. The cup volume is provided as one of the parameters and in eyes suspicious of glaucoma or progressive loss of neuro-retinal rim we can see an increase in cup volume. The cup shape measure is an overall value of three-dimensional representation of cupping and the values are negative in an ocular healthy eye and more positive in an eye suspicious of glaucoma.

The rim details provided are rim area and rim volume both will see a decline with progression of glaucomatous optic neuropathy (see Section C Figure 1). Additionally once the outline of optic disc is marked the device automatically generates Moorfields Regression Analysis. This is arguably the single most important parameter and is discussed in greater detail below. HRT also provides RNFL which is measured 360 degrees just outside the disc margin (see Section D Figure 1). This location of measurement differs from the location of measurement of both the Scanning Laser Polarimeter-GDx-Pro and Optical Coherence Tomograph. Thus the RNFL measured using one technology will not match the values obtained by other and should not be used interchangeably.

All HRT parameters are given symbols of green check mark, yellow exclamation point, or red X which represents statistical limits of normality that is within normal limits, borderline or outside normal limits respectively.

2.2. Moorefield's regression analysis

The Moorfields Regression Analysis was developed by Dr. David Garway-Heath and colleagues [7 8] at the Moorfields hospital, London England. The Moorfields Regression Analysis (MRA) provides an ability to perform cross-sectional analysis, thus classifying an eye as at risk or within normal limits. The analysis exploits prior knowledge that the neuro retinal rim area is positively correlated with the disc size that is the larger the disc size greater is the rim area[9 10] and additionally the rim area narrows in eyes with glaucomatous optic neuropathy[11 12]. The MRA provides information if the rim area of an eye is within 95%, 99% or 99.9% of population. The optic nerve is divided into six sectors, superior 90 degrees is divided into superior nasal and superior temporal, similarly inferior 90 degrees are divided into inferior nasal and inferior temporal. The nasal and temporal 90 degrees form the remaining two sectors. If a rim area falls between 95 to 99% or greater than 99% of predicted population interval it is labeled as borderline or outside normal limits respectively. If any sector falls in either of these two categories the MRA is classified as Outside Normal Limits.

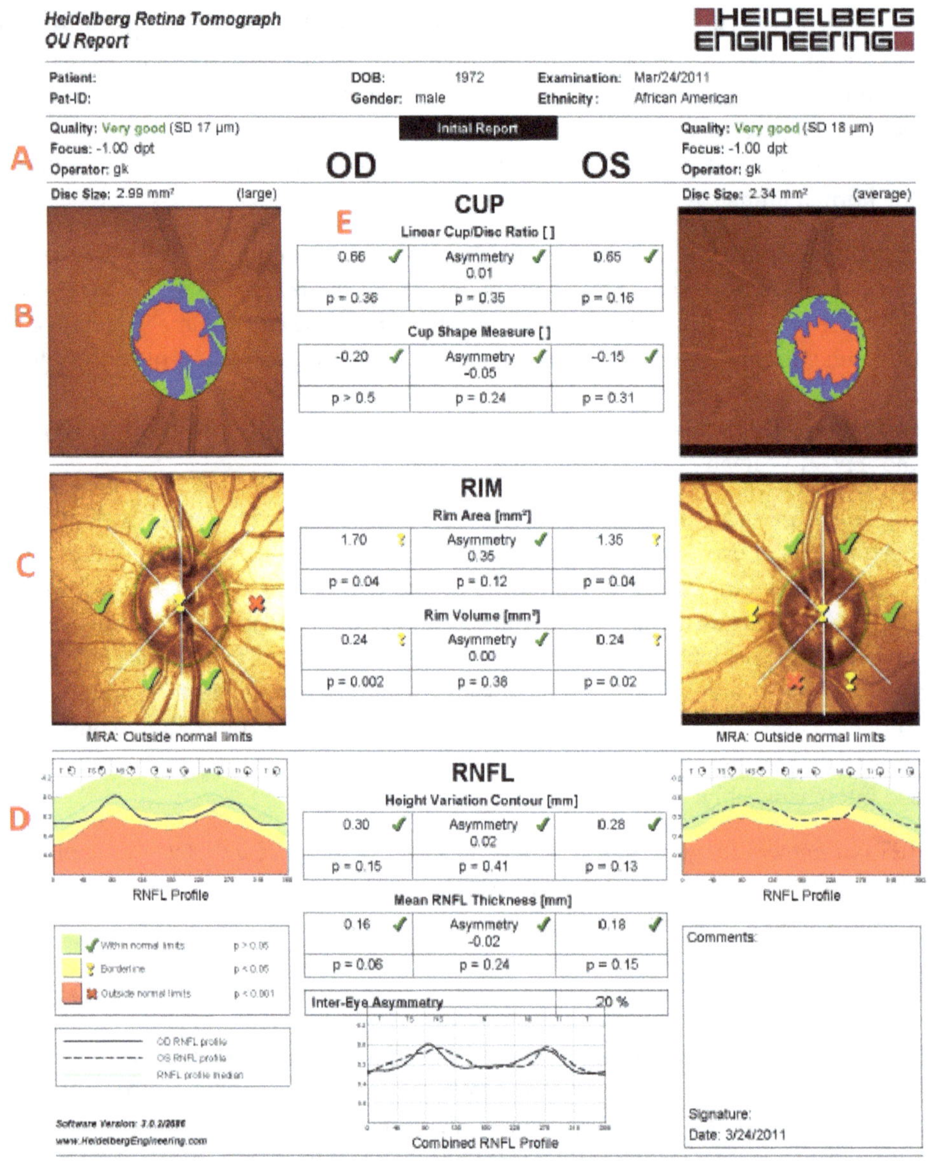

Figure 1. An OU report obtained using HRT III. Section A shows that reliability of the scan and the size of the disc which is obtained once the operator outlines the disc margin. Section B is a courtesy pseudo-isochromatic fundus image that shows the rim and cupping. Red color represents the cupping whereas the blue and the green are rim tissue. Section C shows the Moorfields regression analysis of various sectors of optic disc and section D shows RNFL in the TSNIT region. The section E provides the right eye and left eye information of various parameters measured and its asymmetry analysis along with statistical significance

This parameter was investigated in an Ancillary Study to Ocular Hypertension Treatment Study and was found to be a significant predictor of future development of glaucomatous optic neuropathy in a group of ocular hypertensive eyes.[13] Additionally a more recent report from the same study indicates that these parameters are as effective as stereo photographs at estimating risk of development of primary open angle glaucoma in a group of ocular hypertensive eyes. [14]

3. Scanning laser polarimetry

Carl Zeiss Meditec manufactures the GDx-Pro which is the current generation scanning laser polarimeter. The scanning laser polarimeter uses near infrared laser (780 nm) in a raster pattern to image both the macula and peripapillary region. Details about the working principles can be found in detail elsewhere. [15] Birefringence is optical property that split a light wave by a polar material into two components. These components travel at different velocities which creates a relative phase shift. The phase shift is termed retardation. A few ocular structures, cornea, lens and retinal nerve fiber layer that are highly organized and parallel structures are birefringent. The scanning laser polarimeter is a confocal scanning laser ophthalmoscope that is capable of measuring retardation. It is shown that the RNFL retardation measured using the scanning laser polarimeter correlates well with the retinal RNFL determined by histology. [16 17]

3.1. Measurement and Interpretation of GDx — Pro output

The scanning laser polarimeter as a first step calculates anterior segment birefringence. This procedure is needed only once when examining the patient for the first time as anterior segment birefringence remains similar throughout life If there is a significant change in anterior segment like refractive or cataract surgery it is recommended to re-calculate the anterior segment birefringence. [18-20] Second part of the test is to obtain the brirefringence of the peripapillary retina. Clinicians can choose to scan the eye once or thrice. Obtaining more than one scan during the visit and averaging the scans decreases the variability in measurements obtained.

The output of optic nerve head and peripapillary images are divided into three parts the fundus image, retinal nerve fiber layer map and deviation map (see Figure 2 section A, B and C respectively). The fundus image (Figure 2 section A) in a GDx-Pro printout is a misnomer because the device uses a monochromatic light to capture the image. This image is only utilized to evaluate the focus, centration of scan and to be certain that the scan is evenly illuminated. The retinal nerve fiber layer map provides information about the thickness of retinal nerve fiber layer in a 20-degree image with the optic nerve in the center (Figure 2 section B). It is expected that in healthy eyes inferior and superior retinal nerve fiber layer is thick and represented with bright red and yellow where as the nasal and temporal regions are thinner and is represented with cooler colors like blue. The deviation map provides information if the retinal nerve fiber layer thickness points on the 20 degree image is within statistical limits of normality or has a less than 5%, 2%, 1% or 0.5% chance of being normal (Figure 2 section C).

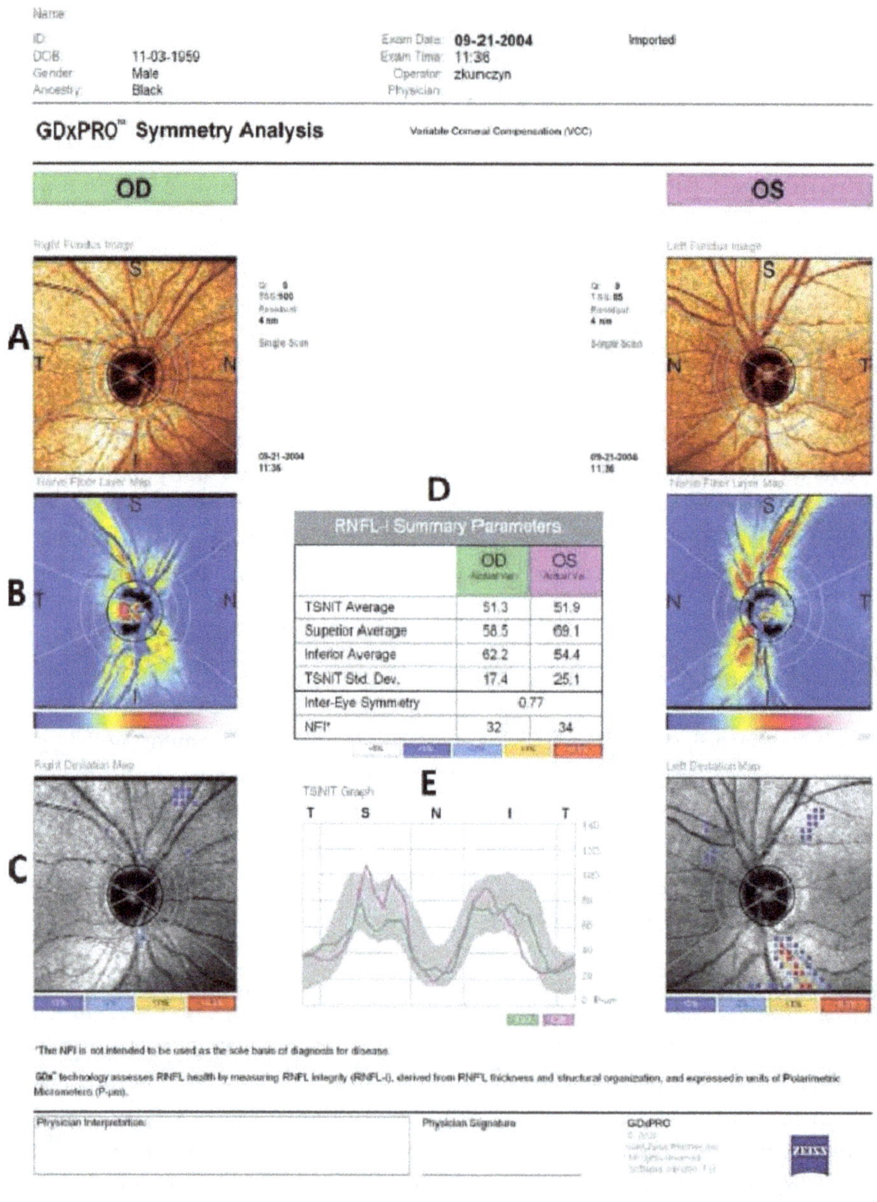

Figure 2. An output obtained using the GDX-Pro scanning laser polarimeter. Section A, B and C represents the courtesy pseudo-isochromatic fundus image, RNFL thickness plot and the deviation plot respectively. The Section C left eye shows a cluster of superpixels in the inferior temporal region that possibly indicates early damage. Section D and E provide the various parameters and TSNIT RNFL plot that can be used diagnostically. Image Courtesy Dr. Joseph Sowka OD, Professor, Nova Southeastern University, College of Optometry.

The two white rings shown on the three image maps is the region where the RNFL is measured to provide the various parameters (figure 2 D) and the thickness profile of the retinal nerve fiber layer in the temporal, superior, nasal, inferior and temporal (TSNIT) region in the peripapillary retina of both eyes (Figure 2 E). The more similar the profiles are the less likely they are glaucomatous, however one has to remember the two eyes of an individual although similar most definitely will have differences.

There are various thickness parameters like TSNIT average, inferior average, superior average are provided along with color coding to indicate if they are within statistical limits of normality. The GDx-Pro also provides with a classifier the Nerve Fiber Indicator (NFI) that ranges 0 to 100 and a higher number is likely suggestive of damage. The manufacturers recommend that a NFI value of less than 30 has a low likelihood of glaucoma, a value between 30 and 50 should be considered a suspect and a value greater than 50 has a high likelihood of glaucoma. Numerous studies have shown that the NFI is the best GDx parameter at differentiating ocular healthy and glaucoma eyes. [21-24]

4. Optical coherence tomography

It is indeed an understatement to say that optical coherence tomography (OCT) has revolutionized clinical imaging in eye care. It was one of the fastest accepted technologies in eye care which is capable of obtaining micron resolution cross-sectional or tomographic scans of biological tissue in vivo. The principles of OCT are similar to ultrasound devices. The OCT uses light instead of sound thus providing excellent resolution (5-10 microns and 15 microns transverse). The echo time delay (that is the delay in time from when the ray of light leaves the device till the reflected light is received back) is calculated thus measuring distance that is an axial scan (A-scan). This is done at about 400 times per second. The axial scans are added to obtain the B-scan of the location being measured. The OCT principles described above is a "Time-domain (TD) OCT". The TD OCT devices are manufactured by Carl Zeiss Meditec. Although a phenomenal breakthrough in itself it was limited by number of scans it was capable of measuring. The scan regions measured were small and time taken was much larger. This was remedied by the "Fourier-Domain" technology. The Fourier domain technology uses a broader band width light source than the time domain OCT with a spectrometer to obtain the spectral interferogram that when analyzed using Fast-Fourier Transformation obtains the A-scan. The A-scans are obtained at a rate of 26,000 to 40,000 per second. Thus large amounts of data can be obtained in a short duration which was not possible accurately using the Time-domain OCT.

Numerous companies' manufacture the Fourier-domain OCT. This article will discuss general parameters output by all OCTs. Furthermore the OCT is capable of measuring both anterior segment and posterior segment. This article is going to restrict to analyzing output of posterior segment scan.

The OCT outputs the retinal nerve fiber layer thickness map and a deviation map (Figure 3 sections A and B). The RNFL thickness map (Figure 3 section A) is similar in interpretation as GDx-Pro which is color coded and it is expected that the inferior and superior region will show thicker RNFL compared to nasal and temporal regions in healthy eyes. The deviation map (Figure 3 section B) provides information if the given region is within statistical limits of normality. It also doubles as a fundus image; a careful look at this region is a must, to evaluate centration, focus and identify any errors in imaging (see next section for further details). The section B, similar to other devices and should not be utilized as a substitute to fundus photography.

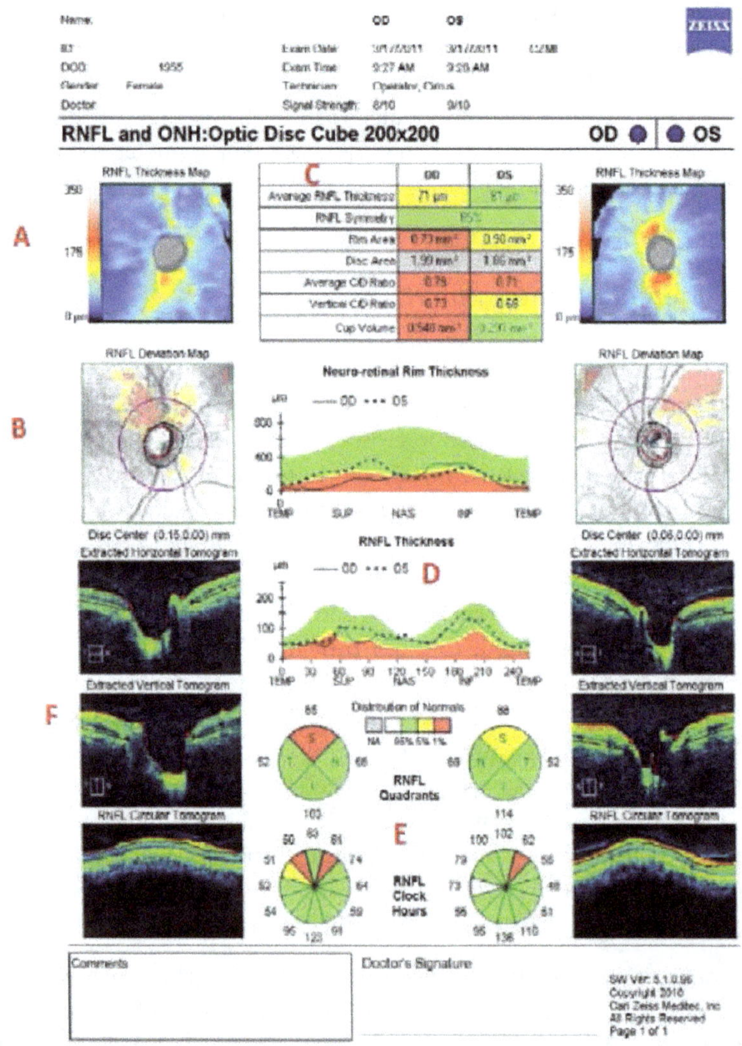

Figure 3. An output of RNFL analysis of Cirrus OCT. Section A shows the thickness map and section B shows the fundus image and highlights regions that are not within statistical limits of normality. Section C provides with the table of various parameters. Section D provides the TSNIT RNFL thickness profile and Section E provides thickness in various sectors and clock hours respectively. The section B,C, D and E are color coded to give an idea if the thickness measurement region or a parameter are within statistical limits of normality or outside normal limits. Section F provides with the vertical and horizontal tomogram obtained at the 12 and 6 O'clock & 3 and 9 O'clock of disc and peripapillary retina providing layer by layer thickness profile of retina and optic disc. The Circular tomogram in Section F is the cross-sectional thickness profile taken on the region of purple ring in section B.

The purple ring in Figure 3 Section B denotes the region where the RNFL is measured on the Temporal Superior, Nasal, Inferior and Temporal (TSNIT) region. This is utilized to calculate the RNFL parameters like the Average RNFL thickness and symmetry provided in the table (Figure3 Section C). The RNFL thickness profile obtained from the purple ring around the optic nerve is plotted graphically for both eyes to obtain symmetry information (Figure 3 section D). The graph has three color coded regions: 1) green represents 95% of normal distribution. 2) The yellow in RNFL plot represents the population that has less than 5% but greater than 1% chance of being normal and is also called the "borderline" category, whereas, 3) the red in the RNFL plot represents <1% chance of being normal; the "outside normal limits" category. The OCT also provides disc parameters in the table of parameters that includes cup to disc ratio cup volume, disc area and rim area (Figure 3 section C). The OCT also provides the RNFL values in each quadrant and each clock hour (Figure 3 Section E). The analysis reports of Optovue OCT Heidelberg and Engineering Spectralis is very similar to that of explained of Cirrus OCT (See Figure 4 and 5).

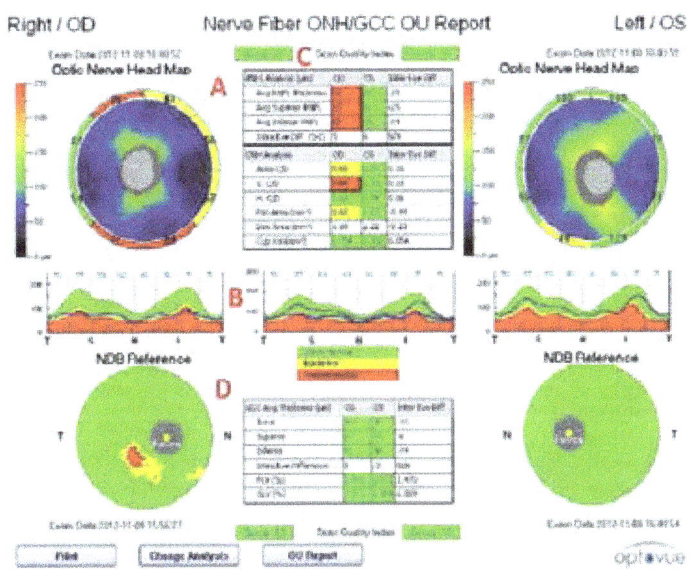

Figure 4. A combined output of retinal nerve fiber layer and ganglion cell complex map obtained by Optovue iVue OCT. The section A provides thickness information around the disc, section B the RNFL thickness in TSNIT region and section C provides the various parameters. The section D provides the ganglion cell complex parameters and the map. The right eye data shows that the infero temporal macula region shows damage that is statistically significant. All sections are color coded to provide information on statistical significance. Image courtesy Dr. Qienyuan Zhou PhD Optovue Inc.

Because OCTs are relatively new technology, automated machine learning algorithms similar to NFI of GDx-Pro and Moorfields regression analysis of HRT III are not available in OCT. It is seen that inferior average consistently shows up as the best parameter in differentiating early glaucoma from ocular healthy eyes.[5 25-32]

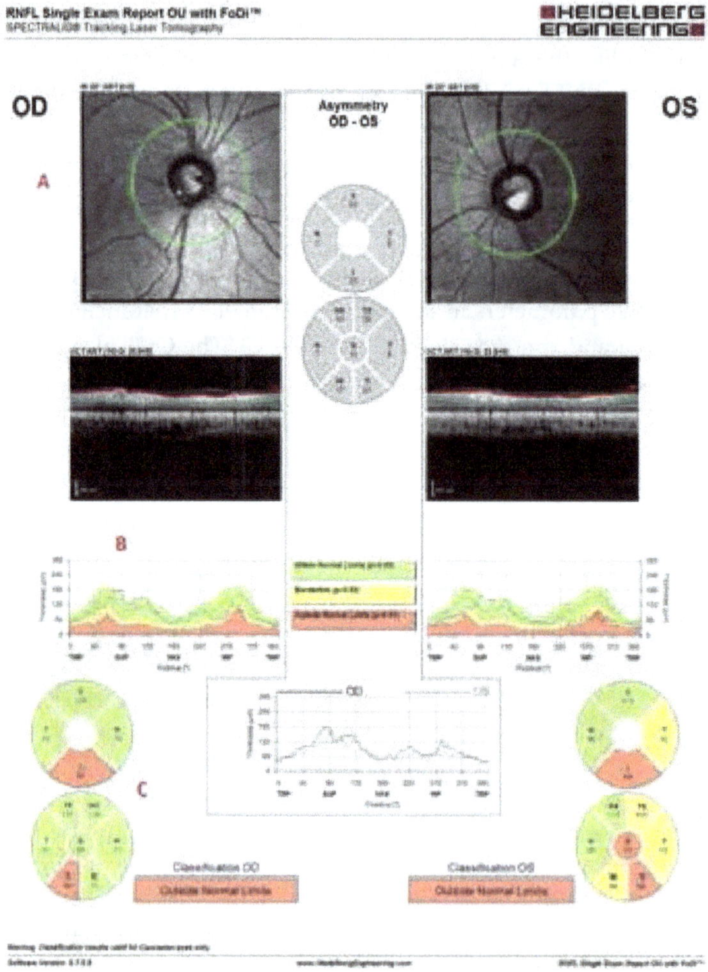

Figure 5. An OU report of RNFL with section A, B and C showing fundus image, RNFL thickness profile in TSNIT region and RNFL thickness in various quadrants respectively. Both the section B and C are color coded to provide information on statistical significance. Image courtesy Mr. Ali Tafreshi of Heidelberg Engineering.

4.1. Macula analysis in glaucoma

A new macula analysis is proposed to evaluate patients at risk of glaucoma. This analysis was proposed by Dr. Sanjay Asrani MD as additional data that might help managing glaucoma patients.[33 34] A separate scanning of the macula region is needed to obtain ganglion cell analysis. Different manufactures perform the analysis with slight variation. The Optovue manufactures of RTvue and iVue OCT call it the Ganglion Cell Complex that includes the nerve fiber layer, ganglion cell layer and the inner plexiform layer (Figure 4 section D). Carl Zeiss Meditec the manufacturers of Cirrus OCT calls it the Ganglion Cell Analysis that includes the

Ganglion cell layer and inner plexiform layer. There is no agreement if one analysis yields better results than the other. Further there is some conflicting reports about the diagnostic accuracy of the macular parameters in glaucoma however they tend to perform at par with other parameters generated by Fourier domain OCT (See review article by Wong et al., [35].)

5. Imaging artifacts

Although invaluable in clinical practice imaging devices like other clinical diagnostic techniques are susceptible to artifacts. Some which can be controlled and some that are not possible to control. When there is reduced signal strength which could possibly be due to image focusing issues, eye movement, tear film issues, or optical quality lowered due to presence of media opacity there is degradation in image quality which leads to errors in measured parameters and diagnostic ability of the devices.

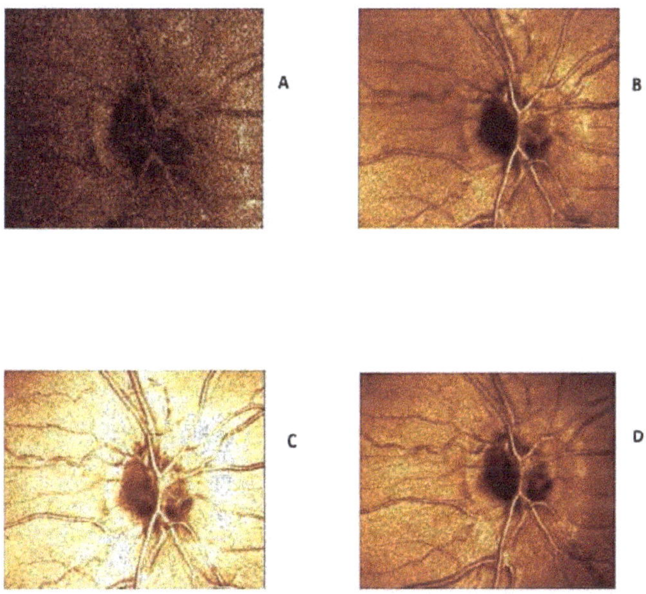

Figure 6. Common errors in imaging, these decrease the signal strength and image quality which in turn decreases the accuracy of parameters obtained. Section A shows an image of a severe dry eye patient that improved upon instil lation of artificial tears (Section B). Section C shows the same patient with 2 diopter myopic defocus. As seen the image is over exposed with imaging artifacts visible. Section D shows the same patient with appropriate focus set.

All imaging devices outcomes would be affected if the image is defocused or if there was image quality degradation. Studies have looked at the effect of dryness and tear film issues that influence the outcome of the imaging. [36-38] It is advisable that patient's blink regularly between scans or artificial tears/lubricants be utilized to form a uniform regular optical surface. It is also be ideal if procedures that require ocular contact be avoided and performed after imaging is complete. Similarly reduced pupil size and optic media can have effect on imaging because the amount of light reaching retina will be decreased thus signal received from the eye will be of decreased leading to missing details.[36] This causes erroneous estimation of parameters measured and also to excessive false positive diagnosis. See figure 6 A-D for error in imaging due to dry eye or defocus and improvement in images when appropriate corrective methods were used.

Involuntary eye movement often leads to measurements obtained not at the intended region.[39] This leads to major errors in imaging. Some of these errors may be obvious to detect however some so subtle and leaving no obvious artifacts (See figure 7A B C and D "eye movement artifacts"). The eye movement artifacts are particularly a serious issue in the case of time domain OCTs slow scans or any scan that takes longer time. The errors in imaging due to eye movements can be avoided in the image acquisition phase as done by re-scanning as done in Spectralis OCT or done post acquisition (post image capture) processing as done in Optovue's OCTs.

The device may also fail in identifying appropriate layers of retinal and thus leading to segmentation errors. The scans should be viewed carefully and imaging performed again if such errors are observed. These errors are becoming less common with advanced instrumentation and algorithms that are in development to provide image registration.

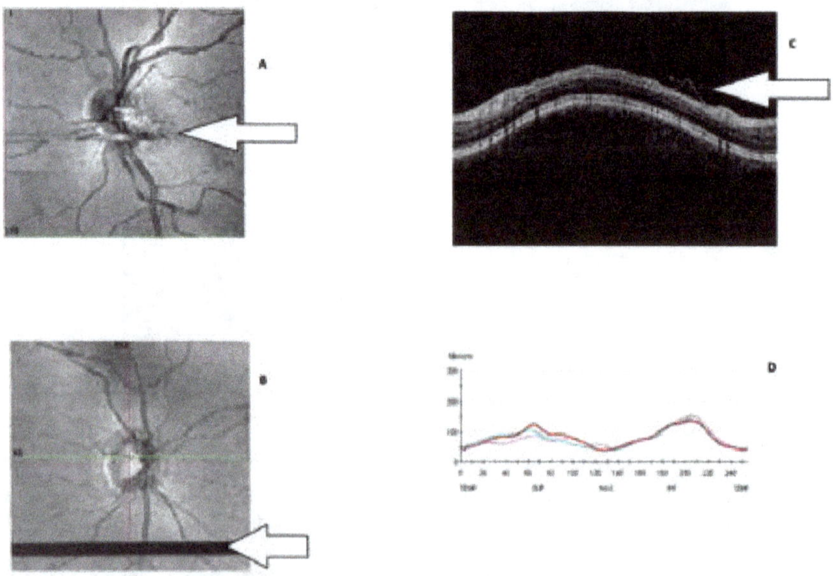

Figure 7. Various errors in imaging marked by an arrow in individual images. Section A shows an eye movement artifact that and is seen as non continuous blood vessels and optic disc. Section B shows blink artifact that is seen as a black band of missing data. Section C shows a segmentation error of RNFL which the machine algorithm has outlined incorrect upper lower layer of RNFL erroneously including the vitreo-retinal interface. Section D shows three consecutive scans obtained using Time domain OCT that were obtained 1-minute apart in a patient moving his eye. Images A,B, C courtesy Miss Kelly Soules Optovue Inc.

Atypical Birefringence pattern is an imaging artifact that affects images obtained in eyes with poor choroidal pigmentation also called "blonde fundus" and influenced results obtained using the prior generation polarimetry device GDx-Variable Corneal Compensator (VCC). These patterns were prevalent in 10-15% of the population when examined with GDx-VCC. [22 40] The images tended to not follow the normal physiological pattern of nerve fiber layer and the RNFL map shows "bicycle spoke like pattern" or "tie dye pattern" (See figure 8). These eyes were deemed not appropriate for imaging using GDx-VCC. With the new generation polarimetr GDx-Pro (Enhanced Corneal Compensator) has dramatically decreased the prevalence of these atypical patterns and long term measurement variability.[41]

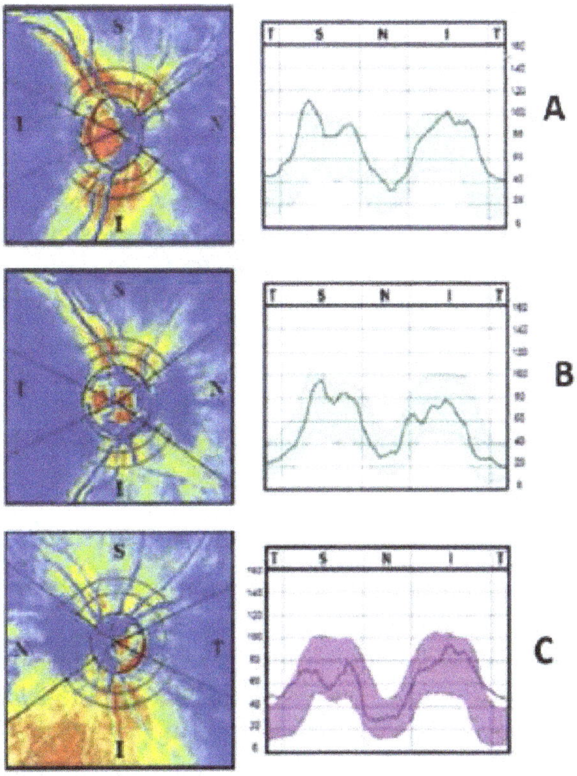

Figure 8. Three eyes with Atypical Retardation Pattern also known as "tie-dye" pattern in RNFL thickness profile map. These are an outcome of poor signal to noise ratio due to poor choroidal pigmentation. These scans are an outcome of an artifact and should not be utilized in managing patients.

6. Diagnostic accuracy and comparison of individual devices

Overall the principles behind the confocal scanning laser ophthalmoscope HRT-I, HRT-II and HRT-III manufactured by Heidelberg engineering are very similar that the data can be transferred from one generation to another. The agreement in stereometric parameters obtained by HRT-I is very similar to HRT-II.[42] Thus as expected the diagnostic accuracy of these different generation devices should be similar.

Whereas where GDx is concerned each generation of technology has fixed an error or problem in the imaging. For example the initial generation device: GDx-Fixed Corneal Compensator (GDx-FCC) used a standard correction factor to correct for anterior segment birefringence. The anterior segment birefringence varies in population thus the technology was changed to GDx Variable Corneal Compensator (GDx-VCC). [43 44] Recently the new generation GDx-Pro was introduced to improve upon the GDx-VCC. It is shown that the GDx-Enhanced Corneal Compensator (ECC now called GDx-Pro) better characterized the RNFL, decreased the number of atypical retardation pattern found in the study population.[45] It is shown by Mai and co-workers that the GDX-Pro has better repeatability, diagnostic ability, and a better structure and function relationship than GDx-VCC.[46-48] Thus it has to be remembered that where polarimetry is concerned newer devices are better than older generation devices.

Similarly the Fourier domain OCT compared to the older generation "time-domain" TD-OCT shows a marked improvement as it tried to address issues related to improved resolution, faster scanning speed. Where glaucoma is concerned the diagnostic accuracy of the TD OCT is similar to FD OCT [49 50], also the population mean RNFL values may not vary significantly however it has to be remembered the RNFL measurements are not comparable and cannot be used interchangeably.[51] The TD OCT RNFL tends to be thicker than FD OCT except for advanced glaucoma.[51] Unlike GDx-Pro and HRT III there are various manufacturers that make the Fourier Domain OCT. Overall comparing various Fourier domain OCT techniques the diagnostic accuracy in identifying individuals with glaucomatous optic neuropathy is very similar in these devices despite having difference in resolution and scanning speed.[52]

7. Comparison of diagnostic accuracy of various devices

Diagnostic accuracy of the imaging devices varies as a function of disease severity.[28 53-57] As the severity of glaucoma increases devices accuracy to detect glaucoma accurately also increases. For various reasons it is difficult to compare all imaging devices and its ability to diagnose glaucoma as there is no large scale population based study that have compared the latest technology that is available. Additionally there are inherent differences in the design and population of the cross-sectional studies that will influence the outcome of the study. For example the nerve fiber layer analysis may better suit than disc topography in evaluating myopes at risk of glaucoma. [58] These factors need to be kept in mind when comparing diagnostic accuracy of various imaging devices.

Studies have compared diagnostic capacity of GDx, OCT and HRT and although slight differences exist in identification of true-positive overall the ROC area which is a function of sensitivity and specificity (true positive and true negative) is similar in all the devices.[32 59] Because both the OCT and GDx provide RNFL data and numerous studies have evaluated its ability in identifying individuals with glaucoma.[5 32 59-62]. Over all these studies report that the diagnostic accuracy of GDx is very similar to OCT in identifying glaucoma eyes from a group of ocular healthy eyes. So in summary it is safe to conclude that although there are differences in diagnostic accuracy of various imaging devices overall they tends to perform quite similar.

8. Progression and imaging

Detecting progression or change over time in eyes at risk of glaucoma or with glaucoma is probably one of the most difficult tasks clinically. Progression in an optic nerve due to open angle glaucoma is subtle, slow and can easily be missed in casual observation. Thus the objectivity and reproducibility of the imaging devices can be of great benefit. All imaging devices have parameters that can be followed over time to monitor progression. These algorithms are overall based on simple regression analysis that is analyzing change in parameters with follow-up over time. This analysis identifies if there is a trend of values lowering or increasing over time was statistically significant also known as trend analysis.

Heidelberg retina tomography has topographical change analysis (TCA). The TCA is a statistical method that compares topographic values in small discrete regions of 4x4 pixels called superpixels. This method is distinctly different than trend analysis as the analysis is performed on raw topography values. The figure 9 shows an optic nerve head with progressive damage compared to the baseline scans. Studies have shown that this may be useful in identifying progressive damage in glaucoma.[63 64]

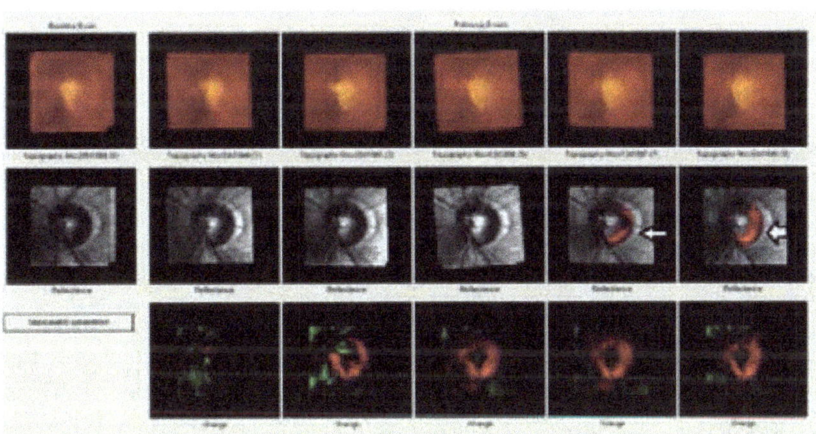

Figure 9. A Topographical Change Analysis output obtained using the HRT. The arrows indicate region of change in thickness particularly thinning in rim area. Image courtesy Mr. Ali Tafreshi of Heidelberg Engineering.

The scanning laser polarimetry GDx-VCC has advanced serial analysis that outputs trend over time in diagnosing progressive change in glaucoma (Figure 10). More recently an advanced

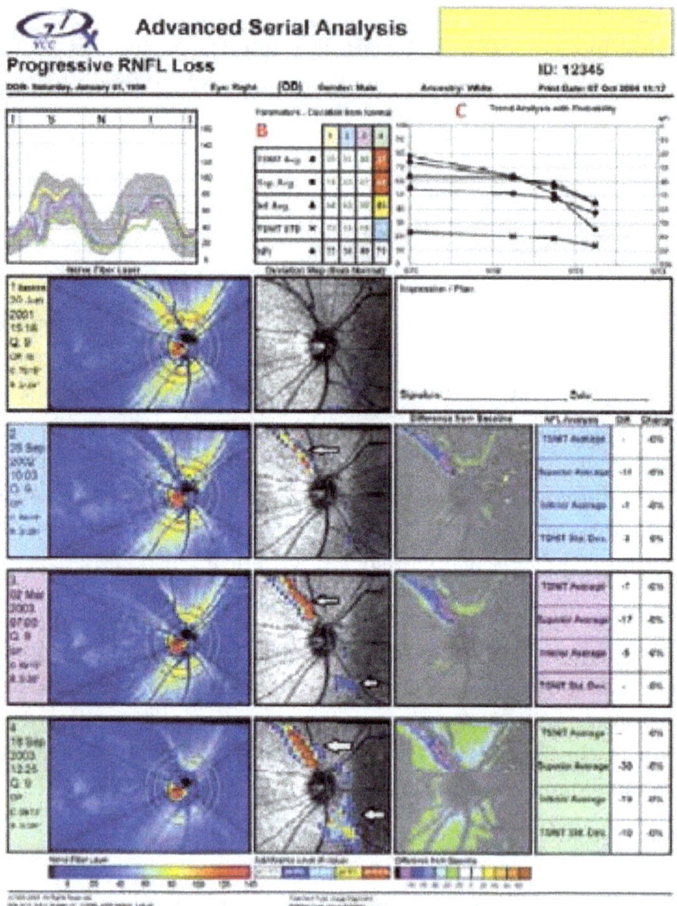

Figure 10. An advanced serial analysis of GDx. The deviation map shows an increase in number of superpixels (see arrow) that are statistically significant showing progressive thinning of retinal nerve fiber layer. The various parameters shown in section B and trend over time shown in section C show progressive decline. Image Courtesy Carl Zeiss Meditec.

"Guided Progression Analysis" that investigates changes in overall 20 degree area of the scan, TSNIT RNFL graph and the thickness parameters. Initial reports show that this may be of advantage in identifying progressive damage. [65-67] This software is however not cleared FDA approval and is not available for sale in USA. The Cirrus optical coherence tomography has a Guided Progression Analysis (figure 11) very similar to that described of GDx is available and is FDA approved. All follow-up scans are compared to baseline data. When two consecutive examinations show loss data the scans are flagged to be "possible loss" and "Likely loss" when three consecutive examinations show damage.

Glaucoma imaging devices have made a long journey from devices of interest in research arena to clinically useful technology. Its place in clinic and its usefulness in managing patients with glaucoma cannot be dismissed. With newer and improved techniques there is also an im-

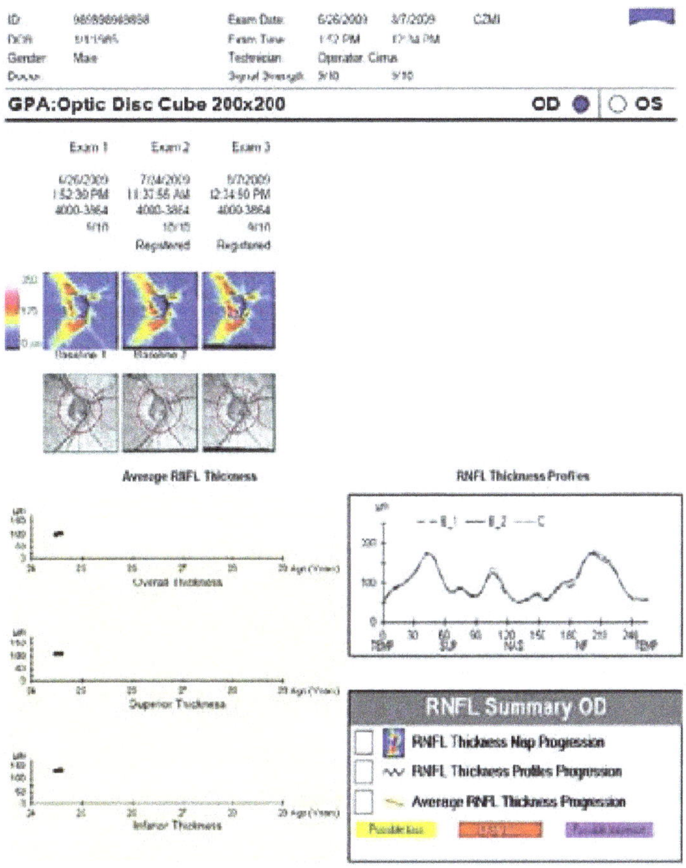

Figure 11. A Guided Progression Analysis (GPA) of Cirrus OCT that is obtained on an ocular hypertensive patient. The scans show no progressive damage in the short duration of follow-up with both RNFL thickness profile and RNFL summary.

provement in correlation of structure-functional loss in eyes with glaucoma.[68-73] This can improve overall diagnostic and prognostic ability in managing patients with glaucoma. With further advance in adaptive optics and improvement in transverse resolution has given us ability to image cones astrocytes, ganglion cells and its dendrites. [74] This should be able to bring the next wave in improvement of patient care and improve understanding of glaucoma pathogenesis.

Author details

Pinakin Gunvant Davey

Western University of Health Sciences, College of Optometry, Pomona CA, USA

References

[1] Gordon MO, Beiser JA, Brandt JD, et al. The Ocular Hypertension Treatment Study: baseline factors that predict the onset of primary open-angle glaucoma. Archives of ophthalmology 2002;120(6):714-20; discussion 829-30

[2] Fingeret M, Mancil L, Bailey IL, et al. Optometric Clinical Practice Guideline: Care of the Patient with Open Angle Glaucoma. Secondary Optometric Clinical Practice Guideline: Care of the Patient with Open Angle Glaucoma 2011.

[3] Prum B, Friedman D, Gedde S, et al. Primary Open Angle Glaucoma. Secondary Primary Open Angle Glaucoma 2010.

[4] Leung CK, Cheung CY, Lin D, et al. Longitudinal variability of optic disc and retinal nerve fiber layer measurements. Investigative ophthalmology & visual science 2008;49(11):4886-92 doi: 10.1167/iovs.07-1187[published Online First: Epub Date]|.

[5] Greaney MJ, Hoffman DC, Garway-Heath DF, et al. Comparison of optic nerve imaging methods to distinguish normal eyes from those with glaucoma. Investigative ophthalmology & visual science 2002;43(1):140-5

[6] Jonas JB, Budde WM, Panda-Jonas S. Ophthalmoscopic evaluation of the optic nerve head. Survey of ophthalmology 1999;43(4):293-320

[7] Garway-Heath DF, Wollstein G, Hitchings RA. Aging changes of the optic nerve head in relation to open angle glaucoma. The British journal of ophthalmology 1997;81(10):840-5

[8] Wollstein G, Garway-Heath DF, Hitchings RA. Identification of early glaucoma cases with the scanning laser ophthalmoscope. Ophthalmology 1998;105(8):1557-63 doi: 10.1016/s0161-6420(98)98047-2[published Online First: Epub Date]|.

[9] Betz P, Camps F, Collignon-Brach C, et al. [Stereophotography and photogrammetry of the physiological cup of the disc (author's transl)]. Journal francais d'ophtalmologie 1981;4(3):193-203

[10] Jonas JB, Gusek GC, Naumann GO. Optic disc, cup and neuroretinal rim size, configuration and correlations in normal eyes. Investigative ophthalmology & visual science 1988;29(7):1151-8

[11] Read RM, Spaeth GL. The practical clinical appraisal of the optic disc in glaucoma: the natural history of cup progression and some specific disc-field correlations. Transactions-American Academy of Ophthalmology and Otolaryngology. American Academy of Ophthalmology and Otolaryngology 1974;78(2):OP255-74

[12] Tuulonen A, Airaksinen PJ. Initial glaucomatous optic disk and retinal nerve fiber layer abnormalities and their progression. American journal of ophthalmology 1991;111(4):485-90

[13] Zangwill LM, Weinreb RN, Beiser JA, et al. Baseline topographic optic disc measurements are associated with the development of primary open-angle glaucoma: the Confocal Scanning Laser Ophthalmoscopy Ancillary Study to the Ocular Hypertension Treatment Study. Archives of ophthalmology 2005;123(9):1188-97 doi: 10.1001/archopht.123.9.1188[published Online First: Epub Date]|.

[14] Weinreb RN, Zangwill LM, Jain S, et al. Predicting the onset of glaucoma: the confocal scanning laser ophthalmoscopy ancillary study to theOcular Hypertension Treatment Study. Ophthalmology 2010;117(9):1674-83 doi: 10.1016/j.ophtha.2010.03.044[published Online First: Epub Date]|.

[15] RNFL analysis with GDx VCC: A primer and a clinical guide. http://www.meditec.zeiss.com/C125679E00525939/EmbedTitelIntern/GDxPrimerChapter2/$File/GDx_Primer_Chapter2.pdf%5Ct_blank, 2004.

[16] Morgan JE, Waldock A, Jeffery G, et al. Retinal nerve fibre layer polarimetry: histological and clinical comparison. The British journal of ophthalmology 1998;82(6):684-90

[17] Weinreb RN, Dreher AW, Coleman A, et al. Histopathologic validation of Fourier-ellipsometry measurements of retinal nerve fiber layer thickness. Archives of ophthalmology 1990;108(4):557-60

[18] Dada T, Behera G, Agarwal A, et al. Effect of cataract surgery on retinal nerve fiber layer thickness parameters using scanning laser polarimetry (GDxVCC). Indian journal of ophthalmology 2010;58(5):389-94 doi: 10.4103/0301-4738.67048[published Online First: Epub Date]|.

[19] Sanchez-Cano A, Pablo LE, Larrosa JM, et al. The effect of phacoemulsification cataract surgery on polarimetry and tomography measurements for glaucoma diagnosis. Journal of glaucoma 2010;19(7):468-74 doi: 10.1097/IJG.0b013e3181c4aed8[published Online First: Epub Date]|.

[20] Zangwill LM, Abunto T, Bowd C, et al. Scanning laser polarimetry retinal nerve fiber layer thickness measurements after LASIK. Ophthalmology 2005;112(2):200-7 doi: 10.1016/j.ophtha.2004.08.019[published Online First: Epub Date]|.

[21] Da Pozzo S, Iacono P, Marchesan R, et al. Scanning laser polarimetry with variable corneal compensation and detection of glaucomatous optic neuropathy. Graefe's archive for clinical and experimental ophthalmology=Albrecht von Graefes Archiv fur klinische und experimentelle Ophthalmologie 2005;243(8):774-9 doi: 10.1007/s00417-004-1118-1[published Online First: Epub Date]|.

[22] Gunvant P, Zheng Y, Toth M, et al. Atypical retardation pattern: can performance of classification be improved? Optometry and vision science : official publication of the American Academy of Optometry 2008;85(6):482-8 doi: 10.1097/OPX.0b013e3181783aa2[published Online First: Epub Date]|.

[23] Iester M, Perdicchi A, De Feo F, et al. Comparison between GDx VCC parameter and achromatic perimetry in glaucoma patients. Journal of glaucoma 2006;15(4):281-5 doi: 10.1097/01.ijg.0000212235.88416.bd[published Online First: Epub Date]|.

[24] Reus NJ, Lemij HG. Diagnostic accuracy of the GDx VCC for glaucoma. Ophthalmology 2004;111(10):1860-5 doi: 10.1016/j.ophtha.2004.04.024[published Online First: Epub Date]|.

[25] Bowd C, Zangwill LM, Berry CC, et al. Detecting early glaucoma by assessment of retinal nerve fiber layer thickness and visual function. Investigative ophthalmology & visual science 2001;42(9):1993-2003

[26] Budenz DL, Michael A, Chang RT, et al. Sensitivity and specificity of the StratusOCT for perimetric glaucoma. Ophthalmology 2005;112(1):3-9 doi: 10.1016/j.ophtha.2004.06.039[published Online First: Epub Date]|.

[27] Chen HY, Huang ML. Discrimination between normal and glaucomatous eyes using Stratus optical coherence tomography in Taiwan Chinese subjects. Graefe's archive for clinical and experimental ophthalmology=Albrecht von Graefes Archiv fur klinische und experimentelle Ophthalmologie 2005;243(9):894-902 doi: 10.1007/s00417-005-1140-y[published Online First: Epub Date]|.

[28] Gunvant P, Zheng Y, Essock EA, et al. Application of shape-based analysis methods to OCT retinal nerve fiber layer data in glaucoma. Journal of glaucoma 2007;16(6):543-8 doi: 10.1097/IJG.0b013e318050ab65[published Online First: Epub Date]|.

[29] Kanamori A, Nakamura M, Escano MF, et al. Evaluation of the glaucomatous damage on retinal nerve fiber layer thickness measured by optical coherence tomography. American journal of ophthalmology 2003;135(4):513-20

[30] Lu AT, Wang M, Varma R, et al. Combining nerve fiber layer parameters to optimize glaucoma diagnosis with optical coherence tomography. Ophthalmology 2008;115(8):1352-7, 57 e1-2 doi: 10.1016/j.ophtha.2008.01.011[published Online First: Epub Date]|.

[31] Medeiros FA, Zangwill LM, Bowd C, et al. Evaluation of retinal nerve fiber layer, optic nerve head, and macular thickness measurements for glaucoma detection using optical coherence tomography. American journal of ophthalmology 2005;139(1):44-55 doi: 10.1016/j.ajo.2004.08.069[published Online First: Epub Date]|.

[32] Zangwill LM, Bowd C, Berry CC, et al. Discriminating between normal and glaucomatous eyes using the Heidelberg Retina Tomograph, GDx Nerve Fiber Analyzer, and Optical Coherence Tomograph. Archives of ophthalmology 2001;119(7):985-93

[33] Asrani S, Zeimer R, Jampel H, et al. Macular symmetry testing for glaucoma detection. Journal of glaucoma 2006;15(2):182; author reply 82

[34] Mathers K, Rosdahl JA, Asrani S. Correlation of Macular Thickness With Visual Fields in Glaucoma Patients and Suspects. Journal of glaucoma 2013 doi: 10.1097/IJG.0b013e31829539c3[published Online First: Epub Date]|.

[35] Wong JJ, Chen TC, Shen LQ, et al. Macular imaging for glaucoma using spectral-domain optical coherence tomography: a review. Seminars in ophthalmology 2012;27(5-6):160-6 doi: 10.3109/08820538.2012.712734[published Online First: Epub Date]|.

[36] Asrani S, Edghill B, Gupta Y, et al. Optical coherence tomography errors in glaucoma. Journal of glaucoma 2010;19(4):237-42 doi: 10.1097/IJG.0b013e3181b21f99[published Online First: Epub Date]|.

[37] Hoh ST, Greenfield DS, Liebmann JM, et al. Factors affecting image acquisition during scanning laser polarimetry. Ophthalmic surgery and lasers 1998;29(7):545-51

[38] Stein DM, Wollstein G, Ishikawa H, et al. Effect of corneal drying on optical coherence tomography. Ophthalmology 2006;113(6):985-91 doi: 10.1016/j.ophtha.2006.02.018[published Online First: Epub Date]|.

[39] Koozekanani D, Boyer KL, Roberts C. Tracking the optic nervehead in OCT video using dual eigenspaces and an adaptive vascular distribution model. IEEE transactions on medical imaging 2003;22(12):1519-36 doi: 10.1109/tmi.2003.817753[published Online First: Epub Date]|.

[40] Toth M, Hollo G. Enhanced corneal compensation for scanning laser polarimetry on eyes with atypical polarisation pattern. The British journal of ophthalmology 2005;89(9):1139-42 doi: 10.1136/bjo.2005.070011[published Online First: Epub Date]|.

[41] Grewal DS, Sehi M, Cook RJ, et al. The impact of retardance pattern variability on nerve fiber layer measurements over time using GDx with variable and enhanced corneal compensation. Investigative ophthalmology & visual science 2011;52(7):4516-24 doi: 10.1167/iovs.10-5969[published Online First: Epub Date]|.

[42] Balasubramanian M, Bowd C, Weinreb RN, et al. Agreement between the Heidelberg Retina Tomograph (HRT) stereometric parameters estimated using HRT-I and HRT-II. Optometry and vision science : official publication of the American Academy of Optometry 2011;88(1):140-9 doi: 10.1097/OPX.0b013e3181fc3467[published Online First: Epub Date]|.

[43] Choplin NT, Zhou Q, Knighton RW. Effect of individualized compensation for anterior segment birefringence on retinal nerve fiber layer assessments as determined by scanning laser polarimetry. Ophthalmology 2003;110(4):719-25 doi: 10.1016/s0161-6420(02)01899-7[published Online First: Epub Date]|.

[44] Zhou Q, Weinreb RN. Individualized compensation of anterior segment birefringence during scanning laser polarimetry. Investigative ophthalmology & visual science 2002;43(7):2221-8

[45] Reus NJ, Zhou Q, Lemij HG. Enhanced imaging algorithm for scanning laser polarimetry with variable corneal compensation. Investigative ophthalmology & visual

science 2006;47(9):3870-7 doi: 10.1167/iovs.05-0067[published Online First: Epub Date]|.

[46] Mai TA, Reus NJ, Lemij HG. Structure-function relationship is stronger with enhanced corneal compensation than with variable corneal compensation in scanning laser polarimetry. Investigative ophthalmology & visual science 2007;48(4):1651-8 doi: 10.1167/iovs.06-1003[published Online First: Epub Date]|.

[47] Mai TA, Reus NJ, Lemij HG. Diagnostic accuracy of scanning laser polarimetry with enhanced versus variable corneal compensation. Ophthalmology 2007;114(11): 1988-93 doi: 10.1016/j.ophtha.2007.01.022[published Online First: Epub Date]|.

[48] Mai TA, Reus NJ, Lemij HG. Retinal nerve fiber layer measurement repeatability in scanning laser polarimetry with enhanced corneal compensation. Journal of glaucoma 2008;17(4):269-74 doi: 10.1097/IJG.0b013e31815c3a6b[published Online First: Epub Date]|.

[49] Chang RT, Knight OJ, Feuer WJ, et al. Sensitivity and specificity of time-domain versus spectral-domain optical coherence tomography in diagnosing early to moderate glaucoma. Ophthalmology 2009;116(12):2294-9 doi: 10.1016/j.ophtha.2009.06.012[published Online First: Epub Date]|.

[50] Chen HY, Chang YC, Wang IJ, et al. Comparison of Glaucoma Diagnoses Using Stratus and Cirrus Optical Coherence Tomography in Different Glaucoma Types in a Chinese Population. Journal of glaucoma 2012 doi: 10.1097/IJG. 0b013e3182594f42[published Online First: Epub Date]|.

[51] Knight OJ, Chang RT, Feuer WJ, et al. Comparison of retinal nerve fiber layer measurements using time domain and spectral domain optical coherent tomography. Ophthalmology 2009;116(7):1271-7 doi: 10.1016/j.ophtha.2008.12.032[published Online First: Epub Date]|.

[52] Leite MT, Rao HL, Zangwill LM, et al. Comparison of the diagnostic accuracies of the Spectralis, Cirrus, and RTVue optical coherence tomography devices in glaucoma. Ophthalmology 2011;118(7):1334-9 doi: 10.1016/j.ophtha.2010.11.029[published Online First: Epub Date]|.

[53] Essock EA, Zheng Y, Gunvant P. Analysis of GDx-VCC polarimetry data by Wavelet-Fourier analysis across glaucoma stages. Investigative ophthalmology & visual science 2005;46(8):2838-47 doi: 10.1167/iovs.04-1156[published Online First: Epub Date]|.

[54] Girkin CA, Liebmann J, Fingeret M, et al. The effects of race, optic disc area, age, and disease severity on the diagnostic performance of spectral-domain optical coherence tomography. Investigative ophthalmology & visual science 2011;52(9):6148-53 doi: 10.1167/iovs.10-6698[published Online First: Epub Date]|.

[55] Leite MT, Zangwill LM, Weinreb RN, et al. Effect of disease severity on the performance of Cirrus spectral-domain OCT for glaucoma diagnosis. Investigative ophthal-

mology & visual science 2010;51(8):4104-9 doi: 10.1167/iovs.09-4716[published Online First: Epub Date]|.

[56] Rao HL, Leite MT, Weinreb RN, et al. Effect of disease severity and optic disc size on diagnostic accuracy of RTVue spectral domain optical coherence tomograph in glaucoma. Investigative ophthalmology & visual science 2011;52(3):1290-6 doi: 10.1167/iovs.10-5546[published Online First: Epub Date]|.

[57] Reddy S, Xing D, Arthur SN, et al. HRT III glaucoma probability score and Moorfields regression across the glaucoma spectrum. Journal of glaucoma 2009;18(5): 368-72 doi: 10.1097/IJG.0b013e31818c6edd[published Online First: Epub Date]|.

[58] Leung CK, Medeiros FA, Zangwill LM, et al. American Chinese glaucoma imaging study: a comparison of the optic disc and retinal nerve fiber layer in detecting glaucomatous damage. Investigative ophthalmology & visual science 2007;48(6):2644-52 doi: 10.1167/iovs.06-1332[published Online First: Epub Date]|.

[59] Medeiros FA, Zangwill LM, Bowd C, et al. Comparison of the GDx VCC scanning laser polarimeter, HRT II confocal scanning laser ophthalmoscope, and stratus OCT optical coherence tomograph for the detection of glaucoma. Archives of ophthalmology 2004;122(6):827-37 doi: 10.1001/archopht.122.6.827[published Online First: Epub Date]|.

[60] Gunvant P, Zheng Y, Essock EA, et al. Comparison of shape-based analysis of retinal nerve fiber layer data obtained From OCT and GDx-VCC. Journal of glaucoma 2009;18(6):464-71 doi: 10.1097/IJG.0b013e31818c6f2b[published Online First: Epub Date]|.

[61] Kanamori A, Nagai-Kusuhara A, Escano MF, et al. Comparison of confocal scanning laser ophthalmoscopy, scanning laser polarimetry and optical coherence tomography to discriminate ocular hypertension and glaucoma at an early stage. Graefe's archive for clinical and experimental ophthalmology=Albrecht von Graefes Archiv fur klinische und experimentelle Ophthalmologie 2006;244(1):58-68 doi: 10.1007/s00417-005-0029-0[published Online First: Epub Date]|.

[62] Leung CK, Chan WM, Chong KK, et al. Comparative study of retinal nerve fiber layer measurement by StratusOCT and GDx VCC, I: correlation analysis in glaucoma. Investigative ophthalmology & visual science 2005;46(9):3214-20 doi: 10.1167/iovs.05-0294[published Online First: Epub Date]|.

[63] Bowd C, Balasubramanian M, Weinreb RN, et al. Performance of confocal scanning laser tomograph Topographic Change Analysis (TCA) for assessing glaucomatous progression. Investigative ophthalmology & visual science 2009;50(2):691-701 doi: 10.1167/iovs.08-2136[published Online First: Epub Date]|.

[64] Chauhan BC, McCormick TA, Nicolela MT, et al. Optic disc and visual field changes in a prospective longitudinal study of patients with glaucoma: comparison of scan-

ning laser tomography with conventional perimetry and optic disc photography. Archives of ophthalmology 2001;119(10):1492-9

[65] Alencar LM, Zangwill LM, Weinreb RN, et al. Agreement for detecting glaucoma progression with the GDx guided progression analysis, automated perimetry, and optic disc photography. Ophthalmology 2010;117(3):462-70 doi: 10.1016/j.ophtha.2009.08.012[published Online First: Epub Date]|.

[66] Grewal DS, Sehi M, Greenfield DS. Detecting glaucomatous progression using GDx with variable and enhanced corneal compensation using Guided Progression Analysis. The British journal of ophthalmology 2011;95(4):502-8 doi: 10.1136/bjo.2010.180810[published Online First: Epub Date]|.

[67] Kjaergaard SM, Alencar LM, Nguyen B, et al. Detection of retinal nerve fibre layer progression: comparison of the fast and extended modes of GDx guided progression analysis. The British journal of ophthalmology 2011;95(12):1707-12 doi: 10.1136/bjophthalmol-2011-300354[published Online First: Epub Date]|.

[68] Kanamori A, Nakamura M, Tomioka M, et al. Structure-function relationship among three types of spectral-domain optical coherent tomography instruments in measuring parapapillary retinal nerve fibre layer thickness. Acta ophthalmologica 2013;91(3):e196-202 doi: 10.1111/aos.12028[published Online First: Epub Date]|.

[69] 69. Lamparter J, Russell RA, Schulze A, et al. Structure-function relationship between FDF, FDT, SAP, and scanning laser ophthalmoscopy in glaucoma patients. Investigative ophthalmology & visual science 2012;53(12):7553-9 doi: 10.1167/iovs.12-10892[published Online First: Epub Date]|.

[70] 70. Medeiros FA, Zangwill LM, Bowd C, et al. The structure and function relationship in glaucoma: implications for detection of progression and measurement of rates of change. Investigative ophthalmology & visual science 2012;53(11):6939-46 doi: 10.1167/iovs.12-10345[published Online First: Epub Date]|.

[71] Naghizadeh F, Garas A, Vargha P, et al. Structure-Function Relationship Between the Octopus Perimeter Cluster Mean Sensitivity and Sector Retinal Nerve Fiber Layer Thickness Measured With the RTVue Optical Coherence Tomography and Scanning Laser Polarimetry. Journal of glaucoma 2012 doi: 10.1097/IJG.0b013e318264cda2[published Online First: Epub Date]|.

[72] Park HY, Park CK. Structure-function relationship and diagnostic value of RNFL Area Index compared with circumpapillary RNFL thickness by spectral-domain OCT. Journal of glaucoma 2013;22(2):88-97 doi: 10.1097/IJG.0b013e318231202f[published Online First: Epub Date]|.

[73] Sato S, Hirooka K, Baba T, et al. Correlation Between the Ganglion Cell-Inner Plexiform Layer Thickness Measured With Cirrus HD-OCT and Macular Visual Field Sensitivity Measured With Microperimetry. Investigative ophthalmology & visual

science 2013;54(4):3046-51 doi: 10.1167/iovs.12-11173[published Online First: Epub Date]|.

[74] Werkmeister RM, Cherecheanu AP, Garhofer G, et al. Imaging of retinal ganglion cells in glaucoma: pitfalls and challenges. Cell and tissue research 2013 doi: 10.1007/s00441-013-1600-3[published Online First: Epub Date]|.

2

Clinical Ocular Electrophysiology

Fatih C. Gundogan and Umit Yolcu

1. Introduction

Ocular electrodiagnostic tests are invaluable tools in most clinical circumstances in routine ophthalmology practice. Sometimes, these tests are the only methods exploring the functional deficits of the patient in otherwise normal structure. In contrast, ocular electrophysiological tests may explore normal function in cases with functional vision loss. In this chapter, we will focus on the clinical use of ocular electrophysiological tests after a short explanation about recording parameters. A basic clinical use of ocular electrophysiological tests will be discussed rather than detailed and theoretical explanations.

2. Full-field electroretinogram

Full-field electroretinogram (ERG) represents a mass-response of the retina to a full-field flash of light. The resultant single waveform is the total response of the retina. The details of full-field ERG recording techniques may be obtained from ISCEV (International Society for Clinical Electrophysiology of Vision) standards [1]. The functions of rod, cones and inner retinal layers may be recorded separately by changing stimulus parameters and the adaptive state of the eye to the light.

In a typical full-field ERG (Figure 1), five recordings are performed. At first, the patient is dark adapted for at least 20 minutes. A dim white or blue flash light [2.0 log unit below the standard flash intensity (Standard flash: 3.0 cds/m^2)] is used to stimulate the retina. This response is shown as 'DA 0.01 response' in the latest ISCEV guideline for full-field ERG recording. At that flash intensity, only rod photoreceptors are stimulated and the resultant waveform belongs to rod functions. In that response, only a positive b wave originated from rod ON-bipolar cells is recorded. This means that DA 0.01 response is an indirect indicator for rod photoreceptor function. Secondly, DA 3.0 response is recorded. A standard flash light is used to stimulate both rod and cone photoreceptors and combined response of rod and cone photoreceptors is recorded. The first negative peak, a-wave is caused by the hyperpolarization of photoreceptors. However, in DA 3.0 response, a-wave has a bifid configuration which makes the evaluation of photoreceptor function problematic. For this reason, ISCEV recommended the use of bright flash ERG recordings (DA 10.0 ERG or DA 30.0 ERG) for photoreceptor function evaluation. In these brighter light levels, a–wave has a clear single peak. Oscillatory potentials, which reflects amacrine cell function is recorded using standard flash light intensity under dark-or light-adapted (LA; at least 10-min of light adaptation using a background luminance of 30cd/m^2) conditions. LA 3.0 response is generated within cone system. LA 3.0 30 Hz flicker response is the most sensitive indicator of cone system however, it arises in the inner retina and cannot be used to localize the level of abnormality within the cone system [2].

Each retina consists of approximately 4-5 million of cone and 100-120 million of rod photoreceptors. The rods contain light-sensitive pigment rhodopsin with a spectral absorption peak at 496 nm. Each cone contains one of three types of color sensitive pigments. L, M and S-cones (L: long wavelength cones, M: middle wavelength cones, S: small wavelength cones) have peak absorption spectra at 558nm, 531nm and 419nm, respectively. L,M and S cones is also named as red cones, green cones and blue cones with respect to colors of peak-sensitized light [3].

It is apparent from the stimulation technique that small areas of retinal dysfunction cannot be explored by full-field ERG, such as cases with Stargardt macular dystrophy or age-related macular degeneration, macular edema, etc. The cone photoreceptors are the most heavily packed in the macula, however 85-90 percent of cone photoreceptors reside in extra-macular retina. For this reason, full-field ERG is not a good way to investigate functional status or follow-up of retinal diseases known to be restricted to the macular area. Full-field ERG should be used for generalized retinal dysfunction.

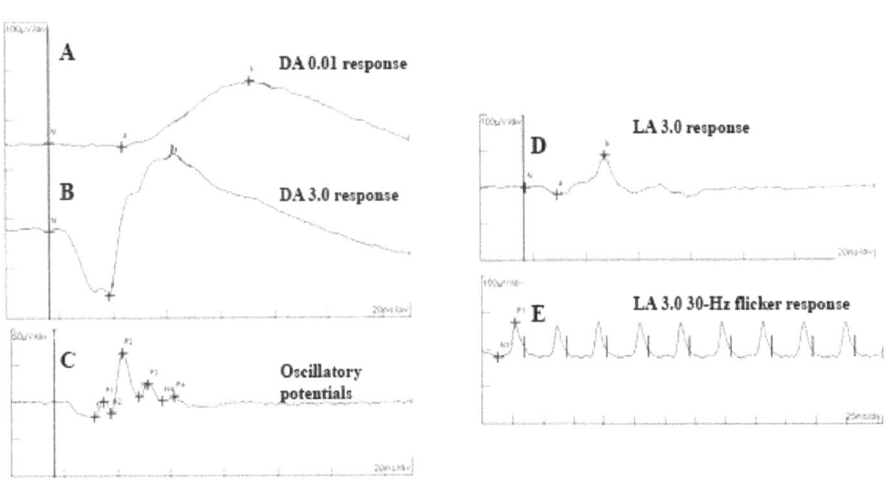

Figure 1. A representative full-field ERG response from a healthy subject.

Retinitis Pigmentosa: Retinitis pigmentosa refers to a large group of genetically heterogeneous disorders characterized by rod dysfunction in the early stages of the disease and progressive rod-cone dysfunction. In typical retinitis pigmentosa, full-field ERG is almost non-recordable in most clinical situations. Rod functions are generally deteriorated earlier and more severely than cone functions. Figure 2 shows a full-field ERG recording belonging to a 21-year-old male patient with retinitis pigmentosa.

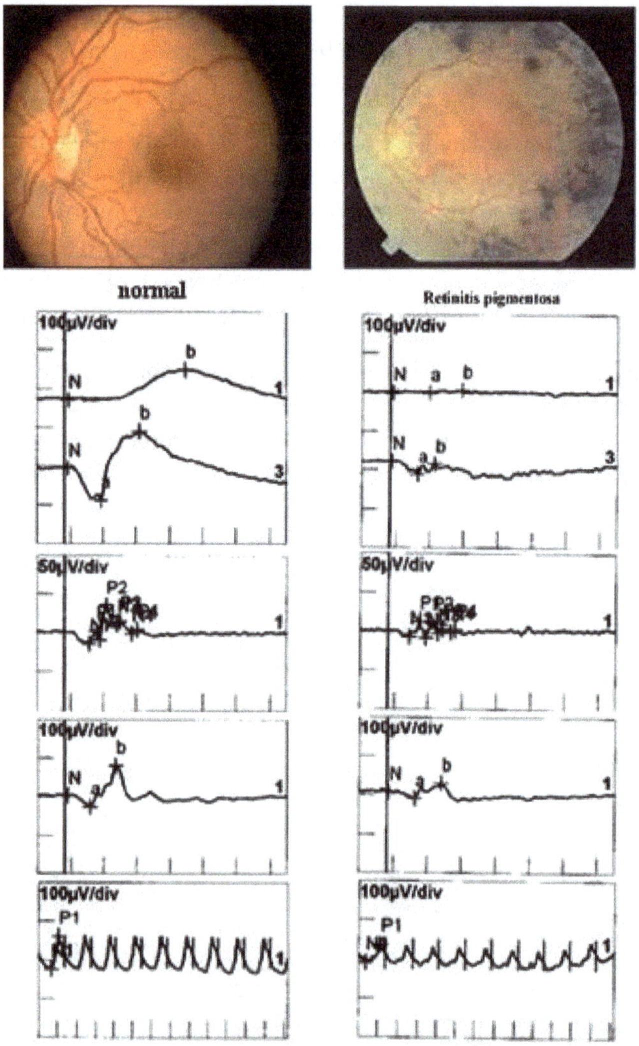

Figure 2. Full-field ERG responses belonging to a healthy subject and a 21-year old male with retinitis pigmentosa. DA 0.01 response is non-recordable. DA 3.0 response has a very low b wave amplitude. LA 3.0 and LA 3.0 30 Hz responses are reduced.

The original report of the ERG in primary retinitis pigmentosa revealed nondetectable or very small responses but these patients usually had advanced disease with attenuation of retinal vessels and extensive pigmentary changes in the retina. However, later studies showed that in the early stages of the disease, the ERG amplitudes are generally subnormal when the patient is asymptomatic. In that stage, however, delays in the implicit times helps in the establishing of widespread progressive forms of retinitis pigmentosa [4].

Retinitis pigmentosa has mainly three types of genetic transmission, autosomal dominant, autosomal recessive and X-linked recessive forms. Almost 50% of patients are sporadic retinitis pigmentosa patients which means that the most common form is this form of the disease. The worst prognosis is seen in X-linked recessive inheritance. These patients generally have non-recordable rod and cone ERG until the end of first decade. However, autosomal dominant type has the best prognosis, and patients with autosomal dominant inheritance may have good rod and cone functions until the fourth and fifth decades [4].

In cases with non-recordable full-field ERG, the follow-up of the macular function may be performed with multifocal ERG, focal ERG or pattern ERG. This will be discussed in the next parts of this chapter.

Cone dystrophies: Cone dystrophy refers to a large group of genetically heterogeneous disorders characterized by progressive diffuse cone dysfunction. Patients have progressive visual acuity loss, decreased color vision and, aversion to bright light. In cone dystrophies, rod function is normal in the early stages of the disease, however may deteriorate in the late stages. Combined rod-cone bright flash ERG shows a mild to moderately reduced a wave and b wave with variable prolongation and oscillatory potentials are also reduced. Single cone responses and 30 Hz cone responses are reduced and prolonged (Figure 3) [5].

Congenital Stationary Night Blindness (CSNB): In contrast to retinitis pigmentosa which is characterized by progressive night vision blindness and photoreceptor loss, CSNB refers to a group of congenital hereditary retinal diseases with non-progressive night blindness and no structural photoreceptor damage. The patient even may not recognize night blindness if the symptoms are mild. Schubert-Bornschein type of CSNB is the most frequent type and is characterized by negative full-field ERG. Negative ERG is told to occur when a b-wave amplitude lower than a-wave amplitude in combined rod-cone response. That is, the peak of the b-wave is under the isoelectric line of the full-field ERG and b/a ratio is under 1 (Figure 4). CSNB represents only one of the stationary night blinding disorders. Others are fundus albipunctatus, Oguchi disease and fleck retina of Kandori. However, CSNB may be said to be the only one with normal fundus, except myopic fundus changes in some subgroups.

Negative ERG is seen in stationary night blidness but is not limited to this condition. A normal a wave and reduced b wave means that there is problem in the transmission of electrical biopotential from the photoreceptors to the inner retinal layers. The retina has a dual circulation. Photoreceptors are nourished by choroidal circulation while inner retinal layers are nourished by retinal circulation. The biopotential cannot be transferred to inner retinal layers if a problem exist in the retinal circulation. For this reason, central retinal artery obstruction, central retinal vein obstruction may cause negative ERG. Similarly, juvenile retinoschisis is one of the causes of negative ERG.

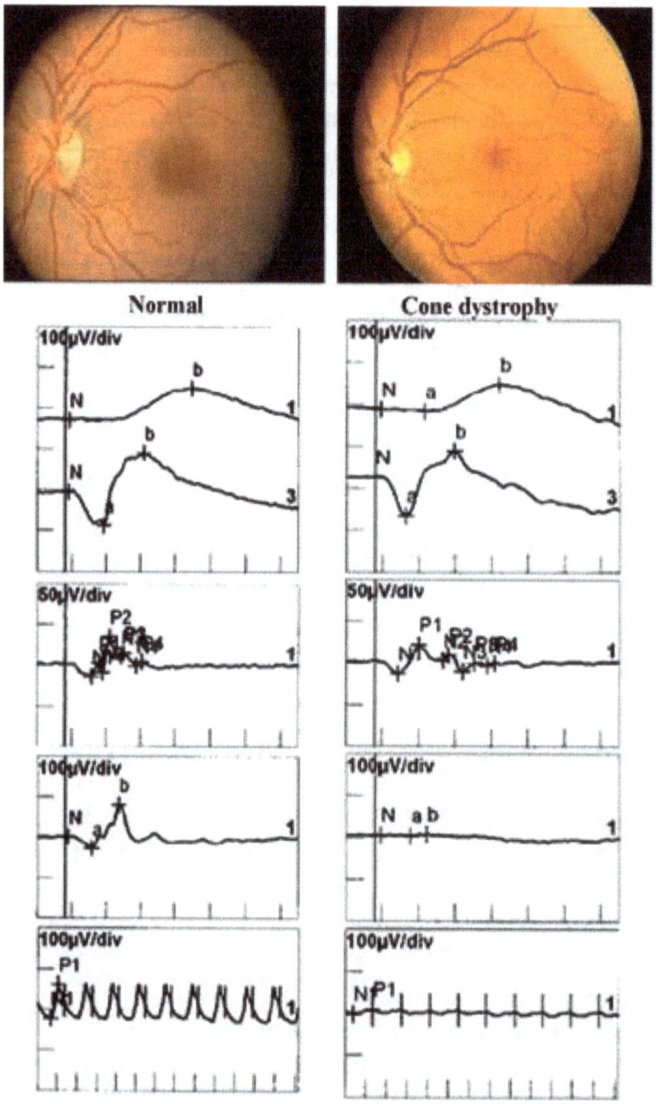

Figure 3. Full-field ERG responses belonging to a healthy subject and a 23-year old male with cone-dystrophy. DA 0.01 and DA 3.0 responses are normal. LA 3.0 response is almost non-recordable. LA 3.0 30 Hz responses are very much reduced.

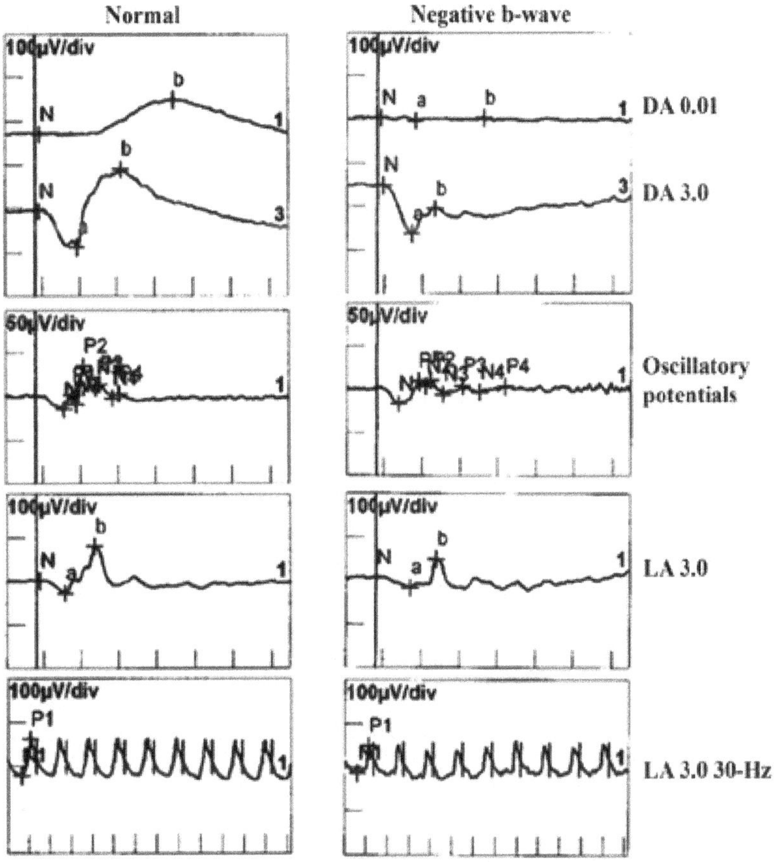

Figure 4. Full-field ERG responses belonging to a healthy subject and a 20-year old male with congenital stationary night blindness. DA 0.01 is non-recordable, DA 3.0 response has a negative configuration that is b-wave amplitude is lower than a-wave amplitude. LA 3.0 response and LA 3.0 30 Hz responses are mildly reduced.

Cone dystrophy with supernormal rod ERG. Cone dystrophy with supernormal ERG was first described by Gouras et al. in 1983 [6]. This autosomal recessively inherited syndrome is characterized by reduced visual acuity, abnormal color vision, discrete macular changes, and specific alterations of ERG responses. Full-field ERG changes are: (1) reduced and delayed cone responses, (2) a reduction and marked delay of rod b-waves at low light intensities, (3) elevated rod b-wave amplitudes at higher light intensities [7]. In the early stages of the disease, the fundus appearance may be normal, however macular pigmentary changes and macular atophy may occur in the later stages [8]. The dystrophy was shown to be caused by KCNV2 gene mutation [9-11]. This gene encodes a subunit of a voltage-gated potassium channel expressed in both rod and cone photoreceptors [9]. It is probable that the rapid increase in b-wave amplitude over a short range of stimulus may result from a 'gated' mechanism, occurring only after an abnormmally high threshold has been exceeded, enabling channel activation and ERG b-wave generation. Robson et al. reported that the ERG to the bright-flash showed a broadened and delayed a-wave through with a rhomboid-like shape [8]. Figure 5 shows a cone dystrophy patient with supernormal rod ERG [12].

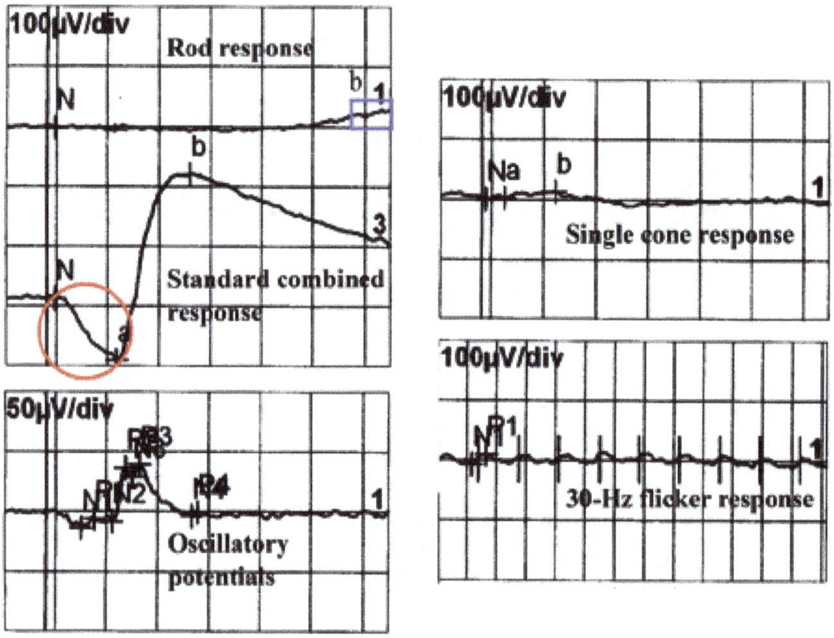

Figure 5. Full-field electroretinogram with very delayed rod response, a rhomboid a-wave and supernormal b-wave in bright-flash rod-cone response and very reduced cone responses in a patient with KCNV2 mutation (Used with permission of Journal of Retina-Vitreus, 2011).

Diabetic retinopathy. Full-field ERG changes are somewhat equivocal in diabetes mellitus. However, there are a number of studies reporting full-field ERG changes in diabetes mellitus. In one study, several ERG changes were reported in diabetics with or without retinopathy From the literature, it is apparent that full-field ERG changes were found in diabetic patients with and without diabetic retinopathy [13]. Holopigian et al. found several ERG parameters to be abnormal in early diabetic retinopathy [14]. Reductions in the oscillatory potentials were reported in diabetic retinopathy, [13, 15, 16] however there was no changes in one study [17]. Bresnick et al. found that oscillatory potential amplitudes predicted the progression of mild nonproliferative diabetic retinopathy to severe proliferative diabetic retinopathy [15, 18].

Toxic effects. Many drugs may have toxic effects on the retina, including choroquine/ hydroxychloroquine, chlorpromazine, thioridazine, indomethacine, quinine, methanol, gentamicin, cisplatin, vigabatrin, desferroxamine, sildenafil,..etc.

Chloroquine/hydroxychloroquine is used in the treatment of rheumatoid arthritis, systemic lupus erithematosis, and malarial fever. Both drugs have an affinity to melanin and tends to accumulate in the choroid, ciliary body, and retinal pigment epithelium. When the degenerative changes are limited to the macular area, normal or subnormal full-field ERG responses are obtained. In the late stages of the toxic effect, peripheral pigmentary changes become apparent. In this stage, minimal or non-recordable responses are obtained. Because full-field ERG responses are minimally affected in the early stages, this test is not recommended to detect early functional deficits. Instead, central 10/2 visual field testing and multifocal ERG is more appropriate for this purpose [19].

Photopic negative response. The photopic negative response is a negative-ongoing wave that occurs following the b-wave in response to a long flash. It is particularly easy to see in red flashes on blue backgrounds. Several studies indicated that the photopic negative response originates from the retinal ganglion cells. The photopic negative response is significantly reduced in patients with primary open-angle glaucoma,[20-24] anterior ischemic optic neuropathy, and other optic neuropathies,[25, 26] consistent with an origin in ganglion cells or their axons [27].

3. Multifocal electroretinogram

Multifocal ERG, first developed by Sutter and Tran in 1991 [28], provides a topographic map of the retinal function. As discussed above, full-field ERG is a mass response of the retina and small areas of retinal dysfunction cannot be explored with full-field ERG. At that point, multifocal ERG has its own advantages. By using a single electrode, multifocal ERG technique allows the recording of the functions of 61, 103 or even more retinal areas in less than 7-8 minutes. The recordings belong to central 30 to 50 degrees of the retina. For this reason, it is an excellent tool in detecting macular function. Multifocal ERG is a reproducible technique although very small responses are produced in each hexagonal area [29].

Multifocal ERG responses may be presented as single waveforms for each hexagonal area, ring analysis beginning from the most central to the periphery of the stimulated area and 3-D presentation (Figure 6).

The multifocal ERG stimulus is displayed on a video monitor. The stimulus consists of a pattern of hexagonal areas which are scaled to produce equal ERG responses from the retina (Figure 7). During stimulation, the display appears to flicker because each hexagon goes through a pseudo-random sequence (the m-sequence) of black and white presentations. Each hexagon has a probability of 0.5 of being white or black on each frame change [30]. Complex mathematical analyses between each retinal response and pseudo-random m sequence provide local retinal responses belonging to each hexagonal area.

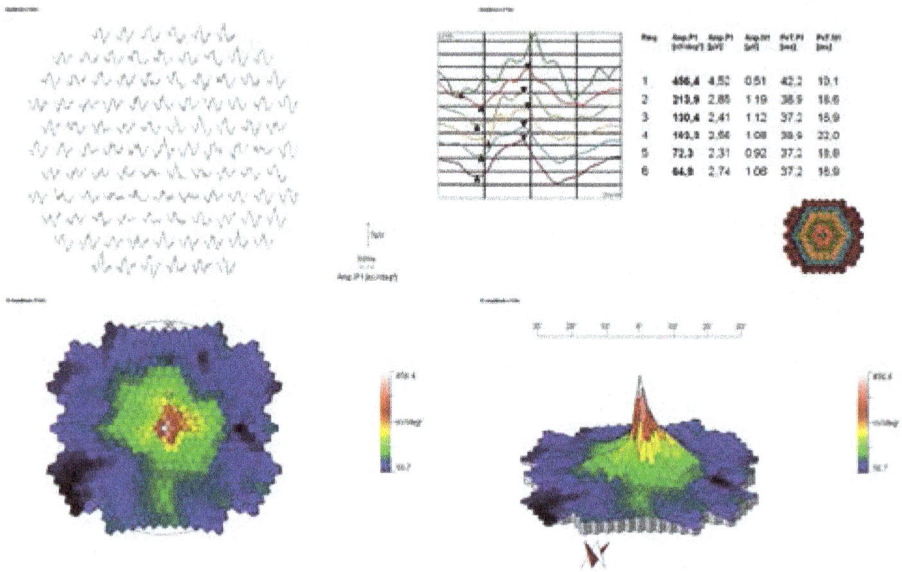

Figure 6. A normal multifocal ERG response output. Upper left: Plots diagram showing single responses from each retinal area. Upper right: Ring analyses. The upper rings show central retinal functions, the lower rings show peripheral functions. Lower right: 2-D amplitudes with color-coded diagram. Lower left: 3-D amplitudes.

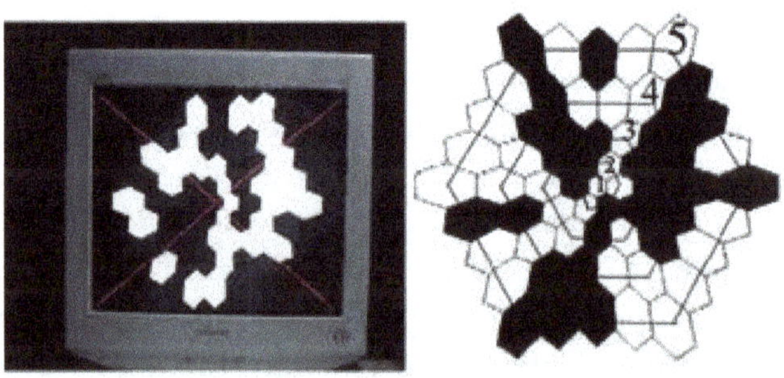

Figure 7. Multifocal ERG stimulus

Macular disease. One of the best uses of multifocal ERG is in Stargardt disease. The central responses are reduced and delayed and the better responses are obtained in the peripheral rings.

Central areolar choroidal dystrophy, first described by Nettleship in 1884, is a macular dystrophy characterized by the development of fine, mottled, depigmented retinal pigment epithelium in the macula. After several decades the pathognomonic zone of circumscript atrophy, affecting retina, retinal pigment epithelium and choriocapillaris, develops in the macular region of the eye [31, 32]. Although, most cases are sporadic, autosomal dominant and recessive inheritance patterns have been reported [33]. In a recent study, we have showed that mfERG responses were reduced corresponding to the areas of ophthalmoscopically visible lesion and there were significant correlations between foveal retinal sensitivity in the Humprey visual field and mfERG P1/N1 amplitudes (Figure 8) [34].

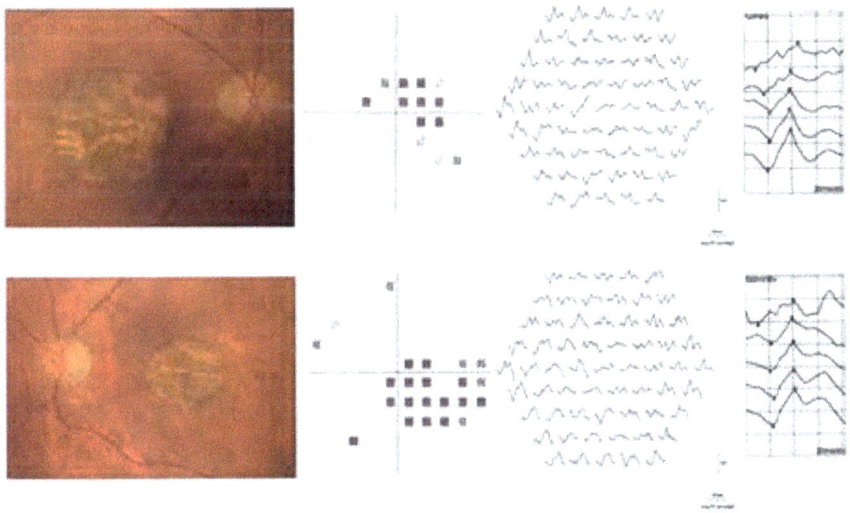

Figure 8. Color fundus photographs, pattern deviation of Humphrey visual fields and multifocal ERG results of four patients with central areolar choroidal dystrophy. Central responses are markedly reduced and delayed in multifocal ERG. (Used with permission of Wichtig Editore. From. 'Multifocal electroretinogram and central visual field testing in central areolar choroidal dystrophy'', Gundogan et al, European Journal of Ophthalmology, Volume 20, Number 5, 2010).

Multifocal ERG was used to evaluate macular function and the response of macular edema to different types of treatment in different types of macular edema. In one of them we showed that multifocal ERG is not a good way to monitor the macular function in *chronic* macular edema [35].

Diabetic retinopathy. One of the important features of early diabetic retinopathy is its focal nature. Full-field ERG is a mass response of all retinal areas. For this reason, full-field ERG recordings cannot detect smaller areas of focal retinopathy in early diabetic retinopathy. Because multifocal ERG records the function of very small retinal areas, it may be used to detect very early local retinal dysfunctions in diabetic retinopathy. Holm et al. showed that hard exudates prolongs the implicit times of the multifocal ERG independent from the macular thickness [36]. In accordance with this finding, Dhamdhere et al. found that local neuroretinal function is not associated with full retinal thickness measured locally in patients with diabetes and no retinopathy, even in abnormal locations. The authors concluded that full retinal thickness measured locally by OCT is not a surrogate for multifocal ERGs in early diabetic retinopathy [37].

Follow-up of retinitis pigmentosa. Multifocal electroretinography is a powerful tool in the follow-up of residual central cone functions in retinitis pigmentosa. In these cases, full-field ERG is generally not reproducible and cone functions are non-recordable. In one study, [38] yearly progression according to the multifocal ERG values was found to be approximately 6% to 10% in the outer three rings. Ring 5 amplitudes of the multifocal electroretinogram correlated well with the scotopic full-field mixed rod-cone ERG response amplitude.

Glaucoma. Glaucoma primarily affects the inner retina, specifically the retinal ganglion cells, most likely with unremarkable signs or symptoms in the early stages. The damage to retinal ganglion cells results in visual field loss. However, approximately 30-35% of ganglion cells should be lost for an evidence of visual field loss. In recent years, retinal nerve fiber layer analysis by optical coherence tomography has become the most common technique for glaucoma detection [39]. Several studies have used multifocal ERG in detecting signs of glaucoma in terms of amplitude [40] and implicit times [41]. The amplitude of the multifocal ERG is also reduced in patients with ocular hypertension [42].

One of the most important studies on the use of multifocal ERG for glaucoma detection was performed by Sutter and Bearse [43]. The authors used a mathematical algorithm to extract a component with a latency, which increased in proportion to the estimated length of the ganglion cell axons from the site of stimulation to the optic nerve head. The authors found that glaucomatous damage may reduce the magnitude of this component (optic nerve head component) [39, 43].

4. Focal electroretinogram

Focal ERG is used to record local ERG response. In contrast to multifocal ERG stimulus, a direct focal light is used over the retinal area being tested, mostly the macular or foveal region. The response to such a stimulus is about a few microvolts, for this reason, signal-to-noise ratio is low in focal ERG. To overcome this issue, hundreds of stimulus should be used to have a reliable average response. Second problem in focal ERG is the scattered light. The original ring-shaped light is scattered in the eye and may easily stimulate the area outside the intended retinal area. For this reason, the stimulating light is encircled by an annulus ring of steady background light that is typically brighter than the test stimulus. However, this is not an unproblematic solution, because it use of a brighter background light prevents the recording of rod functions [44]. Focal ERG is generally not used in routine clinical practice in most electrophysiological units because of these difficulties and the emergence of multifocal ERG in 1992.

5. Pattern electroretinogram

Pattern ERG is a retinal response to a checkerboard pattern stimulus with alternating black and white squares. In low temporal frequencies (<6 reversals per second), a positive component, P50 (positive peak around 50th milliseconds), and a negative component, N95 (negative component around 95th milliseconds), are observed. Sometimes, a negative component around 35 milliseconds may be recorded (N35).This response to low-frequency stimulus is called 'transient PERG. (Figure 9)

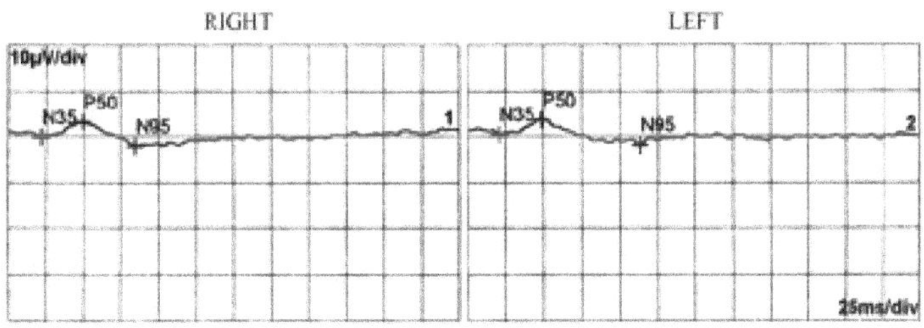

Figure 9. A typical pattern ERG recording.

In high temporal frequencies (>7 reversals per second), P50 and N95 peaks are merged into a sinusoidal waveform, dominated by the N95 component. This response is called 'steady-state pattern ERG'. In steady-state pattern ERG, it is impossible to distinguish the original P50 and N95 peaks [45].

Initially it was thought that PERG is almost totally originated from ganglion cell functions. However, later studies showed that P50 peak has an earlier component originated from cells distal to the ganglion cells and reflecting mostly the macular function [46-49]. In two reports [50, 51], it has been detected that some pattern ERG response still may be recorded after post-traumatic and surgical optic nerve section despite no light perception. In one of them, P50 amplitude reduction with P50 latency shortening was observed. These findings too imply that pattern ERG is not completely originated from ganglion cells. In addition, shortening of the P50 latency caused the theory that a later part of the P50 response is related with ganglion cell function and P50 latency shortens if ganglion cell function extinguishes.

It is apparent from the Figure 9 that P50 amplitude reduction is accompanied by a secondary N95 reduction, as N95 amplitude is measured from P50 peak to N95 trough. However, this is not the same for N95 amplitude reduction. N95 amplitude reduction may be selective. For this reason, the ratio of N95 amplitude to P50 amplitude has an importance in detecting whether the visual loss is related to macular disease or ganglion cell disease. If N95/P50 ratio is normal, then it may be thought that the visual loss may be attributed to macular disease. If the ratio is lower than normal (which is called as 'selective N95 reduction'), visual loss may be attributed to ganglion cell disease. N95/P50 ratio is about 1.5 in the author's electrophysiology laboratory.

5.1. Chronic effect of optic nerve disease to pattern ERG.

The first reports about N95 in optic nerve demyelination were presented by Holder. Holder reported that pattern ERG abnormalities could be limited to N95 component. The author also reported that there was a 40% pattern ERG abnormality among 200 patients with optic nerve demyelination, however 85% of the abnormalities were detected in N95 [52, 53].

Figure 10 and figure 11 show P50 and N95 results of 382 patients with optic nerve demyelination. As shown in Figure 10, most of the patients have normal P50 amplitudes despite prolonged P100 latency in pattern VEP. However Figure 11 shows that N95/P50 ratio decreases as P100 latency increases [52].

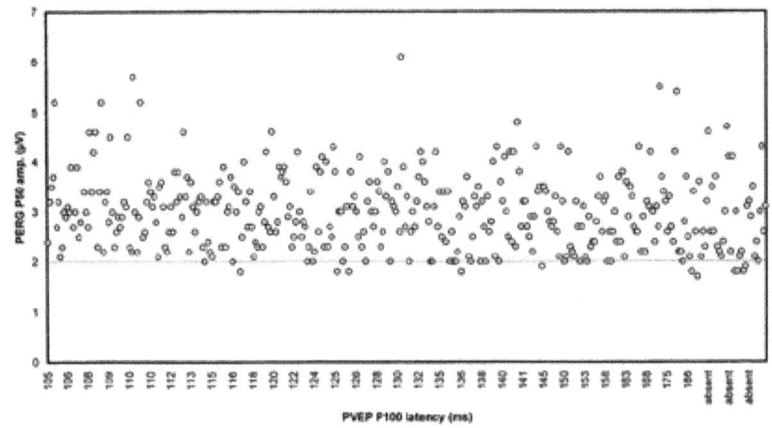

Figure 10. Pattern ERG P50 amplitudes in patients with optic nerve demyelination. (Used with permission of Pergamon. From. 'Pattern Electroretinography (PERG) and an Integrated Approach to Visual Pathway Diagnosis '', Holder GE, Progress in Retinal and Eye Research, Volume 20, Number 4, 2001).

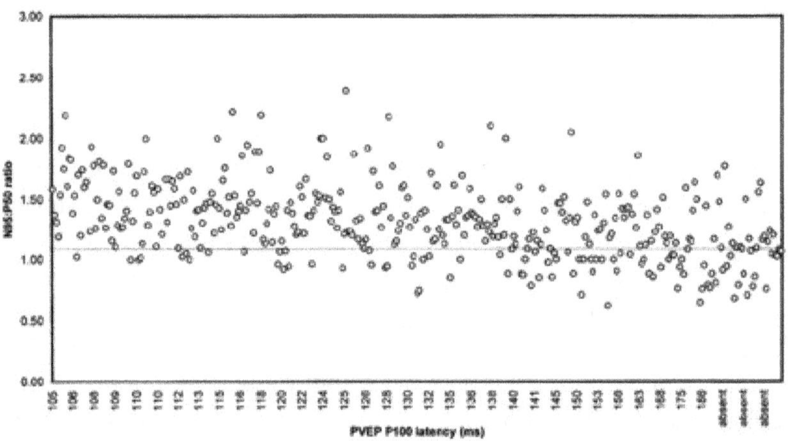

Figure 11. Pattern ERG N95/P50 ratio in patients with optic nerve demyelination. (Used with permission of Pergamon. From. 'Pattern Electroretinography (PERG) and an Integrated Approach to Visual Pathway Diagnosis '', Holder GE, Progress in Retinal and Eye Research, Volume 20, Number 4, 2001).

Acute effects of optic nerve disease on pattern ERG. Pattern ERG changes in the acute phase of the optic nerve inflammation is not simply as mentioned above. In the acute phase of the inflammation, P100 amplitude in pattern VEP is reduced with less latency changes while P50 in pattern ERG is also reduced. A few weeks later, as the inflammation subsides P50 amplitude in pattern ERG and P100 amplitude in pattern VEP recover, however, ganglion cell dysfunction or demyelination begin to appear. N95 is reduced (selectively as mentioned above) while P100 is delayed. N95/P50 ratio is lowered in the chronic phase of the inflammation. MRI findings in the acute and chronic phase of the inflammation was shown to be consistent with this theory [52, 54].

Glaucoma and pattern ERG. Hood et al. [55] studied pattern ERG in glaucoma patients with confirmed visual field deficits. The authors included 21 eyes of 15 patients with glaucoma. Pattern ERG was within normal limits for 4 of the worse eyes of 15 glaucoma patients. Overall, 6 of the 21 eyes that met the criteria for glaucomatous damage had normal pattern ERGs on both N95 amplitude and N95/P50 ratio. Second, the N95 amplitude was nonlinearly related to visual field sensitivity. Small field losses were associated with disproportionately large losses in pattern ERG amplitude. Third, the PERG from both eyes of a patient were very similar, even when the visual fields suggested very different levels of damage.

Ventura et al.[56] investigated the steady-state pattern ERG responses with PERGLA paradigm in 200 glaucoma suspects with increased optic disc cupping and normal visual field and in 42 patients with early manifest glaucoma. The PERG was abnormal in amplitude, phase, or inter-ocular asymmetry in amplitude and phase in 52% of glaucoma suspect patients and 69% of EMG patients. The pattern ERG amplitude was correlated weakly with both mean deviation and vertical C/D (p=0.05). The correlation between pattern ERG amplitude and MD and C/D was stronger for inter-ocular differences rather than absolute measures. Inter-ocular pattern ERG amplitude asymmetry was positively correlated with the severity of the disease. Compared to white glaucoma suspects, a lower pattern ERG amplitude was found in black glaucoma suspects and early manifest glaucoma patients, but not in black glaucoma controls.

6. Electro-oculogram

Unlike full-field ERG, electro-oculogram (EOG) is not a stimulated response. EOG records the continuous resting potential across the retinal pigment epithelium which is named as 'trans-epithelial potential'. This potential is only about a few millivolts. Transepithelial potential is mainly generated by retinal pigment epithelium. However, as well as the integrity of the retinal pigment epithelium, photoreceptor and interphotoreceptor matrix integrity and function should be intact. For this reason, EOG is decreased in photoreceptor diseases, retinal detachment and other generalized outer retinal damages in addition to primary retinal pigment diseases such as Best disease.

The resting potential across the retinal pigment epithelium is not a steady potential. In the dark-adaptation, transepithelial potential is decreased to a minimum value (dark trough) after about 12 minutes. In the light-adaptation, the transepithelial potential increases to a peak value (light-peak) after about 7-12 minutes [57]. The ratio of light-peak to dark-trough is called Arden ratio or 'EOG ratio'. This value should be 1.8 or greater in normal subjects and considered abnormal under 1.6. In the author's institution, Arden ratio is 2.35±0.44 (mean±SD) [58]. Figure 12 shows EOG recordings of a patient with Best disease. There is almost no light peak with light stimulation in EOG. Arden ratios are 1.18 in the right eye and 1.17 in the left eye.

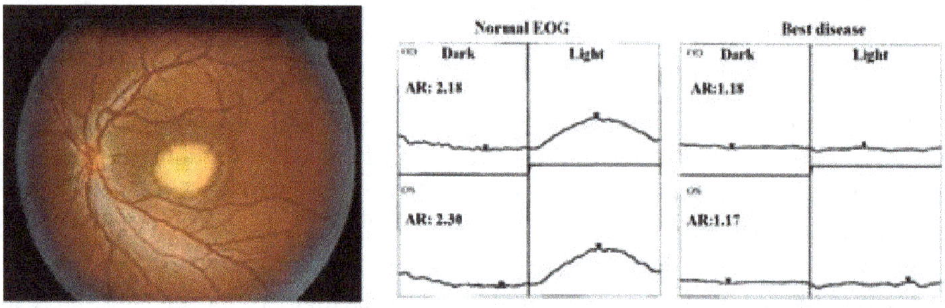

Figure 12. Fundus photo of a patient with Best disease and EOG recordings. Arden ratio is 1.18 in OD and 1.17 in OS. This implies very small change in transepithelial potential with light stimulation.

7. Visual evoked potential

Visual evoked potential (VEP) represents the cortical response to a checkerboard-pattern stimulus (pattern VEP) or a flash stimulus (flash VEP). Pattern VEP components that are commonly measured are N75, P100 and N135 peaks (Figure 13).

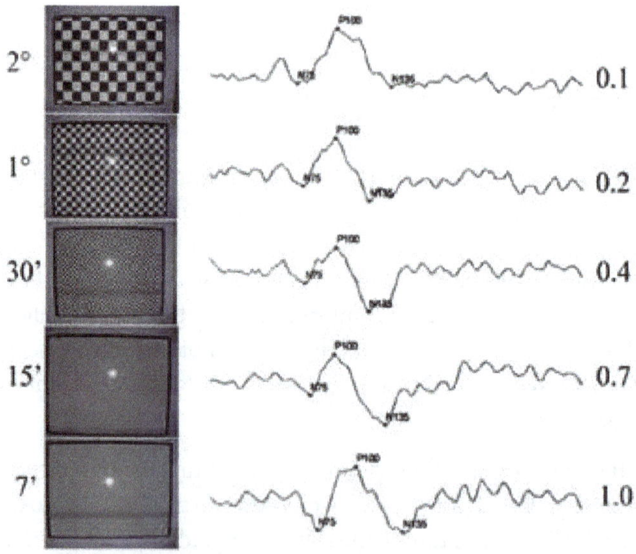

Figure 13. Representative pattern VEP waveforms to five consecutive check sizes.

The amplitudes of the peaks are measured from the peak of the one component to the trough of the preceding component. P and N refer to positive and negative voltages recorded at the occipital electrode with respect to the voltage at the reference electrode.

Flash VEP components are defined as N1, P1, N2, P2, etc (Figure 14).

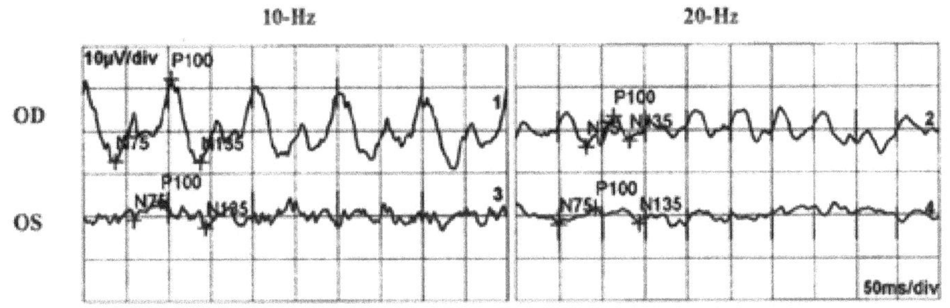

Figure 14. Flash VEP responses in a patient with intravitreal hemorrhage in the left eye. Left-eye flash VEP responses are very much reduced.

VEP response primarily reflects the central retinal function although the stimulated retinal area in pattern VEP and flash VEP is about 50 degrees and full retinal areas, respectively. There are three main reasons for this contribution of the central retina [59]. (1).The central visual field is represented at the outer surface of the visual cortex while peripheral retina is represented at the deep surfaces of the calcarine sulcus. Active electrode in VEP recordings is placed approximately 2 cm above the protuberentia occipitalis externa which is the nearest point to the surface of the visual cortex. (2) Cortical magnification phenomenon. In the central retina each photoreceptor transmits its signal almost to one ganglion cell, while many photoreceptors converges on a single ganglion cell in the peripheral retina. Thus, more than 50% of the cells in the visual cortex represent approximately central 10 degrees of the retina. (3) In PVEP testing, small checkerboard stimuli may be used. These small sized stimuli may only be resolved by the central retina which has the highest concentration of photoreceptors.

Because of the reflection of the central retinal function, pattern VEP is used to estimate visual acuity in many clinical situations besides optic nerve function [60]. An impaired VEP is anatomically non-specific. However, a through ocular examination including the retina, optic nerve and brain frequently explores the localization of the problem [61]. Pattern VEP is more valuable than flash VEP in the clinical evaluations of the visual pathway. However, flash VEP is valuable in the situations of fixation problem, mature cataract, intravitreal hemorrhage, ocular trauma or any other circumstance that prevents patient cooperation. In these situations, flash VEP gives important knowledge about visual status.

Pattern VEP recording requires fixation to a point in the screen. Impaired VEP responses may be produced by deliberate poor fixation, defocusing to the fixation point, or conscious suppression.[61-64] This is an important issue in the evaluation of patients with functional visual loss. Voluntary flash VEP suppression is more difficult, because it does not require fixation.

Optic nerve disease. VEP is commonly used to detect visual pathway deficits in patients with no apparent objective signs of ocular dysfunction. In a study on MS patients with no clinical history of optic nerve involvement, we showed that 21 of 39 patients had delayed P100 latency [65]. Figure 15 shows PVEP recording of an MS patient included in that study. Snellen visual acuity was 1.0 in both eyes although P100 latency was clearly prolonged in the left eye.

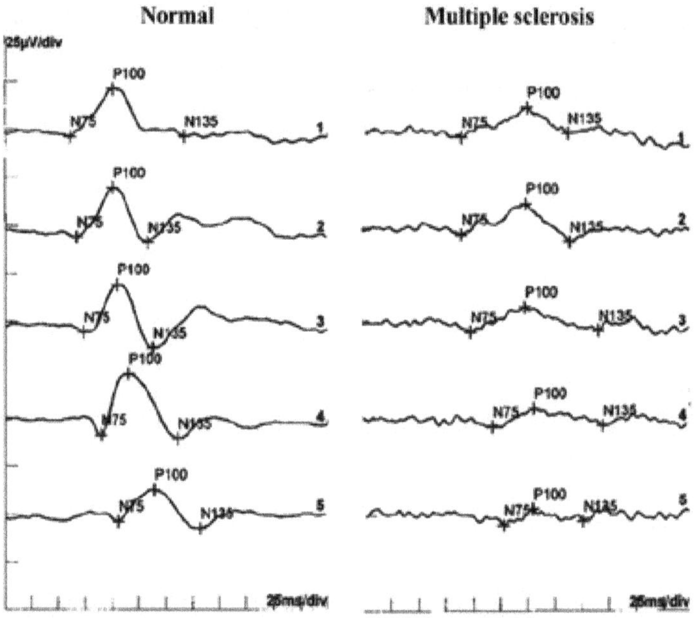

Figure 15. Pattern VEP traces belonging to a –normal and a multiple sclerosis patient. P100 latency to 2 degree check size is about 150 ms in the left eye while it is about 100 ms in the right eye.

Functional Visual Loss. The term 'functional visual loss' is used when the visual loss cannot be explained with organic lesions in the visual pathway. 'Vision' is a cortical function and the bio-potential change in the visual cortex after a visual stimulus is evaluated with visual evoked potentials. In a study, we showed that pattern VEP recordings to five check sizes (2 degree, 1 degree, 30 minute, 15 minute and 7 minute) may be used objectively to estimate visual acuities of the patients with suspected functional visual loss [66].

Figure 16 shows PVEP recordings to 5-consecutive check sizes of an African woman with no light perception in the left eye for 2 years. Biomicroscopic and fundoscopic examinations were unremarkable. No relative afferent pupillary defect was detected. Pattern VEP responses in both eyes were totally in the normal limits in terms of P100 amplitude and latency values. In this patient, we were able to show that the patient was capable of reading at least 0.3 in Snellen chart from 6 meters with the use of polaroid glasses.

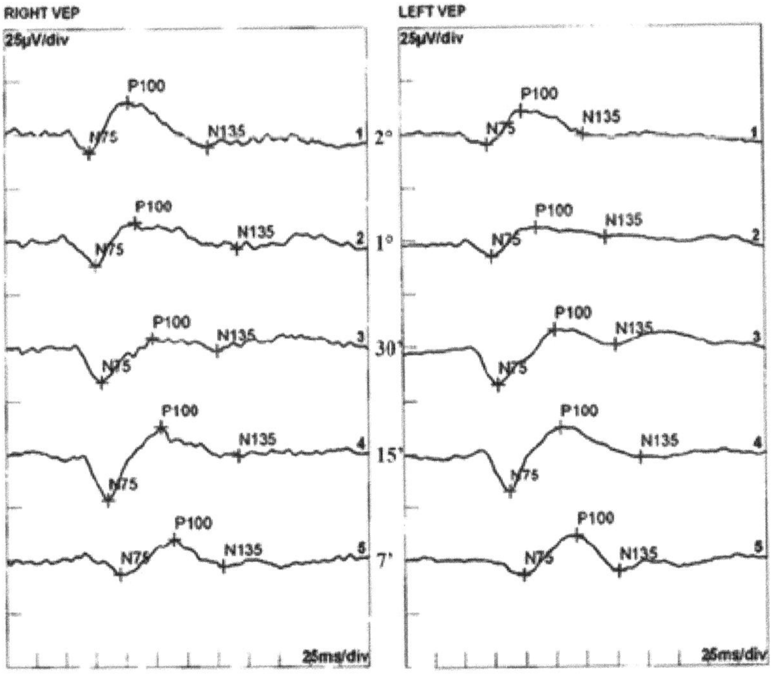

Figure 16. PVEP response to five consecutive check sizes in a malingerer who claimed no light perception in the left eye.

8. Conclusion

Full-field ERG is invaluable in generalized retinal diseases. Pattern ERG is complimentary test for full-field ERG, because it may localize the problem to macula or ganglion cells. Multifocal ERG is used to evaluate central retinal function. EOG is the recording of transepithelial potential. VEP is a cortical potential that is the end of visual pathway, for this reason it gives important knowledge about the 'vision' itself. The ophthalmologist can localize the visual problem with a thorough understanding of the origins of these tests.

Author details

Fatih C. Gundogan[1*] and Umit Yolcu[2]

*Address all correspondence to: fgundogan@yahoo.com

1 GATA Medical School, Ophthalmology, Ankara, Turkey

2 Siirt Military Hospital, Ophthalmology, Siirt, Turkey

References

[1] Marmor MF, Fulton AB, Holder GE, Miyake Y, Brigell M, Bach M, et al. ISCEV Standard for full-field clinical electroretinography (2008 update). Doc Ophthalmol 2009;118(1):69-77.

[2] Vincent A, Robson AG, Holder GE. Pathognomonic (diagnostic) ERGs. A review and update. Retina 2013;33(1):5-12.

[3] Lam BL. Full-field electroretinogram. In: Lam BL, editor. Lam, Byron L. Boca Raton: Taylor & Francis; 2005. p. 1-64.

[4] Berson EL. Retinitis pigmentosa and allied diseases: applications of electroretinographic testing. Int Ophthalmol 1981;4(1-2):7-22.

[5] Lam BL. Macular disorders. In: Lam BL, editor. Electrophysiology of vision : clinical testing and applications. Boca Raton: Taylor & Francis; 2005. p. 277-330.

[6] Gouras P, Eggers HM, MacKay CJ. Cone dystrophy, nyctalopia, and supernormal rod responses. A new retinal degeneration. Arch Ophthalmol 1983;101(5):718-24.

[7] Wissinger B, Dangel S, Jagle H, Hansen L, Baumann B, Rudolph G, et al. Cone dystrophy with supernormal rod response is strictly associated with mutations in KCNV2. Invest Ophthalmol Vis Sci 2008;49(2):751-7.

[8] Robson AG, Webster AR, Michaelides M, Downes SM, Cowing JA, Hunt DM, et al. "Cone dystrophy with supernormal rod electroretinogram": a comprehensive genotype/phenotype study including fundus autofluorescence and extensive electrophysiology. Retina 2010;30(1):51-62.

[9] Wu H, Cowing JA, Michaelides M, Wilkie SE, Jeffery G, Jenkins SA, et al. Mutations in the gene KCNV2 encoding a voltage-gated potassium channel subunit cause "cone dystrophy with supernormal rod electroretinogram" in humans. Am J Hum Genet 2006;79(3):574-9.

[10] Thiagalingam S, McGee TL, Weleber RG, Sandberg MA, Trzupek KM, Berson EL, et al. Novel mutations in the KCNV2 gene in patients with cone dystrophy and a supernormal rod electroretinogram. Ophthalmic Genet 2007;28(3):135-42.

[11] Ben Salah S, Kamei S, Senechal A, Lopez S, Bazalgette C, Bazalgette C, et al. Novel KCNV2 mutations in cone dystrophy with supernormal rod electroretinogram. Am J Ophthalmol 2008;145(6):1099-106.

[12] Gundogan FC, Tas, A., Sobaci, G. Cone Dytrophy with Rod Supernormal Electroretinogram: KCNV2 Mutation. Journal of Retina-Vitreus 2011;19(4):282-84.

[13] Juen S, Kieselbach GF. Electrophysiological changes in juvenile diabetics without retinopathy. Arch Ophthalmol 1990;108(3):372-5.

[14] Holopigian K, Seiple W, Lorenzo M, Carr R. A comparison of photopic and scotopic electroretinographic changes in early diabetic retinopathy. Invest Ophthalmol Vis Sci 1992;33(10):2773-80.

[15] Bresnick GH, Korth K, Groo A, Palta M. Electroretinographic oscillatory potentials predict progression of diabetic retinopathy. Preliminary report. Arch Ophthalmol 1984;102(9):1307-11.

[16] Bresnick GH, Palta M. Oscillatory potential amplitudes. Relation to severity of diabetic retinopathy. Arch Ophthalmol 1987;105(7):929-33.

[17] Wanger P, Persson HE. Early diagnosis of retinal changes in diabetes: a comparison between electroretinography and retinal biomicroscopy. Acta Ophthalmol (Copenh) 1985;63(6):716-20.

[18] Bresnick GH, Palta M. Predicting progression to severe proliferative diabetic retinopathy. Arch Ophthalmol 1987;105(6):810-4.

[19] Fischman GA. The electroretinogram. In: Fishman GA, Sokol S, Holder GE, Brigell M, editors. Electrophysiologic testing in disorders of the retina, optic nerve, and visual pathway. San Francisco, CA: American Academy of Ophthalmology; 2001. p. 1-156.

[20] Machida S, Tamada K, Oikawa T, Gotoh Y, Nishimura T, Kaneko M, et al. Comparison of photopic negative response of full-field and focal electroretinograms in detecting glaucomatous eyes. J Ophthalmol 2011;2011.

[21] Kiszkielis M, Lubinski W, Penkala K. The photopic negative response as a promising diagnostic tool in glaucoma. A review. Klin Oczna 2012;114(2):138-42.

[22] Gotoh Y. [Photopic negative response of eyes with normal-tension glaucoma]. Nihon Ganka Gakkai Zasshi 2002;106(8):481-7.

[23] Viswanathan S, Frishman LJ, Robson JG, Walters JW. The photopic negative response of the flash electroretinogram in primary open angle glaucoma. Invest Ophthalmol Vis Sci 2001;42(2):514-22.

[24] Colotto A, Falsini B, Salgarello T, Iarossi G, Galan ME, Scullica L. Photopic negative response of the human ERG: losses associated with glaucomatous damage. Invest Ophthalmol Vis Sci 2000;41(8):2205-11.

[25] Gotoh Y, Machida S, Tazawa Y. Selective loss of the photopic negative response in patients with optic nerve atrophy. Arch Ophthalmol 2004;122(3):341-6.

[26] Miyata K, Nakamura M, Kondo M, Lin J, Ueno S, Miyake Y, et al. Reduction of oscillatory potentials and photopic negative response in patients with autosomal dominant optic atrophy with OPA1 mutations. Invest Ophthalmol Vis Sci 2007;48(2):820-4.

[27] Frishman LJ. Origins of the electroretinogram. In: Heckenlively JR, Arden GB, editors. Principles and practice of clinical electrophysiology of vision. Cambridge, Mass.: MIT Press; 2006. p. 139-84.

[28] Sutter EE, Tran D. The field topography of ERG components in man--I. The photopic luminance response. Vision Res 1992;32(3):433-46.

[29] Gundogan FC, Sobaci G, Bayraktar MZ. Intra-sessional and inter-sessional variability of multifocal electroretinogram. Doc Ophthalmol 2008;117(3):175-83.

[30] Hood DC. Assessing retinal function with the multifocal technique. Prog Retin Eye Res 2000;19(5):607-46.

[31] Carr RE. Central Areolar Choroidal Dystrophy. Arch Ophthalmol 1965;73:32-5.

[32] Hoyng CB, Deutman AF. The development of central areolar choroidal dystrophy. Graefes Arch Clin Exp Ophthalmol 1996;234(2):87-93.

[33] Nagasaka K, Horiguchi M, Shimada Y, Yuzawa M. Multifocal electroretinograms in cases of central areolar choroidal dystrophy. Invest Ophthalmol Vis Sci 2003;44(4): 1673-9.

[34] Gundogan FC, Dinc UA, Erdem U, Ozge G, Sobaci G. Multifocal electroretinogram and central visual field testing in central areolar choroidal dystrophy. Eur J Ophthalmol 2010;20(5):919-24.

[35] Durukan AH, Memisoglu S, Gundogan FC. Is multifocal ERG a reliable index of macular function after triamcinolone acetonide injection in diffuse diabetic macular edema? Eur J Ophthalmol 2009;19(6):1017-27.

[36] Holm K, Ponjavic V, Lovestam-Adrian M. Using multifocal electroretinography hard exudates affect macular function in eyes with diabetic retinopathy. Graefes Arch Clin Exp Ophthalmol 2010;248(9):1241-7.

[37] Dhamdhere KP, Bearse MA, Jr., Harrison W, Barez S, Schneck ME, Adams AJ. Associations between local retinal thickness and function in early diabetes. Invest Ophthalmol Vis Sci 2012;53(10):6122-8.

[38] Nagy D, Schonfisch B, Zrenner E, Jagle H. Long-term follow-up of retinitis pigmentosa patients with multifocal electroretinography. Invest Ophthalmol Vis Sci 2008;49(10):4664-71.

[39] Chan HH, Ng YF, Chu PH. Applications of the multifocal electroretinogram in the detection of glaucoma. Clin Exp Optom 2011;94(3):247-58.

[40] Frishman LJ, Saszik S, Harwerth RS, Viswanathan S, Li Y, Smith EL, 3rd, et al. Effects of experimental glaucoma in macaques on the multifocal ERG. Multifocal ERG in laser-induced glaucoma. Doc Ophthalmol 2000;100(2-3):231-51.

[41] Hasegawa S, Takagi M, Usui T, Takada R, Abe H. Waveform changes of the first-order multifocal electroretinogram in patients with glaucoma. Invest Ophthalmol Vis Sci 2000;41(6):1597-603.

[42] Chan HH, Brown B. Pilot study of the multifocal electroretinogram in ocular hypertension. Br J Ophthalmol 2000;84(10):1147-53.

[43] Sutter EE, Bearse MA, Jr. The optic nerve head component of the human ERG. Vision Res 1999;39(3):419-36.

[44] Lam BL. Focal Electroretinogram. In: Lam BL, editor. Electrophysiology of vision : clinical testing and applications. Boca Raton: Taylor & Francis; 2005. p. 67-8.

[45] Holder GE. The Pattern Electroretinogram. In: Fishman GA, Birch DG, Holder GE, Brigell MG, editors. Electrophysiologic testing in disorders of the retina, optic nerve, and visual pathways. San Francisco, CA: American Academy of Ophthalmology; 2001. p. 197-237

[46] Berninger T, Schuurmans RP. Spatial tuning of the pattern ERG across temporal frequency. Doc Ophthalmol 1985;61(1):17-25.

[47] Schuurmans RP, Berninger T. Luminance and contrast responses recorded in man and cat. Doc Ophthalmol 1985;59(2):187-97.

[48] Trick GL, Wintermeyer DH. Spatial and temporal frequency tuning of pattern-reversal retinal potentials. Invest Ophthalmol Vis Sci 1982;23(6):774-9.

[49] Kirkham TH, Coupland SG. The pattern electroretinogram in optic nerve demyelination. Can J Neurol Sci 1983;10(4):256-60.

[50] Sherman J. Simultaneous pattern-reversal electroretinograms and visual evoked potentials in diseases of the macula and optic nerve. Ann N Y Acad Sci 1982;388:214-26.

[51] Harrison JM, O'Connor PS, Young RS, Kincaid M, Bentley R. The pattern ERG in man following surgical resection of the optic nerve. Invest Ophthalmol Vis Sci 1987;28(3):492-9.

[52] Holder GE. Pattern electroretinography (PERG) and an integrated approach to visual pathway diagnosis. Prog Retin Eye Res 2001;20(4):531-61.

[53] Holder GE. The incidence of abnormal pattern electroretinography in optic nerve demyelination. Electroencephalogr Clin Neurophysiol 1991;78(1):18-26.

[54] Youl BD, Turano G, Miller DH, Towell AD, MacManus DG, Moore SG, et al. The pathophysiology of acute optic neuritis. An association of gadolinium leakage with clinical and electrophysiological deficits. Brain 1991;114 (Pt 6):2437-50.

[55] Hood DC, Xu L, Thienprasiddhi P, Greenstein VC, Odel JG, Grippo TM, et al. The pattern electroretinogram in glaucoma patients with confirmed visual field deficits. Invest Ophthalmol Vis Sci 2005;46(7):2411-8.

[56] Ventura LM, Porciatti V, Ishida K, Feuer WJ, Parrish RK, 2nd. Pattern electroretinogram abnormality and glaucoma. Ophthalmology 2005;112(1):10-9.

[57] Lam BL. Electro-oculogram. In: Lam BL, editor. Electrophysiology of vision : clinical testing and applications. Boca Raton: Taylor & Francis; 2005. p. 105-22.

[58] Gundogan FC, Uysal Y, Erdem U, Sobaci G, Bayraktar MZ. Our normal values of electrooculogram. Gulhane Medical Journal 2006;48(2):79-82.

[59] Brigell M. The visual evoked potential. In: Fishman GA, Birch DG, Holder GE, Brigell M, editors. Electrophysiologic testing in disorders of the retina, optic nerve, and visual pathway. San Francisco, CA: American Academy of Ophthalmology; 1990. p. 237-81.

[60] Gundogan FC, Mutlu FM, Altinsoy HI, Tas A, Oz O, Sobaci G. Pattern visual evoked potentials in the assessment of objective visual acuity in amblyopic children. Int Ophthalmol 2010;30(4):377-83.

[61] Lam BL. Visual Evoked Potential. In: Lam BL, editor. Electrophysiology of vision : clinical testing and applications. Boca Raton: Taylor & Francis; 2005. p. 123-50.

[62] Ladenson PW, Stakes JW, Ridgway EC. Reversible alteration of the visual evoked potential in hypothyroidism. Am J Med 1984;77(6):1010-4.

[63] Tan CT, Murray NM, Sawyers D, Leonard TJ. Deliberate alteration of the visual evoked potential. J Neurol Neurosurg Psychiatry 1984;47(5):518-23.

[64] Sumskii LI, Guppa NS, Sklovskaia ML. [Alteration of the visual evoked potential following concussion]. Vopr Neirokhir 1976 (5):25-30.

[65] Gundogan FC, Demirkaya S, Sobaci G. Is optical coherence tomography really a new biomarker candidate in multiple sclerosis?--A structural and functional evaluation. Invest Ophthalmol Vis Sci 2007;48(12):5773-81.

[66] Gundogan FC, Sobaci G, Bayer A. Pattern visual evoked potentials in the assessment of visual acuity in malingering. Ophthalmology 2007;114(12):2332-7.

3

Ocular Aberrations and Image Quality, Contact Lens and Myopia Progression

Jie Shen

1. Introduction

The eye as an optical instrument is imperfect with defocus, astigmatism and higher-order aberrations being common. The image formed on the retina is affected by these optical deficiencies. Refractive errors (myopia, hyperopia and astigmatism) are the most common ocular aberrations, and they are called lower-order aberrations. There are numerous higher-order aberrations, of which spherical aberration and coma are most of clinical interest. Refractive errors have been studied for many years and clinicians devote themselves to correct these focusing errors.

Compared to the efforts to understand and optimize the central vision, peripheral vision is not well understood. However, peripheral vision is important for motion and pattern detection and fundus imaging. Also, interest in studying the off-axis optical performance and image quality of humane eye has increased dramatically in recent years because the previous studies suggest a possibility that off-axis aberrations in human eye is important for the development of central refractive error.

Given the hypothesis that off-axis aberrations and image quality may affect central refractive error development, it is important to understand how ordinary ophthalmic lenses, which are used to correct foveal vision, influence the peripheral optics of human eye.

In this chapter, we will describe and discuss the following six major topics: 1) control of ocular growth, 2) axial ocular aberrations, 3) off-axis aberrations, 4) contact lens and myopia progression, 5) peripheral refractions and contact lens correction, and 6) peripheral image quality and contact lens correction.

2. Control of ocular growth

Animal studies have demonstrated that the eyes growth is controlled by local retina mechanism. [1-3] Local retinal mechanism refers to a condition that local retina could minimize the image degradation on the corresponding retinal location by changing the axial eye growth rate. [4] The homeostatic control signals of the eyes growth try to keep the image sharply focused on the retina ("grow to clarity" model). [5] If the eye is in myopic status, the image of a distant object falls in front of the retina and if the eye is hyperopic, the image falls behind the retina. These two situations are simulated in Fig. 1A, inserting a positive lens put the image in front of the retina (myopic focus) and negative lens focus the image behind the retina (hyperopic focus). By increasing the thickness of choroids or slowing the rate of eye's elongation, the eye can grow to counteract the effect of the lens, regaining a sharp focus (for small amount of myopic defocus). For hyperopic defocus, the choroids will become thinning and the rate of eye's elongation will increase in order to focus the image on retina again (Fig. 1B). [6-8] These were proved by previous animal studies. [9-13] For example, animals, like birds, consistently experience near objects in their inferior visual field have longer superior ocular length. [14, 15]

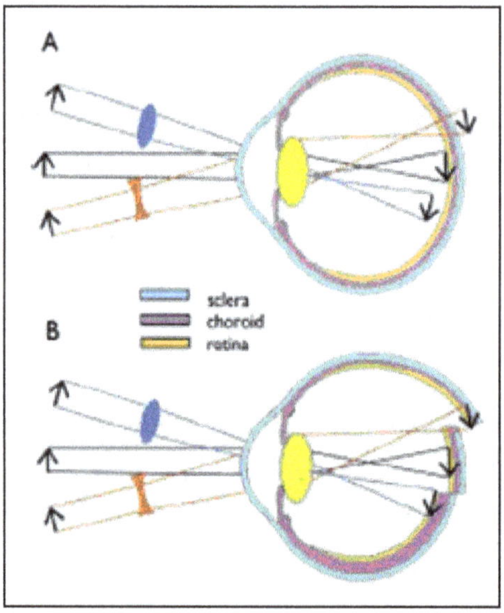

Figure 1. Ocular Compensation for lens-Induced Defocus

a. A positive lens (blue, convex) causes the image to form in front of the retina (myopic defocus), whereas a negative lens (red, concave) pushes the image plane behind the retina (hyperopic defocus). With no lens (black rays), the image of a distant objects is focused on the retina.

b. The eye compensates for positive lenses by slowing its rate of elongation and by thickening the choroid, pushing the retina forward toward the image plane. It compensates of negative lenses by increasing the rate of elongation and thinning the choroid, pulling the retina back toward the image plane. The emmetropic eye is intermediate in length and in choroid thickness. (Figure and legend from [1])

As a development of local retina mechanism model in animal study, data from human beings also suggested that peripheral refractive error can influence the ocular growth. [16-19] For example, young pilots that had relatively hyperopic refractive status in both horizontal and vertical meridian, which potentially contributes to the eye's elongation, were more likely to develop adult-onset myopia than those who showed myopic refractive status at least in one meridian. [16] More recently, Smith and colleagues [20] have tested the hypothesis that the peripheral visual experiences contribute for the ocular growth and central refractive development in primates. Their study provided strong evidence that the peripheral retinal mechanism can influence the refractive development at the fovea and this, most likely, also happens in human beings.

3. Axial ocular aberration

Aberrations are classified as monochromatic and chromatic aberrations. Chromatic aberrations occur when light source has multi-wavelength components. Monochromatic aberrations occur when only one wavelength light source is refracted. The aberration discussed in this chapter is monochromatic aberration.

3.1. Representation of aberration

It is useful to understand wavefront and wavefront aberration before we discuss the measurement and representation of aberration. A wavefront is a surface which is orthogonal to light rays. The wavefront aberration is the distance, in optical path length (product of the refractive index and path length), from the reference plane to wavefront plane at the exit pupil (Figure 2).

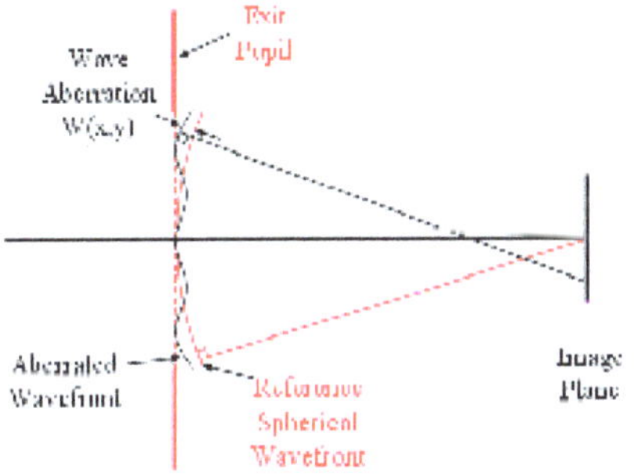

Figure 2. The concept of wavefront aberration: wavefront aberration is the departure of the measured wavefront from the ideal spherical wavefront at the exit pupil.

There are different ways to represent wavefront aberrations such as Taylor series and Zernike polynomials. The Taylor series are rarely used these days since each individual term are not orthonormal. [21] People usually use Zernike series which were recommended by Optical Society of America to describe the eye's wavefront error (Figure 3 & Table 1). [22]

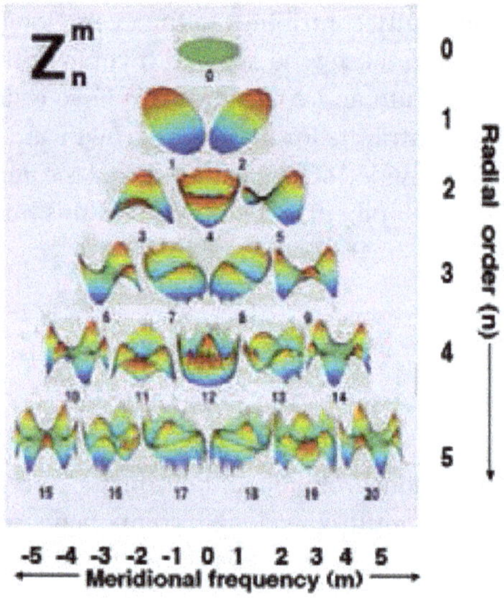

Figure 3. Zernike polynomials: Each row is a radial order. Each column is a meridional frequency. Each function is defined over the circular domain of the pupil and is mathematically orthogonal to all other functions in the table.

The normalized Zernike polynomial has two major advantages when applied to quantify the optical aberrations. First, the magnitude of the Zernike coefficient represents the wavefront error in that mode and usually given in the unit micrometers (μm). Second, in the Zernike series, each mode is orthogonal to the other mode, so the coefficients are independent of each other. This will allow us to manipulate each mode individually. RMS (root mean square) error is widely used to indicate the human eyes' wavefront error in each mode or combined modes. RMS is defined as

$$RMS = \sqrt{\sum_{n>1,m} (C_n^m)^2} \tag{1}$$

First and second order aberrations are regarded as lower-order aberrations. 1st-order Zernike terms are tilts which do not cause image blur therefore are usually ignored. Traditional refractive errors refer to 2nd-order Zernike terms. The relationship between 2nd-order Zernike coefficients and sphero-cylindrical components M, J_0, J_{45} (M: the spherical equivalent, J_0: with-the-rule (WTR) and against-the-rule (ATR) astigmatism, J_{45}: oblique astigmatism with axes at 45 deg and 135 deg) is given by the following equations. [23]

mode j	order n	frequency m	$Z_n^m(\rho,\theta)$
0	0	0	1
1	1	-1	$2\rho\sin(\theta)$
2	1	1	$2\rho\cos(\theta)$
3	2	-2	$\sqrt{6}\rho^2\sin(2\theta)$
4	2	0	$\sqrt{3}(2\rho^2-1)$
5	2	2	$\sqrt{6}\rho^2\cos(2\theta)$
6	3	-3	$\sqrt{8}\rho^3\sin(3\theta)$
7	3	-1	$\sqrt{8}(3\rho^3-2\rho)\sin(\theta)$
8	3	1	$\sqrt{8}(3\rho^3-2\rho)\cos(\theta)$
9	3	3	$\sqrt{8}\rho^3\cos(3\theta)$
10	4	-4	$\sqrt{10}\rho^4\sin(4\theta)$
11	4	-2	$\sqrt{10}(4\rho^4-3\rho^2)\sin(2\theta)$
12	4	0	$\sqrt{5}(6\rho^4-6\rho^2+1)$
13	4	2	$\sqrt{10}(4\rho^4-3\rho^2)\cos(2\theta)$
14	4	4	$\sqrt{10}\rho^4\cos(4\theta)$
⋮	⋮	⋮	⋮

Table 1. List of Zernike Polynomials

$$
\begin{aligned}
M &= \frac{-4\sqrt{3}}{r^2} C_2^0 \\
J_0 &= \frac{-2\sqrt{6}}{r^2} C_2^2 \\
J_{45} &= \frac{-2\sqrt{6}}{r^2} C_2^{-2}
\end{aligned}
\quad (2)
$$

Where C_{20}, C_{22}, C_{2-2} are Zernike coefficients for defocus, WTR/ATR astigmatism and oblique astigmatism terms, and r is pupil radius. We can also use the following equation to convert rectangular Fourier form (M, J_0, J_{45}) to conventional clinical negative-cylinder form. [24]

$$
\begin{aligned}
S &= M + \sqrt{{J_0}^2 + {J_{45}}^2} \\
C &= -2\sqrt{{J_0}^2 + {J_{45}}^2} \\
\alpha &= \frac{1}{2}\tan^{-1}(J_{45} / J_0)
\end{aligned}
\quad (3)
$$

Start from 3rd order Zernike terms, aberrations are referred as higher-order aberrations. Coma ($C_{3\pm1}$) and spherical aberration (C_{40}) are the most important higher-order aberrations since they present in higher amounts than the other higher-order aberrations in the population. [25, 26]

3.2. Measurement of aberrations

As a development of autorefractors, aberration measuring instruments bear the same principle (Scheiner disc principle) which illustrated in Figure 4. [27, 28] Aberrations can be measured by "into-the-eye" or "out-of-the-eye" aberrometry technique. [28, 29] "Into-the-eye" aberrometry means an image is formed on the retina and re-imaged out of the eye for analysis, like laser ray tracing and Tscherning aberrometer. "Out-of-the-eye" aberrometry refers to an instrument which project a narrow beam into the eye and trace the rays from the retina out of the eye, like Hartmann-Shack wavefront sensor. [28] Aberrometer measure aberrations either sequentially or simultaneously. Sequential aberrometry, like laser ray tracing, measures aberration in one location of the pupil once a time but simultaneous aberrometer (Hartman-Shack wavefront aberrometer) can measure aberration at multiple locations of the pupil at the same time.

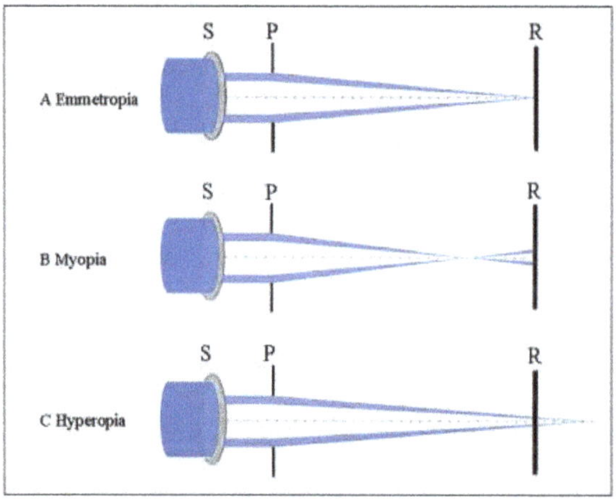

Figure 4. Scheiner disc principle: Light comes from a distant object reduce to two small bundles of light by two pinholes on Scheiner disc. These two rays focus to be a single image on the retina if the eye is emmetropia (Figure 4 a). Double images will be sensed if the eye is myopia or hyperopia (Figure 4 b&c). By adjusting the position of the object until on image is seen, the far point and refractive error of the patient's eye can be determined. S: Scheiner disc; P: Pupil; R: Retina

Most commercial aberrometers use Hartmann-Shack wavefront sensor. Hartmann-Shack technology can be tracked back to early 20th century when Hartmann test was used to measure aberration of optical system. [30, 31] Shack and Platt modified Hartmann technique to invent the Hartmann-Shack aberrometer. [32] This technique was originally developed by astronomers for improving the image quality of the stars and satellites and Liang et al. [33] adapted it to measure conventional refractive errors as well as higher-order aberrations of the eyes. The principle of operation of the Hartmann-Shack aberrometer is shown in Figure 5.

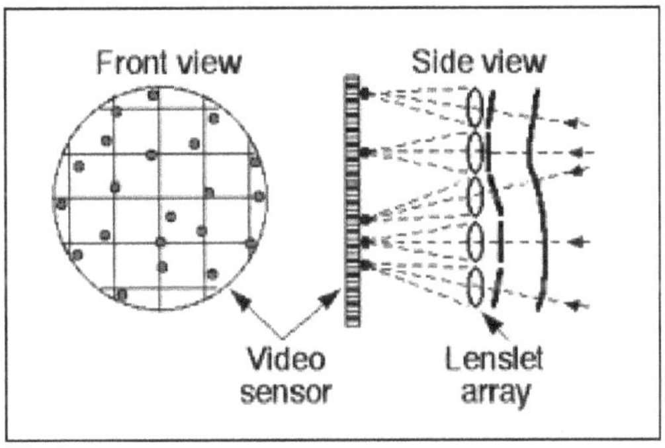

Figure 5. Principle of the Hartmann-Shack (HS) wavefront sensor. HS sensor subdivides the wavefront into hundred small beams which are focused on to a CCD video sensor by an array of small lenses. The displacement of each image relative to the grid of optical axes is determined by the local slope of the wavefront in x-and y-direction at the face of the corresponding lenslet. [Adapted from Thibos [34]]

The critical part of Hartmann-Shack wavefront sensor is a micro-lenslet array. A CCD video sensor is placed in one focal length of those small lenses behind the lenslet array. The reflected wavefront of light emerging from the eye will be partitioned to hundred smaller wavefront and will be focused on the CCD sensor. If the measured eye is a perfect optical system, the wavefront emerging from the eye will be a plane and will be focused perfectly on the intersections of the grids. In the real situation, the aberrated wavefront coming back from the eye will be focused by each lenslet on CCD sensor with displacement corresponding to lenslet axis. The local slopes of the wavefront can be deduced from this displacement.

Hartmann-Shack aberrometer have been widely used to measure aberrations in different area of clinical research [34-40] due to its fast measuring and less affected by scattering of light compared to most other aberrometers. [41] Hartmann-Shack wavefront aberrometer has been reported as a robust and reliable instrument to measure both lower and higher order aberrations. [34, 42, 43]

4. Off-axis aberration

While previous studies concentrated on foveal aberrations, investigations of off-axis (peripheral) vision increased dramatically in recent years because the quality of off-axis optics is important for retina imaging, motion and orientation detection, and development of refractive error. [20, 44-48]

4.1. Measurement of Off-axis aberration

Little is known about off-axis wavefront aberrations and image quality in the eccentric visual fields, for which most studies only reported the changes of defocus and astigmatism in the peripheral visual angle. [16, 46, 47, 49-51] Different techniques, such as retinoscopy, [46, 49, 51, 52] subjective refraction, [47, 50],photorefraction [53] and autorefraction, [54] were used to measure these lower-order aberrations in the peripheral visual field.

The published studies on peripheral refraction [16, 17, 28, 53, 55-58] suggested that hyperopes had relative less hyperopic error in the periphery, while myopes usually had relative less myopic error in periphery. These experimental data was consistent with the previous predictions made by Charman and Jennings [59] and Dunne et al. [60, 61] which used simple models with ray tracing technique on the schematic eye.

In 1998, Navarro et al. first measured higher-order aberrations in four naked eyes using laser ray-tracing method and described aberrations using Zernike polynomials. [62] They measured nasal visual field only and reported that despite large variation between subjects, the four subjects showed the same pattern of the change of the aberrations across the visual field. They found both 3rd-and 4_{th}-order aberrations increasing from center to periphery. Atchison and Scott were the first to use Shack-Hartmann wavefront aberrometer to measure off-axis higher-order aberrations in human eye. [63] They measured aberrations both in nasal and temporal visual field up to 40_0. Like Navarro's study, Atchison's data also showed large between-subject variability. They reported that 3rd-order aberration increased to both nasal and temporal visual field and with nasal-temporal asymmetry. Unlike Navarro's study, they didn't report the large change of 4_{th}-order aberration across the horizontal visual field. Both these two studies only recruited small number of subjects.

In the previous studies, [62-67] researchers didn't attempt to quantify the image quality in the peripheral visual field. Most researchers talked about the peripheral image quality, speculated that off-axis IQ would drop fast and become worse based on the measurements of peripheral refraction (defocus and astigmatism). They neglected the complex interaction between these lower-order and the higher-order aberrations in eyes. [68] In order to investigate the off-axis image quality, to study the interaction between lower-order aberrations and higher-order aberrations in the large visual angle and to study the potential contributions of the off-axis image quality to the whole eyes refractive development, the first step is to measure the monochromatic aberrations in the peripheral visual field accurately.

4.2. Peripheral vision and development of refractive error

The rationale that peripheral refraction can influence the development of refractive error is pointed out by Wallman [1] that if the peripheral retina is relatively hyperopic, this relatively hyperopic defocus will cause the elongation of the eyeball no matter what the foveal refractive status is. As mentioned above, the homeostatic signals from the hyperopic periphery will guide the eye to elongate. If the fovea retina is emmetropic or myopic, the homeostatic signals from the central retina will direct the eye to elongate less. These two signals, from central retina and from the peripheral retina, will try to keep balance. Although the neurons density is higher in the central than in the peripheral retina, considering the total area of the central retina is quite small, the homeostatic signals from peripheral retina directing the eye to elongate more will be stronger than the signals from central retina that directing the eye to elongate less if these signals have spatial summation. If the larger area of the retina become elongated surrounding the fovea area, the mechanical constrains in eye growth will also make the fovea axially elongated. [1] This mechanism has been hypothesized by several studies. [53, 58, 69]

The critical step to understand the above mechanism is that the peripheral retina has the capacity to detect the changes of image quality which are produced by the off-axis aberrations.

[47, 70, 71] Peripheral vision is limited by two factors: the optical image quality and the neurons density in the periphery. It is already known that in large visual angles, the oblique astigmatism increases dramatically. However, these refractive errors can be corrected by ordinary ophthalmic lenses. There are other higher-order aberrations such as coma and spherical aberrations in the off-axis visual field which can also deteriorate the image quality but are difficult to correct. [72] The neurons density (including cones and ganglion cells) is at maximum near the fovea and drops quickly in the periphery. [73] This neurons density constitutes an upper limit of the visual acuity at higher retinal field angles when the off-axis optics is corrected.

The resolution acuity becomes worse with the increasing of the retina eccentricity, but the detection acuity remains high at large eccentricities given the peripheral optics are well corrected. [71, 74] Detection acuity is significantly influenced by the optical defocus and is lower when the retina image is formed by the eye's natural optics, these suggest that the detection acuity is optically limited. [74, 75] But after correct the major off-axis aberrations (defocus and astigmatism), the detection acuity becomes quite good in the peripheral visual field. [70, 76]

Besides evidences supported by other human studies, [16, 17, 19, 77] Smith and colleagues [20] provided further evidence that visual experience in peripheral retina can influence the refractive development at the fovea. And as a development, other studies made a hypothesis that high level of aberrations will guide ocular elongation by degradation of the retinal image. [78-82] Growth of the eye tends to minimize the image blur on the most part of the retina (known as "grow to clarity" model). [5] Thus peripheral vision is closely related with development of central refractive error.

5. Contact lens and myopia progression

Contact lenses are widely used treatments for refractive errors. They had long been used as an optical correction since their introduction by Eugen Fick in 1888. [83] A large number of studies investigated the effect of different types of contact lenses (silicone acrylate contact lenses, hydrophilic contact lenses, hydrogel lenses) on the progression of myopia had been done. [84-90] Though most of the studies had small sample size or were not randomized, they did suggest that wearing soft contact lenses induced increasing in myopia progression. [84, 91, 92] Another large sample size, randomized study done by Horner et al. suggested that there were no significant different in the rate of myopia progression between the children who wore SCLs and spectacles. [93]

Hard contact lenses have longer history than the SCLs. PMMA (polymethyl methacrylate) hard contact lenses were widely prescribed in the clinic although they have side effects caused by low oxygen permeability. After 1970', Rigid-Gas-Permeable (RGP) lens becomes popular. These lenses have higher oxygen permeability than soft contact lens, clinically proved to be a suitable and safer alternative for correcting refractive error. [89] In a three years study, 100 children with myopia were fitted with RGP and compared with control group who wore spectacles, significant reduction of myopia progression was found. [94] Another study also reported a similar results. [95]

Although in 2003, a larger randomized clinical trial of rigid contact lenses conducted in Singapore Children didn't report significant difference of myopia progression between RGP wearers and spectacles wearers, [96] the more recent CLAMP (Contact Lens and Myopia Progression) study [18] has shown that RGP produced a significant slower rate of progression of myopia in children, although this was largely due to flattening of the cornea rather than slowing of axial elongation. [97]

No matter whether the SCLs or RGP lenses can slow the progression of myopia or not, all of the SCLs and RGP studies above tried to relate the lens' efficacy with the ocular physiological changes. No studies have examined the peripheral optical quality after these ophthalmic corrections although there were attempts to evaluate on-axis optical performance of these lenses. [39, 98] Since the peripheral vision is an important factor to contribute for the development of myopia, experimentally measure the monochromatic off-axis aberrations with these ophthalmic lenses on-eye is my proposed experiment and will discussed in detail in later chapters.

5.1. Contact lens and on-axis ocular aberration

The on-axis optical quality after wearing RGP lenses has been well studied both by theoretically calculation and experimental measurements. [99-101] It is widely accepted in clinic that RGP lenses provided the best optical performance for the central vision compared to SCLs and spectacles. RGP lens can smooth the irregularities of the corneal front surface with its rigidity and smooth lens surface. With the correction of moderate astigmatism by the tear lens between RGP and cornea, RGP lenses provide the best on-axis optical performance. Due to the conformity of SCLs, the corneal astigmatism and corneal irregularity will be preserved in some extent for the SCLs wearer (Fig. 6). Theoretically calculation of the on-axis aberrations of RGP lenses always ignores the interaction between the cornea and contact lenses, also without considering the contribution of inner components of the eye to the total optical aberrations. Only Hong et al. [100] and Dorronsoro et al. [98] have measured aberrations in subjects wearing RGP lenses, finding that RGP lenses provided lower aberrations than SCLs and spectacle lenses. They concluded that wearing RGP lenses can significantly reduce the ocular aberrations, not only defocus and astigmatism, but also higher-order aberrations.

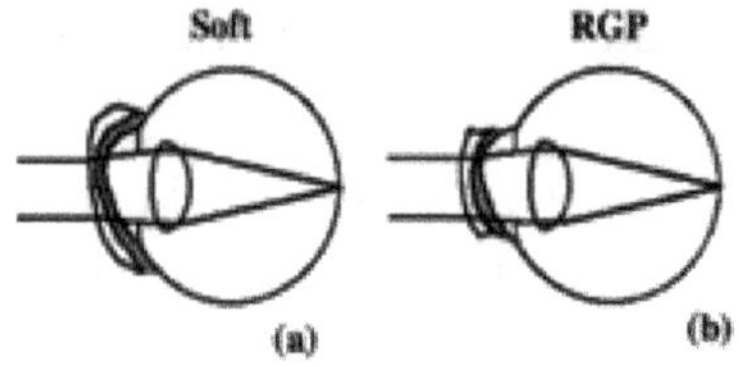

Figure 6. Schematic diagram of the eye with a) soft contact lens, b) rigid gas-permeable (RGP) contact lens. The shaded regions indicated the tear layer. Corneal distortions are exaggerated to illustrate the differences between different optical corrections. [Adapted from [39]]

5.2. Contact lens and off-axis aberrations

Since contact lens correct central refractive error by adding an appropriate compensating power across the entire eye, it will affect the peripheral vision as well while foveal refractive errors are corrected. And due to the potential role of peripheral vision in the development of central refractive error, it is possible that the ophthalmic corrective methods which only correct the central vision but ignoring peripheral image quality will be less successful for controlling myopia progression. Since the myopic eyes have a relative hyperopic periphery, correcting the central myopic will leave the periphery hyperopic (if the correcting lenses have the same power everywhere across the lens piece). The hyperopic periphery will continue to guide the elongation of the eye and the progression of myopia will not stop. Thus the contact lens correction which only corrects the central vision might actually have no effect or even increase the progression of myopia. However, we lack the knowledge of how contact lenses affect peripheral optics of the eye. Although knowledge of off-axis aberrations of CL in isolation is important to help understanding the effect of CLs on peripheral optics of the eye, [102] to obtain a definitive result of how the peripheral refractive error and image quality changes across the visual field with CLs correction requires that the CLs be worn by a human eye.

6. Peripheral refractions and contact lens correction

Multiple studies [53, 103-105] have shown that hyperopic and emmetropic eyes tend to have peripheral refractive errors that are myopic relative to the fovea. The image shell from a distant, extended object is therefore more curved than the retinal surface, resulting in an increasing amount of myopic blur at greater retinal eccentricities. In this chapter, we will refer to this condition as "myopic field curvature" or "relative peripheral myopia". By contrast, myopic eyes tend to have less myopia in the peripheral visual field than foveally. Most authors agree on this point for the horizontal field, but there is some controversy regarding the generality of the finding at the other meridian. [53, 54, 106] The image shell from a distant, extended object is less curved than the retinal surface in myopic eyes, resulting in a decreasing amount of myopic blur at greater retinal eccentricities. Thus, relative to foveal refractive error, the eye has an increasing amount of hyperopic blur at greater retinal eccentricities. In this chapter, we will refer to this condition as "hyperopic field curvature" or "relative peripheral hyperopia".

The rationale that peripheral refraction can influence the development of refractive error is that if the peripheral retina is relatively hyperopic, this relatively hyperopic defocus will cause the elongation of the eyeball no matter what the foveal refractive status is. As mentioned above, the homeostatic signals from the hyperopic periphery will guide the eye to elongate. If the fovea retina is emmetropic or myopic, the homeostatic signals from the central retina will direct the eye to elongate less. These two signals, from central retina and from the peripheral retina, will try to keep balance. Although the neurons density is higher in the central than in the peripheral retina, considering the total area of the central retina is quite small, the homeostatic signals from peripheral retina directing the eye to elongate more will be stronger than the signals from central retina that directing the eye to elongate less if these signals have spatial summation. If the larger area of the retina become elongated surrounding the fovea area, the mechanical constrains in eye growth will also make the fovea axially elongated. This also demonstrated by the local retina mechanism. [58, 69, 107].

More recently, Smith and colleagues [108] have tested the hypothesis that the peripheral visual experiences contribute for the ocular growth and central refractive development in primates. Their study provided strong evidence that the peripheral retinal mechanism can influence the refractive development at the fovea and this, most likely, also happens in human beings.

6.1. Curvature of field and peripheral astigmatism for the naked eye

Consistent with most previous studies, emmetropic eyes showed myopic shift into the periphery (Fig.7 a & b) whereas myopic subjects showed relatively hyperopic shift (Fig.8 a & b). Greater myopia and higher astigmatism in the nasal visual field than in the temporal visual field were found in most of the subjects in the study (Fig.7, 8, 9, 10 & Fig.11). This asymmetry of the changes of M, J_0 and J_{45} across horizontal visual field has been noted in previous, large-scale studies of peripheral refraction. However, the larger error bar indicated that there were considerable differences occur among the subjects. (Within-subject variance was small as indicated from the Fig.7a and Fig.8a, but this might be due to the lack of necessary realignments of the instrument between the measurements in each visual angle position.) A more apparent hyperopic shift beyond 20 degree eccentricity was found (Fig.7). (Previous, Atchison et al. reported a subtle changes in refraction across the central 10º of the retina, with changes in M varying by up to half a diopter and with smaller changes in astigmatism [109].)

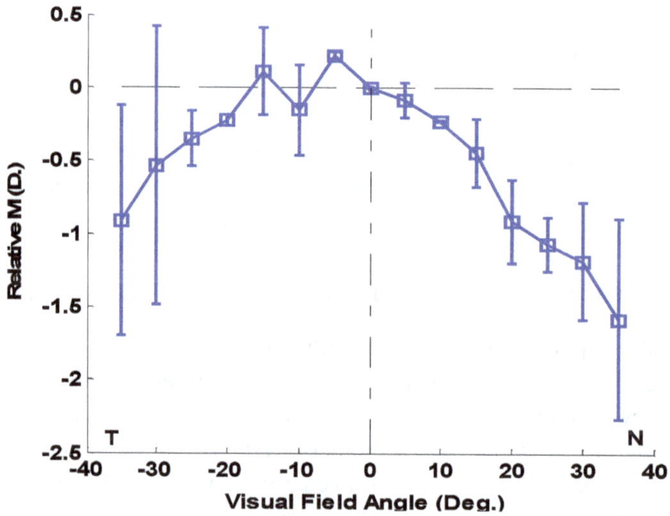

Figure 7. a) Spherical equivalent refractive error (M) relative to the fovea as a function of visual field angle for Sub.1 and Sub.2. Both of these two subjects are emmetropes. Symbols show the means and Error bar indicate the standard deviation of 5 repeated measurements. b) The mean value of Spherical equivalent (M) as a function of visual field angle for the two emmetropes. Error bar indicate the standard deviation of the two emmetropic subjects.

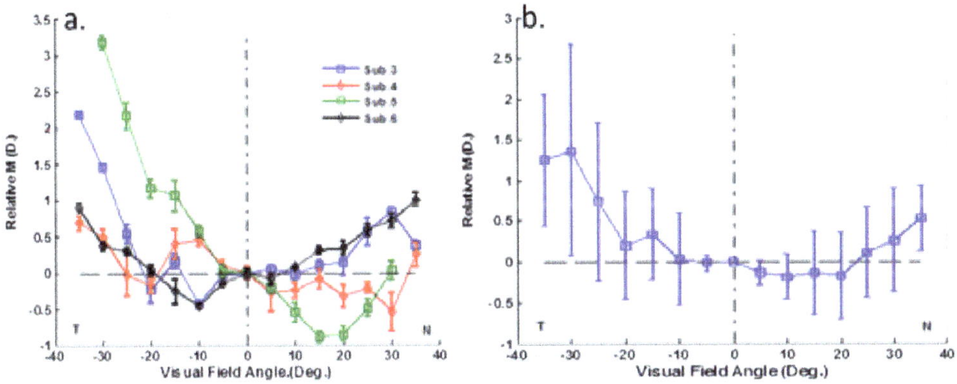

Figure 8. a) Relative M as a function of visual field angle for the naked eye of 4 myopic subjects separately. Error bar indicate the within-subject variance of 5 repeated measurements. b) Relative M as a function of retina eccentricity for myopes. Error bar indicate the standard deviation of the four myopic subjects.

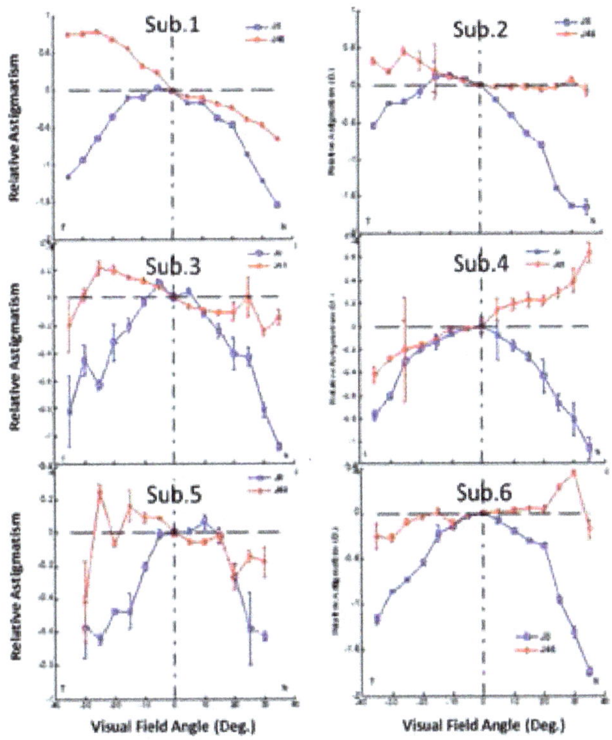

Figure 9. a) Relative J_0 and J_{45} as a function of visual field angle for the six naked eye. Symbols show the mean and error bar indicate the standard deviation of 5 repeated measurements. b) Mean value of the relative J_0 and J_{45} of the six subjects. Error bar indicate the standard deviation of these six subjects.

In another published study, the mean data show a monotonic increase in PRM with eccentricity that is approximately linear with a slope of 0.01 diopters/deg of eccentricity. Thus for an eccentricity of E degrees, PRM is approximately E percent of foveal refractive error in the naked eye. [110]

6.2. Effect of contact lenses on field curvature and peripheral astigmatism

In the group with 4 myopic subjects, the mean value of the change of mean spherical and astigmatism across the horizontal visual field without any correction and with full SCLs correction were shown in Fig. 10 and Fig. 11. With the SCLs corrections, which rendered the fovea conjugate to infinity, the M component still showed a relatively hyperopic shift to the peripheral visual field away from the center. In most of the measurement positions, spherical equivalent had larger hyperopic value after subjects wearing SCLs than their naked eye's data. This suggested that using Acuvue 2 SCLs in this experiment to fully correct the foveal refractive error might cause more hyperopic shift in the peripheral visual field. The nasal-temporal asymmetry after wearing the SCL was not apparent anymore (Fig.10). This result suggested that either corneal shape was responsible for the asymmetry or it was an artifact of CL movement. In the new experiment, the measurements will be taken by rotate subject's head instead of eye rotation. This can eliminate the artifact of SCLs movement and will give us answer about this issue. J_0 was the major contributor for the increase of astigmatism in large visual angle. After full correction with SCLs, J_{45} did not change much across the horizontal visual field, but greater J_0 (more negative) was found in the experiment (especially across the temporal retina) (Fig.11). However, large between-subject differences were found. Only 4 subjects who had very different center refractive error participated in the study. Hopefully, the variance will be reduced by recruiting more subjects who have similar central refractive status in the future study.

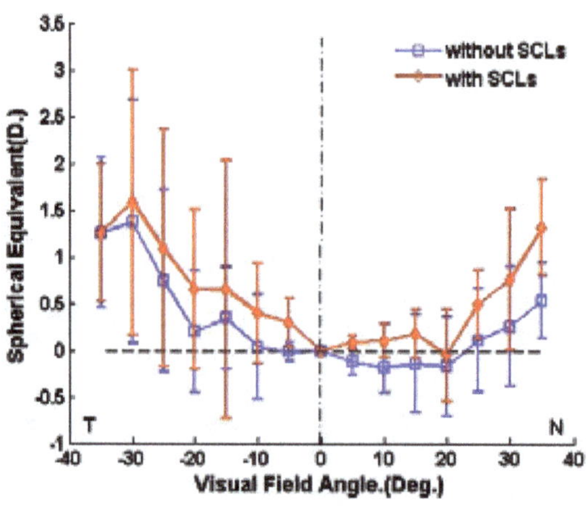

Figure 10. The effect of SCLs on relative M as a function of visual field angle with and without SCLs correction. Error bar indicate the standard deviation.

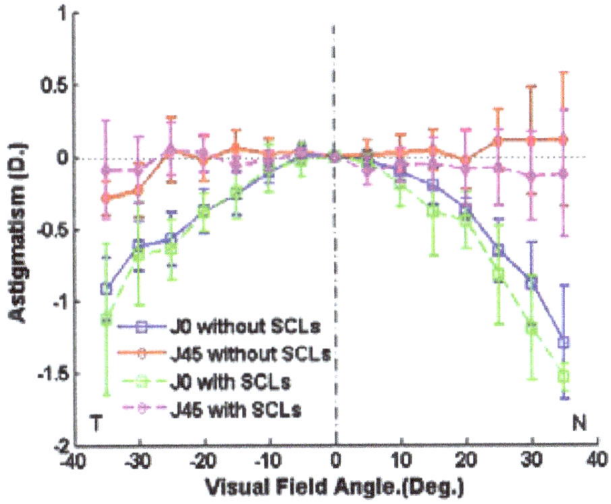

Figure 11. The effect of SCLs on relative J_0 and J_{45} across the horizontal visual field with and without SCLs. Red lines are $J_{45,}$ blue lines are $J_{0.}$ Dash lines indicate the astigmatisms after subjects wear the SCLs. Error bar shows the standard deviation.

Compared to the naked eye, curvature of field was reduced, and in some cases reversed in sign, by contact lenses.

6.3. Contact lens effect on total sphero-cylindrical blur

The results described above show that defocus (M) and astigmatism (J_0) both vary across the visual field. If image quality is a driving force for myopia progression as suggested previously, [78-82] then it is important to determine the combined effects of M and J_0. The effect of contact lenses may be complex because, as shown above, relative hyperopic defocus is reduced by contact lenses, but peripheral astigmatism increases. Therefore, to determine the effect of contact lenses on peripheral image quality, we need to quantify and compare the total sphero-cylindrical image blur on the peripheral retina before and after wearing contact lenses.

In one of our published studies, [110] the average image blur caused by sphere and cylinder in naked eye increased to 2 D at 35° periphery relative to the eye's optical axis. SCLs did not have a consistent effect on sphero-cylindrical blur but RGP lenses consistently reduced the blur across the visual field ($p < 0.01$, non-parametric sign test) by approximately 0.25 diopter.

7. Peripheral image quality and contact lens correction

7.1. Variation of higher-order aberrations with visual field eccentricity

The data was also analyzed in Zernike coefficient terms in order to study the change of high-order aberrations as a function of the visual field angle. Coefficients from 2nd-to 6th-order were used to describe the wavefront aberrations. The change of mean (all 6 subjects) relative 2nd-

order aberration as a function of visual field angle was shown in Fig.12. The 2nd-order aberration increased with the visual field angle. Across the horizontal visual field, C_2^2 was the major contributor for the change of 2nd-order aberration (Fig.13 b). Since positive value of C_2^2 indicates Against-The-Rule (ATR) astigmatism and negative value of C_2^2 indicates With-The-Rule (WTR) astigmatism, mean value of C_2^2 in this experiment suggested that the astigmatism changed from WTR to ATR with the increasing of visual field angle from center to periphery (Fig.13 a). Considerable differences occurred among the 6 subjects. This might partly due to the different center refractive error of these six subjects had effects on the peripheral refraction shift.

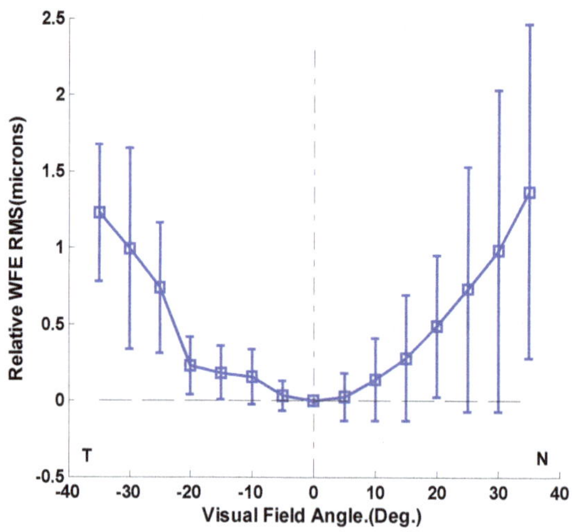

Figure 12. Relative RMS in 2nd-order aberration across the horizontal visual field of the naked eye. Error bar indicate the standard deviation among the six subjects.

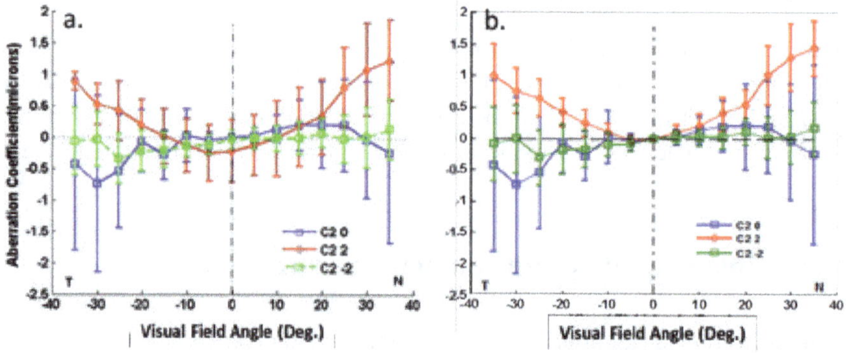

Figure 13. a) The change of Zernike coefficients in the 2nd-order aberration without any correction with the increasing of visual field angle. The data is the mean value of six subjects. Error bar indicate the standard deviation. b) Relative Zernike coefficients in 2nd-order aberration as a function of visual field angle. Error bar indicate the standard deviation.

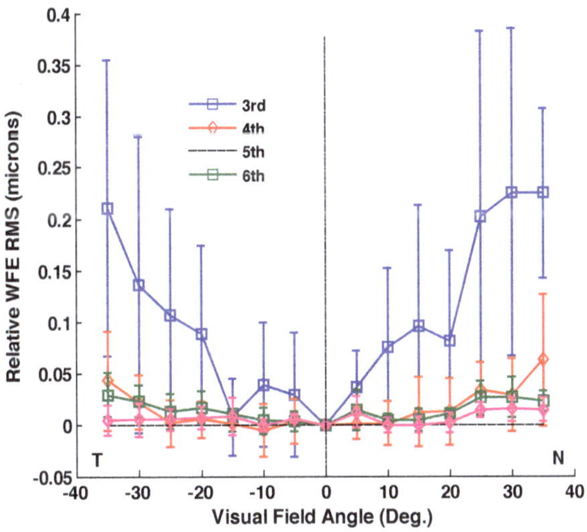

Figure 14. Relative RMS value of high order aberrations' change across the horizontal visual field without any correction for the all six subjects. Error bar indicate the standard deviation.

The high order aberrations (3rd-to-6th-, in this experiment) basically showed the same pattern with Atchison & Navarro's data [62, 111]. The 3rd-, 4th-and 5th-order aberrations showed an increasing magnitude with the visual field angle. Changes of 6th-order aberration were quite small across the horizontal visual field. The nasal-temporal asymmetry of 3rd-order aberration was not as apparent as Atchison's data. In the nasal visual field, there was a factor of 2.8 increasing in 3rd-order aberration. Which reported by Atchison was 5 and by Navarro was 2.5. For temporal visual field, there was a factor of 2.6 for 3rd-order aberration, which reported by Atchison was 3. For 4th-and 5th-order aberrations, a small increase of magnitude with the increasing visual field angle was also noticed. Big individual variance was found in our data as well as in Atchison and Navarro's data (Fig. 14). The sample size was small both in this experiment and previous studies.

Horizontal coma (C_3^1) was a major contributor to the increase of 3rd-order aberration in the peripheral visual field and it showed a linear dependence on the visual field position. This contrasted with changes of vertical coma (C_3^{-1}) and trefoils (C_3^3 and C_3^{-3}), which were quite flat across the visual field. This linear relationship between horizontal coma and retina eccentricity was predicted by Seidel theory [112], and both Atchison's data and my data showed this relationship in the human eye (Fig.15). Although there were large individual variances, both spherical aberrations (C_4^0) and secondary astigmatism (C_4^2) showed a quadratic dependence on visual field position. This relationship between C_4^0, C_4^2 and visual field position was also predicted by Seidel Theory. The spherical aberration (C_4^0) showed a positive value in the fovea (most people have positive spherical aberration in the un-accommodated state for foveal vision [28]). However, the magnitude of spherical aberration reduced into the horizontal periphery and finally became negative (Fig. 16).

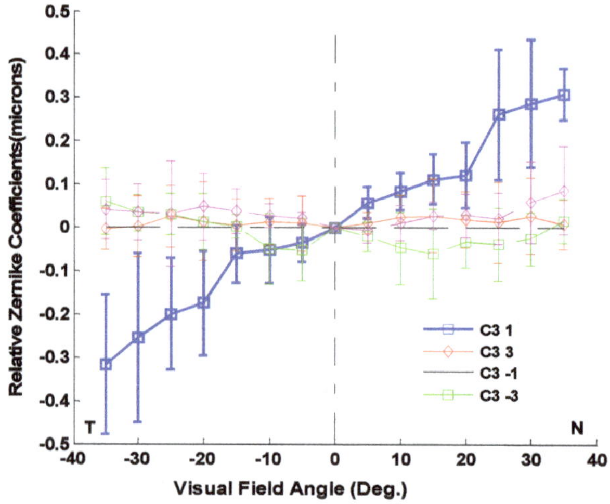

Figure 15. Relative Zernike coefficients in 3rd-order aberration across the horizontal visual field without any correction. Data is mean value of 6 subjects. The blue line is the horizontal coma (C_3^1). Error bar indicate the standard deviation.

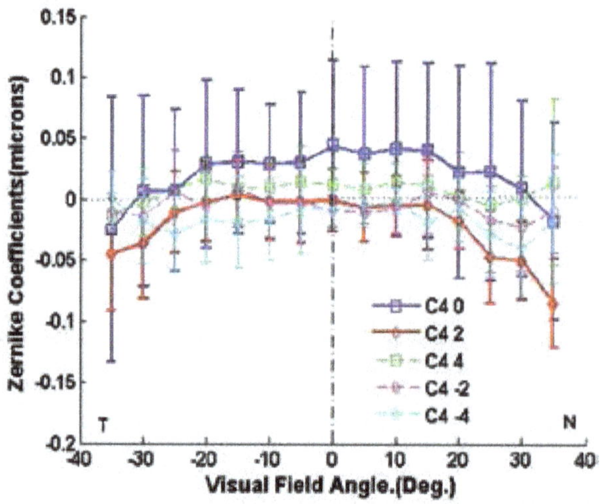

Figure 16. a) The change of Zernike coefficients in 4th-order aberration across the horizontal visual field without any correction. Blue line and red line are spherical aberration (C_4^0) and secondary astigmatism (C_4^2), respectively. Data is mean value of 6 subjects. Error bar indicate the standard deviation. (From the figure, we can notice the C_4^0 is positive value in the fovea and finally become negative in the far periphery) b) Relative Zernike coefficients in the 4th-order aberration. Error bars was omitted in order only to show the change pattern of C_4^0 and C_4^2 more clearly.

After wearing SCLs, the changes of 2nd-to 6th-order aberrations kept the similar pattern from center to periphery as those uncorrected eyes. Large individual variances still existed, and the 2nd-to 5th-order aberration increased with the visual field angle. The nasal-temporal asymmetry was not apparent as well. In the 3rd-order aberration, after wearing soft contact lens, the horizontal coma still somehow showed a linear dependence with the horizontal visual angle. The spherical aberration and secondary astigmatism continued to show quadratic dependences on the visual field positions after soft contact lenses wearing. (Fig. 17 a, b, c & d)

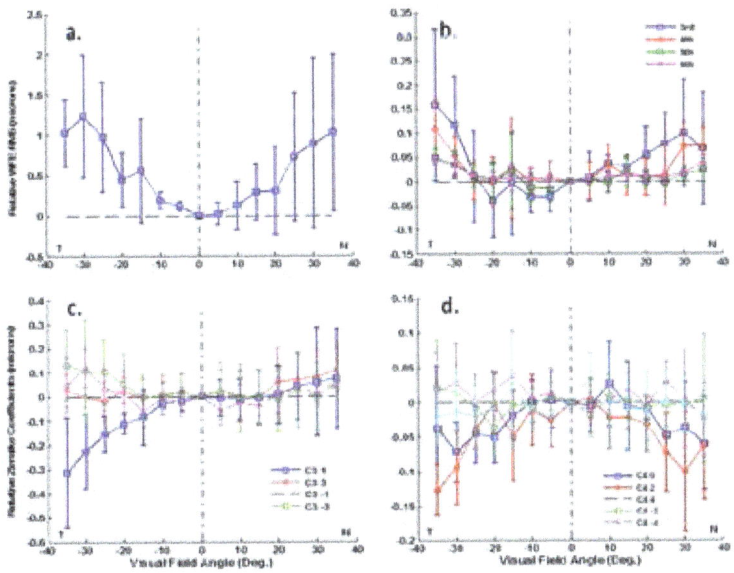

Figure 17. The relative value of 2nd-to 6th-order aberrations and Zernike coefficients across the horizontal visual field with SCLs fully corrected the subjects' foveal vision. Error bar indicate the standard deviation of the 4 SCL wearer subjects. a). Mean relative value of 2nd-order aberration. b). Mean relative value of 3rd-to 4th-order aberrations. c). Relative Zernike coefficients in the 3rd-order aberration. d). Relative Zernike coefficients in the 4th-order aberration.

7.2. Effect of contact lens correction on ocular higher-order aberrations

After wearing SCLs to fully correct the foveal refractive error, 2nd-order aberration increased in the most positions in temporal visual field but decreased in most positions in nasal visual field (Fig. 18 a & b). This was consistent with the data shown in Fig.7 & 8.

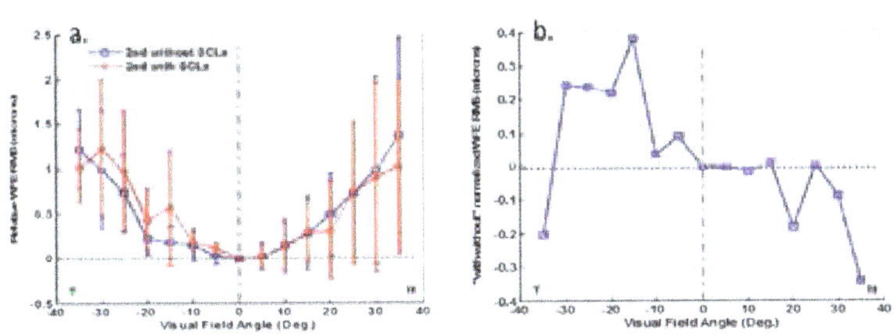

Figure 18. a) The change of 2nd-order aberrations across the horizontal visual field with and without SCL correction. Error bar indicate the standard deviation. b) By subtracting the naked eye's data, the curves in the figure indicate the effect of SCLs on relative wavefront RMS of the subjects. Negative value means the RMS becomes smaller after wearing SCL.

When comparing 3rd-to 6th-order aberrations before and after wearing soft contact lenses, we found that the magnitude increasing rate of 3rd-order aberration decreased after SCLs correction compared to that in the naked eyes, especially beyond 20 degree nasal visual field (Fig. 19 a & b). A 1.4 fold increase in 3rd-order aberration of the nasal visual field after wearing soft contact lenses compared to the 2.5 fold before wearing the soft contact lenses was found. Since the irregular corneal anterior surface contributed significantly to the asymmetric aberrations, the eye with soft contact lenses more or less smoothed the anterior corneal surface, thus the reduction of 3rd-order aberration after contact lens fitting was anticipated. Another more possible reason might be the movement of SCLs in the eye. When the eye turned around to the far periphery to fixate on the target, SCLs would move in the opposite direction, thus the measurements taken by aberrometer in these visual angles would not be the exact reading taken if the SCLs could move with the eyes perfectly but this might be a great advantage of SCLs in real life. RGP lens can probably reduce 3rd-order aberration more since RGP lenses have larger movement than SCLs (if the measurements are still taken in the same way with the eye rotation to fixate on target in different visual angle). After wearing SCLs, the 4th-order aberration increased to the far horizontal periphery beyond center 50 degrees. This, again, might be caused by the movement of the contact lenses. The 5th-and 6th-order aberrations also slightly increased after wearing soft contact lenses in the temporal visual field (Fig. 19 a & b).

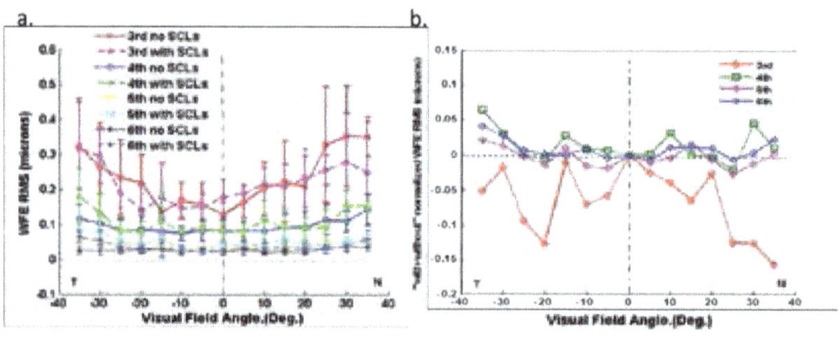

Figure 19. a) The change of 3rd-to 6th-order aberrations across the horizontal visual field with and without SCLs correction. Error bar indicate the standard deviation. b) Data after wearing SCLs subtract naked eye's data. Negative value means after wearing SCLs, the RMS wavefront error become smaller.

Only horizontal coma was shown in Fig. 20a), because the other coefficients were quite small across the horizontal visual field comparing to horizontal coma in both before and after SCLs fitting. After wearing SCLs, the slope of that linear relationship between the C_3^1 and visual field angle became flatter (Fig.20 a). This contributed to the overall decrease of 3rd-order aberration after wearing SCLs. For the 4th-order aberration, since the spherical aberration (C_4^0) and secondary astigmatism (C_4^2) were the two major components which contributed to the 4th-order aberration change across the horizontal visual field, data were plotted of these two coefficients only with and without SCLs correction (Fig.20 b & c). The spherical aberration (C_4^0) did not show significant differences across all the retina eccentricity before and after contact lenses fitting. However, secondary astigmatism (C_4^2) showed larger magnitudes to the horizontal periphery compared to the uncorrected eye (Fig.20 b & c). This might help to explain the increase in the magnitude of 4th-order aberration in the far periphery. Both the primary astigmatism and secondary astigmatism became larger in the large off-axis visual angle after wearing SCLs, but there was no adequate explanation currently to explain this.

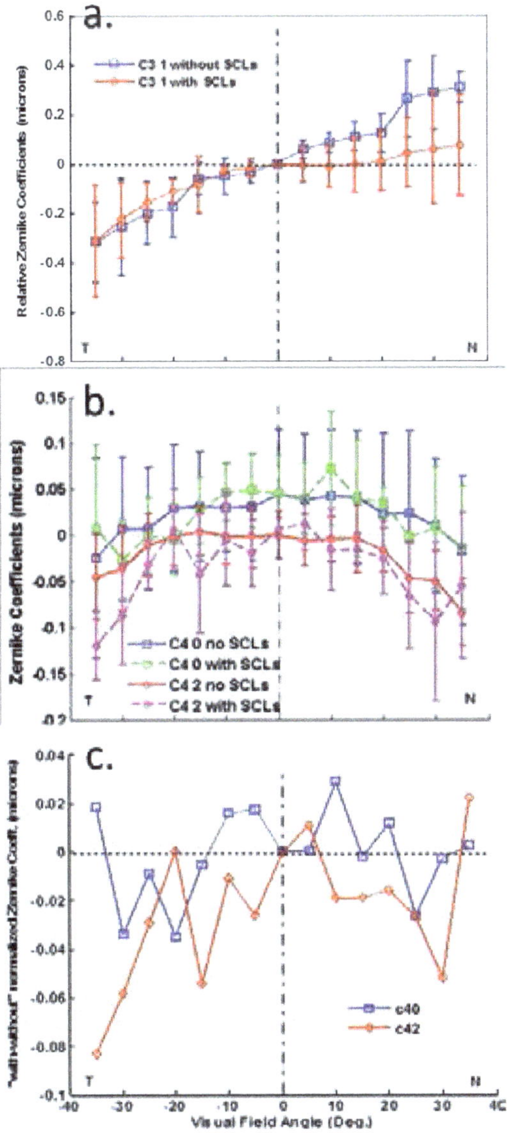

Figure 20. The change of Zernike coefficients as a function of visual field angle. The data are the mean value got from 4 myopic subjects with and without SCL correction. Error bar indicate the standard deviation. a). Change of the relative horizontal coma (C_3^1) across the horizontal visual field before and after SCLs correction. b). Change of spherical aberration (C_4^0) and secondary astigmatism (C_4^2) across the horizontal visual field before (solid lines) and after (dash lines) SCLs correction. c). Data after wearing SCLs subtract naked eye's data. Negative value means Zernike coefficients of C_4^2 became larger after wearing SCLs comparing to naked eyes.

7.3. Peripheral image quality with and without contact lens correction

Image quality was assessed with the VSOTF metric [113, 114] for the complete wavefront aberration (including 2nd order aberrations) measured over the full entrance pupil of each eye in another published study Without contact lens correction, VSOTF gradually decreases from center to periphery. With contact lens correction, image quality improves greatly both in the center and in the periphery. This improvement is due mainly to a reduction in 2nd order aberrations. RGP lens correction shows a trend of better image quality than SCLs across the whole visual field. Image quality drops quickly from center to the periphery after contact lens correction.

8. Conclusion

Both SCL and RGP lenses reduce the degree of hyperopic field curvature present in myopic eyes, but only RGPs reduce the relative amount of image blur on the peripheral retina. Although our study was motivated by the myopia question, the results pertain also to the perceptual quality of peripheral vision. The visual benefit of improved image contrast for peripheral vision obtained by RGP lenses should outweigh the visual benefit of SCLs. The tradeoff between reduced field curvature but increased peripheral astigmatism with RGP correction limits the net improvement of image blur on the peripheral retina that might, in turn, limit RGP lens effectiveness for improving vision or controlling myopia progression. Our results suggest that axial growth mechanisms that depend on retinal image quality will be affected more by RGP than by SCL lenses. These results provide some guidance for future designs of contact lenses to control myopia progression.

Contact lens increases higher-order aberrations in the peripheral visual field except 3rd-order Zernike terms. RGP lenses improve peripheral image quality for objects located at the foveal far point. Increased HOA after contact lens correction reduces image quality by an amount that depends on the eye's initial IQ. If the eye has good IQ initially, changes in HOA have a relatively large effect on IQ. But if the eye has poor IQ initially, HOA will have relatively small effect on IQ. These results suggest contact lens designer and manufacturers should aim to improve the capabilities of contact lens for correcting HOA while simultaneously providing best sphero-cylinder correction for the eye across the visual field.

Author details

Jie Shen*

Address all correspondence to: jshen@westernu.edu

College of Optometry, Western University of Health Sciences, USA

References

[1] Wallman, J.J.W., *Homeostasis of Eye Growth and the Question of Myopia.* Neuron, 2004. 43: p. 447-468.

[2] Hodos, W. and W.J. Kuenzel, *Retinal-image degradation produces ocular enlargement in chicks.* Invest Ophthalmol Vis Sci, 1984. 25: p. 652-659.

[3] Diether, S. and F. Schaeffel, *Local changes in eye growth induced by imposed local refractive error despite active accommodation.* Vision Res, 1997. 37 (6): p. 659-68.

[4] Bartmann, M. and F. Schaeffel, *A simple mechanism for emmetropization without cues from accommodation or colour.* Vision Res, 1994. 34 (7): p. 873-6.

[5] Wildsoet, C.F., *Active emmetropization--evidence for its existence and ramifications for clinical practice.* Ophthalmic Physiol Opt, 1997. 17 (4): p. 279-90.

[6] Gentle, A. and N. McBrien, *Modulation of scleral DNA synthesis in development and recovery from induced axial myopia in the tree shrew.* Exp. Eye Res., 1999. 68: p. 155-163.

[7] Wallman, J., et al., *Moving the retina: choroidal moduation of refractive state.* Vision Res, 1995. 35: p. 37-50.

[8] Wildsoet, C. and J. Wallman, *Choroid and scleral mechanisms of compensation for spectacle lenses in chicks.* Vision Res, 1995. 35: p. 1175-1194.

[9] Graham, B. and S.J. Judge, *The effects of spectacle wear in infancy on eye growth and refractive error in the marmoset (Callithrix jacchus).* Vision Res, 1999. 39 (2): p. 189-206.

[10] Hung, L.F., M.L. Crawford, and E.L. Smith, *Spectacle lenses alter eye growth and the refractive status of young monkeys.* Nat Med, 1995. 1 (8): p. 761-5.

[11] Irving, E.L., M.G. Callender, and J.G. Sivak, *Inducing myopia, hyperopia, and astigmatism in chicks.* Optom Vis Sci, 1991. 68 (5): p. 364-8.

[12] Schaeffel, F. and H.C. Howland, *Properties of the feedback loops controlling eye growth and refractive state in the chicken.* Vision Res, 1991. 31 (4): p. 717-34.

[13] Siegwart, J.T., Jr. and T.T. Norton, *Regulation of the mechanical properties of tree shrew sclera by the visual environment.* Vision Res, 1999. 39 (2): p. 387-407.

[14] Hodos, W. and J.T. Erichsen, *Lower-field myopia in birds: an adaptation that keeps the ground in focus.* Vision Res, 1990. 30 (5): p. 653-7.

[15] Fitzke, F.W., et al., *Refractive sectors in the visual field of the pigeon eye.* J Physiol., 1985. 369: p. 33-34.

[16] Hoogerheide, J., F. Rempt, and W.P. Hoogenboom, *Acquired myopia in young pilots.* Ophthalmologica, 1971. 163 (4): p. 209-15.

[17] Mutti, D.O., et al., *Peripheral refraction and ocular shape in children.* Invest Ophthalmol Vis Sci, 2000. 41 (5): p. 1022-30.

[18] Walline, J., et al., *A randomized trial of the effects of rigid contact lenses on myopia progression.* Arch Ophthalmol., 2004. 122: p. 1760-1766.

[19] Schmid, G.F., *Retinal steepness vs. myopic shift in children (Abstract).* Optom Vis Sci, 2004. 12 (suppl) (23).

[20] Smith, E.L., 3rd, et al., *Peripheral vision can influence eye growth and refractive development in infant monkeys.* Invest Ophthalmol Vis Sci, 2005. 46 (11): p. 3965-72.

[21] Atchison, D.A., *Recent advances in representation of monochromatic aberrations of human eyes.* Clin Exp Optom, 2004. 87 (3): p. 138-48.

[22] Thibos, L.N., et al., *Standards for reporting the optical aberrations of eyes.* J Refract Surg, 2002. 18 (5): p. S652-60.

[23] Thibos, L.N., et al., *Accuracy and precision of objective refraction from wavefront aberrations.* J. Vis.,, 2004. 4: p. 329-351.

[24] Thibos, L.N., W. Wheeler, and D. Horner, *Power vectors: an application of Fourier analysis to the description and statistical analysis of refractive error.* Optom Vis Sci, 1997. 74 (6): p. 367-75.

[25] Thibos, L.N., A. Bradley, and X. Hong, *A statistical model of the aberration structure of normal, well-corrected eyes.* Ophthalmic Physiol Opt, 2002. 22 (5): p. 427-33.

[26] Wang, L. and D.D. Koch, *Ocular higher-order aberrations in individuals screened for refractive surgery.* J Cataract Refract Surg, 2003. 29 (10): p. 1896-903.

[27] Thibos, L.N., R.A. Applegate, and S. Marcos, *Aberrometry: the past, present, and future of optometry.* Optom Vis Sci, 2003. 80 (1): p. 1-2.

[28] Atchison, D.A., *Recent advances in measurements of monochromatic aberrations of human eye.* Clin. Exp. Optom., 2005. 88: p. 5-27.

[29] MacRae, S., R. Krueger, and R. Applegate, *Customized Corneal Ablation: The Quest for Super Vision II.* Thorofare: Slack Incorporated, 2001.

[30] Hartmann, J., *Bemerkungen uber den Bau und die Justirung von Spektrographen.* Z Instrumentenkd, 1900. 20 (47).

[31] Hartmann, J., *Objektuvuntersuchungen.* Z Instrumentenkd, 1904. 24 (1).

[32] Shack, R. and B. Platt, *Production and use of a lenticular Hartmann screen.* J Opt Soc Am A., 1971. 61 (656).

[33] Liang, J., et al., *Objective measurement of wave aberrations of the human eye with the use of a Hartmann-Shack wave-front sensor.* J Opt Soc Am A., 1994. 11: p. 1949-57.

[34] Thibos, L.N. and X. Hong, *Clinical applications of the Shack-Hartmann aberrometer.* Optom Vis Sci, 1999. 76 (12): p. 817-25.

[35] Cheng, X., et al., *Relationship between refractive error and monochromatic aberrations of the eye.* Optom Vis Sci, 2003. 80 (1): p. 43-9.

[36] Klein, S.A., *Optimal corneal ablation for eyes with arbitrary Hartmann-Shack aberrations.* J Opt Soc Am A Opt Image Sci Vis, 1998. 15 (9): p. 2580-8.

[37] Miller, J.M., et al., *Higher order aberrations in normal, dilated, intraocular lens, and laser in situ keratomileusis corneas.* J Refract Surg, 2002. 18 (5): p. S579-83.

[38] Guirao, A., et al., *Calculated impact of higher-order monochromatic aberrations on retinal image quality in a population of human eyes.* J Opt Soc Am A Opt Image Sci Vis, 2002. 19 (3): p. 620-8.

[39] Munson, K., X. Hong, and L.N. Thibos, *Use of a Shack-Hartmann aberrometer to assess the optical outcome of corneal transplantation in a keratoconic eye.* Optom Vis Sci, 2001. 78 (12): p. 866-71.

[40] Hong, X. and L.N. Thibos, *Longitudinal evaluation of optical aberrations following laser in situ keratomileusis surgery.* J Refract Surg, 2000. 16 (5): p. S647-50.

[41] Dai, G., *Wavefront optics for vision correction.* Bellingham: SPIE, 2008.

[42] Cheng, X., et al., *Validation of a clinical Shack-Hartmann aberrometer.* Optom Vis Sci., 2003b. 80: p. 587-595.

[43] Cheng, X., et al., *Test-retest reliability of clinical Shack-Hartmann measurements.* Invest Ophthalmol Vis Sci, 2004. 45 (1): p. 351-60.

[44] Atchison, D.A., *Effect of defocus on visual field measurement.* Ophthalmic Physiol Opt, 1987. 7 (3): p. 259-65.

[45] Fankhauser, F. and J.M. Enoch, *The effects of blur upon perimetric thresholds. A method for determining a quantitative estimate of retinal contour.* Arch Ophthalmol, 1962. 68: p. 240-51.

[46] Johnson, C. and H. Leibowitz, *Practice, refractive error, and feedback as factors influencing peripheral motion thresholds.* Percept Psychophys, 1974. 15 (2): p. 276-280.

[47] Wang, Y.Z., et al., *Subjective refraction of the peripheral field using contrast detection acuity.* Journal of the American Optometric Association., 1996. 67: p. 584-589.

[48] Smith, E.L., 3rd, et al., *Effects of foveal ablation on emmetropization and form-deprivation myopia.* Invest Ophthalmol Vis Sci, 2007. 48 (9): p. 3914-22.

[49] Ferree, C., G. Rand, and C. Hardy, *Refraction for the peripheral field of vision.* Arch Ophthalmol., 1931. 5: p. 717-731.

[50] Millodot, M. and A. Lamont, *Refraction of the periphery of the eye.* J. Opt. Soc. Am., 1974. 64: p. 110-111.

[51] Anderson, R.S. and L.N. Thibos, *Relationship between acuity for gratings and for tumbling-E letters in peripheral vision.* J Opt Soc Am A Opt Image Sci Vis, 1999. 16 (10): p. 2321-33.

[52] Rempt, F., Hoogerheide, J., & Hoogenboom, W.P.H., *Peripheral retinoscopy and the skiagram.* Ophthalmologica., 1971. 162: p. 1-10.

[53] Seidemann, A., et al., *Peripheral refractive errors in myopic, emmetropic, and hyperopic young subjects.* J Opt Soc Am A Opt Image Sci Vis, 2002. 19 (12): p. 2363-73.

[54] Atchison, D.A., *Higher order aberrations across the horizontal visual field.* J Biomed Opt, 2006. 11 (3): p. 34026.

[55] Logan, N.S., Gilmartin, B., Wildsoet, C.F., & Dunne, M.C., *Posterior retinal contour in adult human anisomyopia.* Invest Ophthalmol Vis Sci, 2004. 45: p. 2152-2162.

[56] Love, J., Gilmartin, B., & Dunne, M.C.M., *Relative peripheral refractive error in adult and emmetropia.* Invest Ophthalmol Vis Sci, 2000. 41: p. s302.

[57] Millodot, M., *Effect of ametropia on peripheral refraction.* American Journal of Optometry and Physiological Optics., 1981. 58: p. 691-695.

[58] Schmid, G.F., *Variability of retinal steepness at the posterior pole in children 7-15 years of age.* Current Eye Research., 2003. 27: p. 61-68.

[59] Charman, W.N. and J.A. Jennings, *Ametropia and peripheral refraction.* Am J Optom Physiol Opt, 1982. 59 (11): p. 922-3.

[60] Dunne, M.C. and D.A. Barnes, *Schematic modelling of peripheral astigmatism in real eyes.* Ophthalmic Physiol Opt, 1987. 7 (3): p. 235-9.

[61] Dunne, M.C., D.A. Barnes, and R.A. Clement, *A model for retinal shape changes in ametropia.* Ophthalmic Physiol Opt, 1987. 7 (2): p. 159-60.

[62] Navarro, R., E. Moreno, and C. Dorronsoro, *Monochromatic aberrations and point-spread functions of the human eye across the visual field.* J. Opt. Soc. Am. A, 1998. 15: p. 2522-9.

[63] Atchison, D.A. and D.H. Scott, *Monochromatic aberrations of human eyes in the horizontal visual field.* J Opt Soc Am A Opt Image Sci Vis, 2002. 19 (11): p. 2180-4.

[64] Atchison, D.A., N. Pritchard, and K.L. Schmid, *Peripheral refraction along the horizontal and vertical visual fields in myopia.* Vision Res, 2006. 46 (8-9): p. 1450-8.

[65] Guirao, A. and P. Artal, *Off-axis monochromatic aberrations estimated from double pass measurements in the human eye.* Vision Res,, 1999. 39: p. 207-217.

[66] Lundstrom, L., P. Unsbo, and J. Gustafsson, *Off-axis wave front measurements for optical correction in eccentric viewing.* J Biomed Opt, 2005. 10: p. 034002.

[67] Sheehan, M.T., et al., *Population study of the variation in monochromatic aberrations of the normal human eye over the central visual field.* Opt Express, 2007. 15 (12): p. 7367-80.

[68] Applegate, R.A., et al., *Interaction between aberrations to improve or reduce visual performance.* J Cataract Refractive Surg., 2003. 29: p. 1487-1495.

[69] Stone, R.A. and D.I. Flitcroft, *Ocular shape and myopia.* Ann Acad Med Singapore, 2004. 33: p. 7-15.

[70] Thibos, L.N., *Calculation of the influence of lateral chromatic aberration on image quality across the visual field.* Journal of the Optical Society of America, A,, 1987. 4: p. 1673-1680.

[71] Wang, Y.Z., L.N. Thibos, and A. Bradley, *Effects of refractive error on detection acuity and resolution acuity in peripheral vision.* Invest Ophthalmol Vis Sci., 1997. 38: p. 2134-2143.

[72] Williams, D.R., et al., *Off-axis optical quality and retinal sampling in the human eye.* Vision Res, 1996. 36: p. 1103-1114.

[73] Curcio, C.A., et al., *Human photoreceptor topography.* J Comp Neurol, 1990. 292 (4): p. 497-523.

[74] Artal, P., A.M. Derrington, and E. Colombo, *Refraction, aliasing, and the absence of motion reversals in peripheral vision.* Vision Res., 1995. 35: p. 939-947.

[75] Thibos, L.N., D.L. Still, and A. Bradley, *Characterization of spatial aliasing and contrast sensitivity in peripheral visual.* Vision Res., 1996. 36: p. 249-258.

[76] Still, D.L., L.N. Thibos, and A. Bradley, *Peripheral image quality is almost as good as central image quality.* Invest Ophthalmol Vis Sci., 1989. 30 (suppl):52.

[77] Mutti, D.O., et al., *Refractive error, axial length, and relative peripheral refractive error before and after the onset of myopia.* Invest Ophthalmol Vis Sci, 2007. 48 (6): p. 2510-9.

[78] Charman, W.N., *Aberrations and myopia.* Ophthalmic Physiol Opt, 2005. 25 (4): p. 285-301.

[79] Marcos, S., S. Barbero, and L. Llorente, *The sources of optical aberrations in myopic eyes.* Invest. Ophthalmol. Vis. Sci. (suppl.), 2002. 43: p. Abstract 1510.

[80] Thorn, F., et al. *The vision of myopic children: how wavefront aberrations alter the image of school book text..* in *Myopia 2000, Proceedings of the VIII international conference in Myopia.* 2000. Boston.

[81] Wildsoet, C., *Structural correlates of myopia. In: Myopia and nearwork,* M.R.a.B. Gilmartin, Editor. 1998, Butterworth-Heinemann, Oxford. p. 31-56.

[82] Kee, C.S., et al., *Effects of optically imposed astigmatism on emmetropization in infant monkeys.* Invest Ophthalmol Vis Sci, 2004. 45 (6): p. 1647-59.

[83] Haugwitz, T. and F. Blodi, *Hirschberg's history of ophthalmology.* Optical instruments Postage stamps. West Germany, 1986. 11: p. 77.

[84] Dumbleton, K., et al., *Changes in myopic refractive error with nine months' extended wear of hydrogel lenses with high and low oxygen permeability.* Optom Vis Sci., 1999. 76: p. 845-9.

[85] Grosvenor, T., D. Perrigin, and J. Perrigin, *Rigid gas-permeable contact lenses for myoipia control: effects of discontination of lens wear..* Optom Vis Sci., 1991. 68: p. 385-9.

[86] Kemmetmuller, H., *Contact lenses versus spectacles in myopia.* Contact lens Med Bull, 1972. 5: p. 14-17.

[87] Miller, B., *Can progressive myopia be prevented by contact lenses.* Contacto, 1962. 6: p. 196-9.

[88] Nolan, J., *Myopia control with contact lenses.* Contacto, 1967. 11: p. 24-7.

[89] Perrigin, J., D. Perrigin, and e.a. Quintero S, *Silicone-acrylate contact lenses for myopia control: 3-year results.* Optom Vis Sci., 1990. 67: p. 764-9.

[90] Stone, J., *Myopia control after contact lens wear..* Br J Physiol Opt., 1974. 29: p. 93-108.

[91] Harris, M., M. Sarver, and K. Polse, *Corneal curvature and refractive error changes associated with wearing hydrogel contact lenses.* Am J Optom Physiol Optics., 1975. 52: p. 313-9.

[92] Binder, P., *Myopic extended wear with the Hydrocurve 2 soft contact lens.* Ophthalmology., 1983. 90: p. 623-6.

[93] Horner, D., P. Soni, and T. Salmon, *Myopia progression in adolenscent wearers of soft contact lenses and spectacles.* Optom Vis Sci., 1999. 76: p. 474-9.

[94] Grosvenor, T., D. Perrigin, and J. Perrigin, *Do rigid gas permeable contact lenses control the progress of myopia?* Spectrum, 1991: p. 29-35.

[95] Khoo, C., J. Chong, and U. Rajan, *A 3-year study on the effect of RGP contact lenses on myopic children.* Singapore Med J., 1999. 40: p. 230-7.

[96] Katz, J., O. Schein, and B. Levy, *Arandomized trial of rigid gas permeable contact lenses to reduce progression of children's myopia.* Am J Ophthalmol., 2003. 136: p. 82-90.

[97] Walline, J.J., et al., *A randomized trial of the effects of rigid contact lenses on myopia progression.* Arch Ophthalmol, 2004. 122 (12): p. 1760-6.

[98] Dorronsoro, C., S. Barbero, and L. Llorente, *On-eye measurement of optical perfomance of rigid gas permeable contact lenses based on ocular and corneal aberrometry.* Optom Vis Sci., 2003. 80 (2): p. 115-125.

[99] Atchison, D.A., *Aberrations associated with rigid contact lenses.* J Opt Soc Am A., 1995. 12: p. 2267-73.

[100] Hong, X., N. Himebaugh, and L.N. Thibos, *On-eye evaluation of optical performance of rigid and soft contact lenses.* Optom Vis Sci., 2001. 78: p. 872-80.

[101] Lu, F., et al., *Monochromatic wavefront aberrations in the human eye with contact lenses.* Optom Vis Sci., 2003. 80: p. 135-141.

[102] Atchison, D.A., *Aberrations associated with rigid contact lenses.* J Opt Soc Am A Opt Image Sci Vis, 1995. 12 (10): p. 2267-73.

[103] Logan, N.S., et al., *Posterior retinal contour in adult human anisomyopia.* Invest Ophthalmol Vis Sci, 2004. 45 (7): p. 2152-62.

[104] Millodot, M., *Effect of ametropia on peripheral refraction.* Am J Optom Physiol Opt, 1981. 58 (9): p. 691-5.

[105] Schmid, G.F., *Axial and peripheral eye length measured with optical low coherence reflectometry.* J Biomed Opt, 2003. 8 (4): p. 655-62.

[106] Schmid, G.F., *Variability of retinal steepness at the posterior pole in children 7-15 years of age.* Curr Eye Res, 2003. 27 (1): p. 61-8.

[107] Seidemann, A., Schaeffel, F., Guirao, A., Lopez-Gil, N., & Artal, P., *Peripheral refractive errors in myopic, emmetropic, and hyperopic young subjects.* Journal of the Optical Society of America A. Optics and Image Science, 2002. 19: p. 2363-2373.

[108] Smith, E.L., et al., *Peripheral vision can influence eye growth and refractive developement in infant monkeys.* invest Ophthalmol Vis Sci., 2005. 46 (11): p. 3965-72.

[109] Atchison, D.A., et al., *Refraction and aberration across the horizontal central 10 degree of the visual field.* Optom Vis Sci., 2006. 83 (4): p. 213-221.

[110] Shen, J., et al., *Peripheral refraction with and without contact lens correction.* Optom Vis Sci., 2009.

[111] Atchison, D.A. and D.H. Scott, *Monochromatic aberrations of human eyes in the horizontal visual field..* J Opt Soc Am A Opt Image Sci Vis,, 2002. 19 (2180-2184).

[112] Smith, G. and D.A. Atchison, *The eye and visual optical instruments.* Cambridge University Press, New York, 1997: p. 601-606.

[113] Cheng, X., A. Bradley, and L.N. Thibos, *Predicting subjective judgment of best focus* with objective image quality metrics. J Vis, 2004. 4 (4): p. 310-21.

[114] Cheng, X., L.N. Thibos, and A. Bradley, Estimating visual quality from wavefront aberration measurements. J Refract Surg, 2003. 19 (5): p. S579-84.

4

Diabetic Retinopathy – An Update on Pathophysiology, Classification, Investigation and Treatment

Vikas Tah, Sonia Mall, James Myerscough,
Kamran Saha, Elizabeth Emsley, Andrew Swampillai,
Ganeshan Ramsamy, Daren Hanumunthadu and
Mandeep Bindra

1. Introduction

The global prevalence of diabetes was estimated at 285 million in 2010.[1] The countries with the most significant number of sufferers in 2010 were India, China, United States, Russia and Brazil.[1] Countries with a low and middle income experience the worst burden of diabetes, compared with higher income countries.[1]

The total prevalence of diabetes in children and adults in the United States was 25.8 million in 2011, which is 8.3% of the entire population.[2] It is estimated that 18.8 million of this figure are diagnosed and 7 million remain undiagnosed.[2] 79 million individuals in the United States are expected to be at risk of diabetes.[2] The overall cost of diabetes in the United States in 2012 was $245 billion, with $176 being directly related to medical costs and $69 billion related to reduced productivity.[2] In the UK, 2.6 million individuals were diagnosed with diabetes in 2009,[3] and this is expected to exceed 4 million in 2024.[4] It is also expected that up to 500,000 other UK individuals remain undiagnosed.[5] An estimated one in 20 individuals in England have diabetes-both diagnosed and undiagnosed, and this is marginally reduced UK-wide.[1] For adults in the UK it is estimated that 10% of individuals with diabetes mellitus (DM) have Type 1 diabetes mellitus and 90% have type 2 diabetes mellitus.[1, 6]

Effective management of diabetes reduces complication risk.[7] However failure to control the condition can lead to microvascular and macrovascular complications. At the time of diagnosis, 50% of those with type 2 diabetes mellitus face complications.[8] Complications may begin five to six years prior to diagnosis, whilst the onset of diabetes itself may precede the clinical diagnosis by a decade.[9]

Diabetic retinopathy (DR) is the most frequent complication associated with diabetes mellitus, and is the number one cause of blindness in individuals of working age in developed nations.[10] Indeed individuals with diabetes are 10 to 20 times at greater risk of developing blindness than those without the diagnosis.[11] DR prevalence in the Wisconsin Epidemiological Study of Diabetic Retinopathy (WESDR) was identified as 50.1% and 54.2% in the diabetes control and complications trial (DCCT) in insulin-dependent diabetes mellitus (IDDM)[12, 13] DR prevalence in non-insulin dependent diabetes mellitus (NIDDM) was found to be 35-39% in the United Kingdom Prospective Diabetes Study.[14] During 2005-2008, 4.2 million (28.5%) of diabetics in the United States aged 40 years and above suffered from diabetic retinopathy, with 0.7 million (4.4% of these diabetics) experiencing advanced DR, thus risking severe loss of vision.[2] In the WESDR, 1.4% of patients with IDDM were able to achieve a best-corrected visual acuity of 20/80 to 20/160, with 3.6% having an acuity of 20/200 or worse in the better eye.[15] 3% of the older-onset group had vision ranging from 20/80 to 20/160, and 1.6% were 20/200 or worse in the best eye.[15]

1.1. Incidence of visual impairment

10 years following diabetes mellitus (DM) onset, blindness (a visual acuity of equal to or worse than 20/200 in the best eye) was 1.8% in the type 1 cohort, 4.0% in the insulin-treated type 2 group and 4.8% in the non-insulin-treated type 2 patients.[16] Further, in these groups the incidence of visual impairment at 10 years (loss of 15 letters on a 0-70 letter scale) was identified as 9.4, 37.2 and 23.9 respectively.[16]

There appear to be few paediatric cases of DR, though it has been identified in children as young as 5.5 years in an American study, and severe blindness has also been described in adolescents as the microvascular effects of diabetes, including DR, can develop during puberty years.[17]

1.2. Historical developments

The Diabetic Retinopathy Study in the 1970s and the Early Treatment Diabetic Retinopathy Study in the 1980s, identified the major effects of retinal photocoagulation on visual loss associated with proliferative diabetic retinopathy and macular oedema, as well as influencing guideline and screening programme development for early identification and management of diabetic retinopathy.[18, 19, 20] Following this, both the incidence and progression risk of diabetic retinopathy has reduced from an estimated 90% of patients with diabetes, to less than 50%.[20] In the WESDR, which focused on individuals with type 1 diabetes mellitus, the yearly incidence of proliferative diabetic retinopathy reduced by 77% from 1980 to 2007, with a 57% reduction in visual impairment during this same time period.[21] Evidence from a range of international studies, including those from Sweden, Denmark and the United States, indicate that individuals recently diagnosed with type 1 or type 2 diabetes mellitus have a significantly reduced risk of proliferative diabetic retinopathy, macular oedema and visual impairment, compared with those diagnosed in the past.[22, 23, 24, 25, 26] The considerable decrease in the prevalence and incidence of diabetic retinopathy and visual impairment over the previous few decades suggests improved glycaemic, blood pressure and lipid level management.[26]

1.3. A global epidemic

However the number of individuals with diabetes is expected to exponentially increase internationally to 429 million by 2030, attributed to the increased prevalence of obesity, an ageing population and enhanced identification of the disease.[27, 28] This represents a major public health concern. As an exemplar, in India 32 million individuals were diagnosed with diabetes in 2000 and an estimated 79 million will be affected by 2030, and if complication prevalence remains the same, around 0.7 million Indians will suffer from proliferative diabetic retinopathy and 1.8 million with have macular oedema with clinical manifestations.[29] This identifies a large population at risk of visual impairment attributed to their diabetes, and highlights the importance of effective epidemiological surveillance of developing countries as there may be reduced delivery of health care capacity compared with developed nations.[20]

2. Pathophysiology

The DCCT and United Kingdom Prospective Diabetes Study (UKPDS) both support the significant association between a long-term hyperglycaemic status and the establishment, as well as progression, of DR.[36, 37] However the mechanism which result in microvascular injury attributed to hyperglycaemia is uncertain.[36, 37] Several interlinking molecular pathways have been discussed as being possibly involved in the mechanism, and these include enhanced polyol pathway activity, diacylglycerol-(DAG-)PKC pathway activation, enhanced growth factor expression for example vascular endothelial growth factor (VEGF) and insulin-like growth factor-1 (IGF-1), haemodynamic alterations, faster advanced glycation endproducts (AGEs) production, oxidative stress, renin-angiotensin-aldosterone system (RAAS) activation, inflammation and leukostasis.[38] However the final metabolic pathway resulting in the establishment of DR is uncertain.[39]

2.1. Polyol pathway

The polyol pathway is involved in the metabolism of surplus glucose.[38]

Aldose reductase (AR), which exists in the retina, is involved in the reduction of glucose into sorbitol, employing nicotinamide adenine dinucleotide phosphate (NADPH) as a cofactor.[38] Sorbitol is then converted to fructose using sorbital dehydrogenase (SDH).[38] Sorbitol is impermeable to cellular membranes, and therefore there is an intracellular accumulation of it, which is followed by the gradual metabolism of sorbitol to fructose.[40] NADPH is also employed as a cofactor for glutathione reductase in the regeneration of intracellular glutathione, therefore limiting the antioxidant capability of the cells.[38]

Sorbitol accumulation may have multi-injurious effects on retinal cells, such as osmotic injury. [41] Further, the fructose formed in the polyol pathway can undergo a phosphorylation

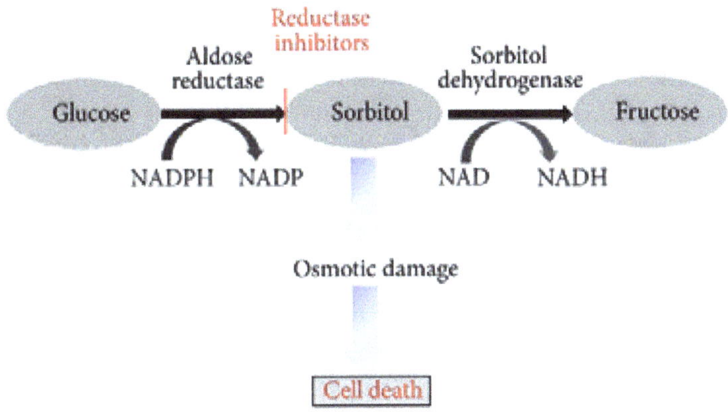

Figure 1. Polyol pathway

reaction, forming fructose-3-phosphate, with the potential for further degradation to 3-deoxyglucosone.[42] Both of these products are potent glycating mediators and can support the production of AGEs.[42] Moreover employment of NADPH in the polyol pathway, reduces NADPH availability for glutathione reductase, thereby preventing the production of reduced glutathione, resulting in reduced protection against oxidative stress.[43]

More recently, evidence suggests that AR is localised in retinal cells such as pericytes,[44] retinal endothelial cells,[45] ganglion cells,[45] Muller cells,[45] retinal pigment epithelial cells and neurons.[45, 46] Enhanced AR activity may be involved in retinal cell destruction.[43] Importantly, pericyte or endothelial cell exposure to enhanced concentrations of glucose or galactose reduces the survivability of these cells,[38] with reversal of this cell death on the administration of ARIs.[47] Generally, electrolye imbalance attributed to high aldose reductase levels results in cellular death, in particular retinal pericytes, which contribute to microaneurysm formation.[48]

The polyol pathway is also associated with other pathophysiological characteristics in DR, including a thickened retinal capillary basement membrane,[49] with ARI preventing this thickening in rat models.[50] ARIs are also effective in reducing leukocyte adhesion in endothelial cells,[51] which results in leukostasis and is discussed later, as well as preventing enhanced vascular permeability and blood retinal barrier breakdown which is a hallmark feature of DR.[46] Genetically, AR may also contribute to DR establishment.[52]

Thus far, ARIs employed in animal models at the onset of diabetes has been useful in preventing DR, though limited clinical benefit has been shown.[38]

2.2. Protein glycation

The establishment and accumulation of AGEs is a significant contributor to DR.[53] AGEs are molecules produced non-enzymatically when sugars are reduced with free amino groups of proteins, lipids and nucleic acids.[38] Normally, AGEs are produced at a constant and gradual rate, commencing at the embryonic stage and accumulating with time.[38] In the context of increased glucose availability in diabetes, their production is accelerated.[54]

AGEs are important in several diabetic complications.[38] For example, they have been identified in the retinal vessels of diabetics, and these AGE levels have been correlated with those found in the serum, as well as retinopathy severity.[55] AGE interaction with certain cell surface receptors such as RAGE, CD36 and the macrophage scavenger receptor have been described in DR development.[55]

Animal studies suggest significantly high AGE exposure is contributory to renal and vascular complications.[56, 57] In rats which developed diabetes, retinal capillaries had enhanced AGE accumulation, as well as a loss of pericytes.[53] Treatment with AGE formation inhibitors considerably reduced AGE accumulation, and stopped microaneurysm formation, acellular capillaries and pericyte loss.[53] In another study, rats with a diabetes duration of 29 weeks, there was an increase in acellular capillaries by more than three times compared to previously, and there was increased thickening of the basement membrane.[56] A thickened capillary basement membrane and enhanced deposition of extracellular matrix components is a contributor to the development of abnormal retinal haemodynamics.[58] Again, treatment with an AGE formation inhibitor prevented capillary dropout and reduced basement membrane protein formation.[56]

These studies, which are still in their infancy, identify AGE formation and activation of their respective receptors as important targets for pharmacotherapeutic strategies.[38]

2.3. Activation of Protein Kinase C (PKC)

PKC is a kinase involved in signal transduction activity in response to a stimulus which may be hormonal, neuronal or growth factor in origin.[38] The Beta1/2 isoform of PKC is associated with DR development.[59] Raised blood glucose increases glucose flux in the glycolysis pathway, thereby increasing diacylglycerol (DAG) production. DAG is a major PKC activator.[60] Clinical and experimental research has identified an increase in DAG and PKC activation in diabetes.[59]

PKC can also influence other physiological pathways therefore having the capability to alter endothelial permeability, retinal haemodynamics and expression of vascular endothelial growth factor (VEGF) in the retina and enhanced leukostasis.[59, 61, 62]

In particular, the expression of the PKC beta1/2 isoform is increased in diabetics, thereby contributing to DR pathogenesis by extracellular matrix (ECM) protein synthesis, remodeling of the ECM, increased angiogenic factor production, endothelial and leukocyte cell abnormalities, ultimately resulting in occluded capillaries and leukostasis, with alterations in retinal blood flow.[38] The PKC pathway also influences other activities such as inflammatory changes, neovascularisation and abberant haemodynamics.[38] This further progresses the pathogenic changes in DR. Experimentally, PKC-beta1/2 inhibitors significantly reduce DR progression.[63] In clinical trials, inhibitors do not prevent DR but considerably reduce the associated vision loss.[64]

2.4. Haemodynamic alterations

Hypertension, which has a high incidence in diabetes, is likely to contribute to DR progression.[38] This may involve the mechanical stretch and sheer stresses associated with hypertension, injuring endothelial cells. Enhanced retinal perfusion and increased blood viscosity can also lead to endothelial dysfunction.[65] Further, the endocrine mechanisms which have regulatory influences over blood pressure are also independently involved in DR pathogenesis.[66]

2.5. Renin-angiotensin-aldosterone system involvement

RAAS is fundamental in blood pressure and fluid regulation, with aberrant changes identified in this system in diabetics.[66] There is an increase in the expression of certain receptors and signaling molecules in the retina, in PDR, including renin, angiotensin converting enzymes (ACE) and angiotensin receptors.[66, 67] This is independent of systemic blood pressure.[38] In experimental studies, ACE inhibitor use prevents neovascularization and several clinical studies suggest that targeting of RAAS reduces the incidence of retinopathy in type 1 diabetes and prevents progression of DR.[68]-[70]

The exact mechanism of RAAS involvement in DR is uncertain, though in vitro evidence identifies association with PKC activation and VEGF signaling.[71]

2.6. Inflammatory changes and Leukostasis

The importance of inflammation, in particular subclinical inflammation in DR development is considerable, though complex.[38] The hyperglycaemic state, oxidative stress, AGE production and hypertension are all contributory to the inflammation. Moreover, the inflammation is self-propagating by means of cytokines, adhesion molecules, VEGF activity, increased RAGE expression, nitric oxide regulatory changes and NF-kB signaling.[38] This subclinical retinal inflammation increases intraocular blood pressure by the involvement of endothelial nitric oxide synthase (eNOS), formation of new but weak vessels and their enhanced VEGF permeability which results in retinal haemorrhages, as well as leukostasis attributed to multiple proinflammatory agents.[38] Leukostasis is crucial in DR pathogenesis, resulting in capillary occlusion, reactive oxygen species (ROS)-related cellular death and local retinal amplification of the inflammatory activities.[72]-[75]

There is a considerable increase in systemic proinflammatory cytokine expression, soluble and cell surface adhesion molecule activation and chemokine expression in the DR retina.[76] The increase in serum proinflammatory cytokines, adhesion agents and immune cell activation in diabetes correlates with DR progression.[77, 78] Endothelial abnormalities, as well as increased proinflammatory cytokines and adhesion molecules, contribute to leukostasis by increasing leukocyte and endothelial cell interaction.[79, 80] Localised inflammation including the activation of microglia, macrophages and immune cells is considered important in DR pathogenesis.[81] This is corroborated by the use of minocycline, an antibiotic and anti-inflammatory agent, which prevents microglial activation and thereby prevents DR.[81]

2.7. Oxidative stress

Oxidative stress occurs when the level of ROS or oxygen radicals increase to a degree where the antioxidant defences are unable to cope.[82] Oxidative stress established by hyperglycaemia is pivotal in microvascular complications.[83] Correlation between hyperglycaemia, alterations in redox homeostasis and oxidative stress is essential in DR pathogenesis.[84, 85] Increased ROS are likely to be involved in both the development and progression of DR.[86] It has been proposed that oxidative stress may be a "unifying mechanism" linking several injurious pathways induced by the hyperglycaemic state in DR.[87] ROS derived from mitochondria cause DNA breaks, which activate poly-(ADP-ribose)-polymerase (PARP).[87] PARP activation results in inhibition of glyceraldehyde phosphate dehydrogenase (GAPDH) activity, causing glycolytic metabolite accumulation.[87] These metabolites cause the activation of AGE, PKC-beta-2, polyol and hexosamine pathways.[87] NADPH oxidase-derived ROS may also be involved in the pathogenesis.[87]

2.8. Growth factor involvement

The importance of growth factors in DR is confirmed by the rare observation of serious DR in growth hormone deficient diabetic dwarfs,[88] and this is further corroborated by slowed DR progression in individuals with pituitary ablation in the 1970s.[89]

The growth factor most frequently considered in DR is VEGF, which promotes angiogenesis, causes blood-retinal barrier breakdown, endothelial cell growth stimulation and neovascularization, as well as increased vascular permeability in an ischaemic retina.[90]-[92] Ischaemia in the retina causes angiogenic factors, such as vascular endothelial growth factor (VEGF) to establish neovascularization, resulting in proliferative diabetic retinopathy (PDR). VEGFs are produced by retinal pigment epithelium, pericytes and retinal endothelial cells.[39] Animal and clinical evidence suggests VEGF, especially the 165 isoform, is important in the development and progression of DR.[93, 94]

Anti-VEGF agents have clinical efficacy in the treatment of DMO, but are not effective in all patients.[38] Further long-term use of anti-VEGF agents should be considered with caution in DR.[38]

2.9. Carbonic Anhydrase (CA)

Enhanced intraocular VEGF concentrations correlates with increased vascular permeability, contributing to haemorrhage, exudate formation, vascular leakage, and ultimately leading to NPDR, angiogenesis and vasculogenesis leading to PDR.[38]

CAs are ubiquitous metalloenzymes which cause conversion of carbon dioxide to bicarbonate and protons.[38] Diabetics have considerably higher CA concentrations than controls,[95] and CA inhibitors reduce DR progression and prevents visual loss in animal and clinical research.[96] The mechanisms involved may include reduced humour secretion, induction of vasodilatation and improved ocular blood flow, platelet aggregation inhibition and reduction in vascular permeability.[95]

2.10. Neurodegeneration in the retina

As well as the changes already described, structural and functional alterations can injure certain non-vascular cells.[38] It is believed that neurodegeneration of retinal neurons and glia may even precede microaneurysm development.[97]

3. Risk factors

Epidemiologic studies have shown several risk factors associated with the incidence of diabetic retinopathy and subsequent macular oedema (table 1). Several other risk factors have also been implicated in disease progression such as sleep apnoea [98], non-alcoholic fatty liver disease, genetic mutations[21, 99] and serum prolactin, homocysteine and adinopectin levels [33, 31, 34]. However the exact contribution of these factors to disease progression remains unknown. The precise association of smoking with diabetic retinopathy appears complex and is unclear.

Type of diabetes
Duration of diabetes
Poor glycaemic control
Hyperlipidaemia
Hypertension
Pregnancy

Table 1. Recognised risk factors associated with diabetic retinopathy

3.1. Type of diabetes

Type 1 diabetic patients are at substantially higher risk than type 2, which is independent of the duration of the disease process[100, 101]. Both severity and prevalence increase with age in the former group but not the later.

3.2. Duration of diabetes

A clear correlation exists between diabetic retinopathy and disease duration[1]. This risk factor has influenced the formation of guidelines for early examination of suspected patients to decrease disease progression. In two studies [100, 102] evidence was shown that after 15 years retinopathy would be present in virtually all type 1 diabetics and up to 75% of type 2 diabetics, with 2% becoming blind and up to 10% developing severe visual impairment. Puberty is now an accepted risk factor for retinopathy in type 1 diabetes, due to the acceleration of microvascular compromise as a result of physiological changes post puberty [103]. One study found that younger post-menarchal subjects were up to 3.2 times more likely to develop retinopathy, in comparison to pre-menarchal subjects[104]. Subjects older than 13 years at the time of diagnosis were more likely to suffer from retinopathy, than those younger. A four year follow-up also showed that the same post-menarchal had greater progression of their retinopathy than pre-menarchal (P=0.06). While the exact mechanism is not known, hormonal factors have been speculated to play a part.

3.3. Glycaemic control

The relationship between glycaemic control and onset/progression of diabetic retinopathy is well documented. Intensive metabolic control has shown a decreased in diabetic related complications [105]. Studies such as the Early Treatment of Diabetic Retinopathy Study (ETDRS) and Diabetes Control and Complication Trial (DCCT)[13] show that risk of progression is reduced with aggressive glycaemic control. Glycosylated haemoglobin levels have shown a relationship with the severity of proliferative diabetic retinopathy[106]. However, while glycosylated haemoglobin remains a formidable risk factor, it only accounted for 11% of all risks for retinopathy in DCCT [107].

3.4. Hyperlipidaemia

Association of hyperlipidaemia and diabetes is well documented [108]. A statistically significant association between elevated serum total cholesterol and low density lipoprotein cholesterol and the severity of retinal hard exudation in patients with diabetic retinopathy was confirmed by the ETDRS group and the Wisconsin Epidemiologic Study of Diabetic Retinopathy (WESDR) found [109]. As reported by Chew found patients with serum cholesterol level more than 240mg/dl were twice as likely to have more hard exudates as those patients with serum cholesterol level 200 mg/dl [110].

3.5. Hypertension

A major risk factor of cardiovascular disease in diabetics is hypertension. An age-adjusted 82% increase in risk of diabetes-related death is thought to come from this risk factor alone.[111] This is accorded with the theory that increased blood pressure is implicated in the onset of diabetic retinopathy [112, 113]. The UK Prospective Diabetic Study (UKPDS) showed that tight blood pressure control (144/82 vs 155/87) was associated with a 34% reduction in retinopathy with a 47% reduction in deterioration of visual acuity of three lines [14]. The use of angiotensin-converting-enzyme (ACE) inhibitors and their role in directly affecting the progression of retinopathy (as opposed to their therapeutic effects in hypertension) was the subject of much debate. ACE inhibitors were found to be associated with reduced levels of vascular endothelial growth factor in diabetic retinopathy patients[114]. However in the UKDPS group demonstrated an overall reduction of blood pressure was proven to be effective in slowing down the progression of retinopathy, rather than the type of antihypertensive drug used [115]. More recently, the '**DI**abetic **RE**tinopathy **C**andesartan **T**rial' (DIRECT) study recently posited that while candesartan did not have any beneficial effect on the progression of retinopathy in type 1 diabetic patients, it did yield improvement in type 2 patients with mild to moderate retinopathy [69, 68].

3.6. Pregnancy

Many studies have concluded that diabetic women in pregnancy have a substantial risk of worsening their retinopathy [116, 117] although resolution of ocular changes in post-partum period is reported [116, 118]. Studies by Phelps et al [119] and the Diabetes in Early Pregnancy Study (DIEP) group [120] concluded that retinopathy was most likely to progress in those who had the poorest control at baseline. DIEP also found that a disease duration of more than 15 years and severity of existing retinopathy were the most important factors in the development and progression of retinopathy in pregnancy. Type 1 diabetic women are most at risk and should be undergo an ophthalmic examination prior to pregnancy and counselled on good glycaemic control. The exact mechanism of progressive retinopathy in pregnant diabetic woman is the subject of much debate. Factors thought to be involved include duration of diabetes, co-existing hypertension, poor glycaemic control and its rapid normalisation during pregnancy [121].

4. Signs

Microaneurysms are out-pouchings of the capillary wall that form by either focal dilatation of the capillary wall in the absence of pericytes, or fusion of the two arms of a capillary loop. Clinically these are seen as tiny red dots. Retinal haemorrhages are divided into intraretinal, retinal nerve fibre layer and deeper dark round haemorrhages. Intraretinal haemorrhages are located in the middle layers of the retina and give rise to dot/blot configuration. Retinal nerve fibre layer haemorrhages are flame-shaped and arise from larger superficial pre-capillary arterioles. Deeper dark round haemorrhages represent retinal infarcts within the middle layers and are marker for progression to retinal neovascularisation. Cotton wool spots result from nerve fibre layer infarcts. Axon disruption causes accumulation of neuronal debris in the nerve fibre layer. Clinically these are seen as small fluffy lesions that can obscure underlying blood vessels. Exudates are composed of lipoprotein and lipid-filled macrophages located within the outerplexiform layer. They are seen as waxy yellow lesions with relatively distinct margins. They tend to progress as retinopathy worsens and can affect the macula resulting in macular oedema. Exudates reabsorb spontaneously when leakage ceases over a period of months. Venous changes include beading of blood vessels, tortuosity, and focal narrowing with dilatation called 'beading'. The extent of venous change correlates well with the proliferative change. IRMA, or intraretinal microvascular abnormalities are arteriolar venous shunts that run from retinal arterioles to venules. They bypass capillary beds and are seen in areas of capillary hypoperfusion. Arteriolar narrowing often can be marker for ischaemic dysfunction. Proliferative retinopathy is seen as new preretinal vessels that may arise at the optic disc or elsewhere in the retina or iris. There are fine fragile vessels that can develop fibrous tissue over time.

Diabetic macula oedema is one of or a combination of focal, diffuse or ischaemia. It is the main reason for visual impairment and represents foveal oedema, exudates or ischaemia. Focal maculopathy has retinal thickening and exudates. Fluoroscein angiogram shows late focal hypofluorescence from leakage. Diffuse maculopathy can be associated with cystoids changes and diffuse retinal thickening. Fluoroscein angiogram shows late hypofluorescence with a flower petal pattern if cystoids macula oedema is present. Ischaemic maculopathy often has a relatively normal looking macula in the presence of reduced visual acuity. Fluoroscein angiogram shows non-perfusion and an enlarged foveal avascular zone.

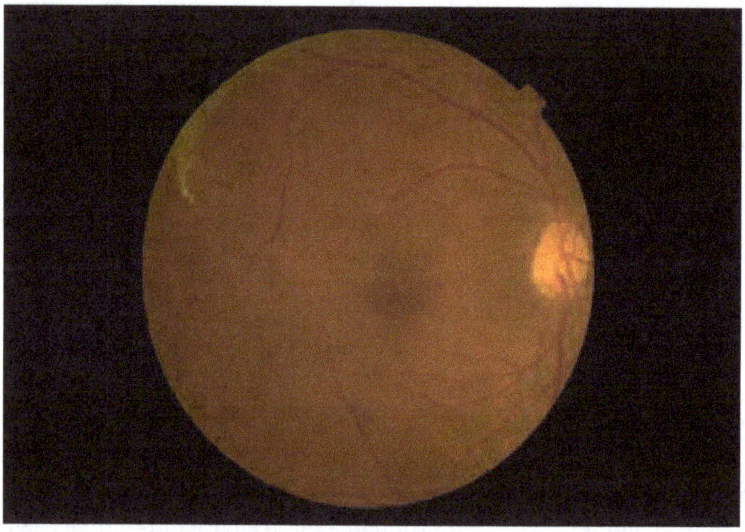

Figure 2. Microaneurysms at the macular and blot haemorrhages temporally

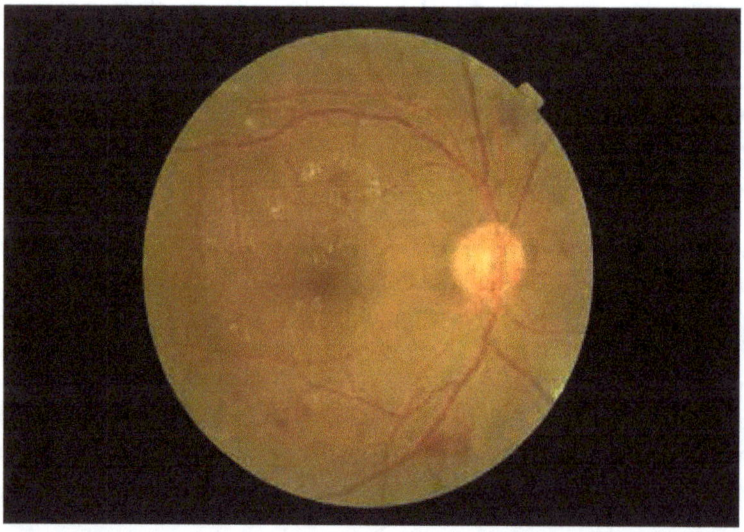

Figure 3. Exudates and microaneurysms at the macula, blot haemorrhages at the arcades, new vessels on the disc and cotton wool spots, IRMA and venous beading supoertemporally.

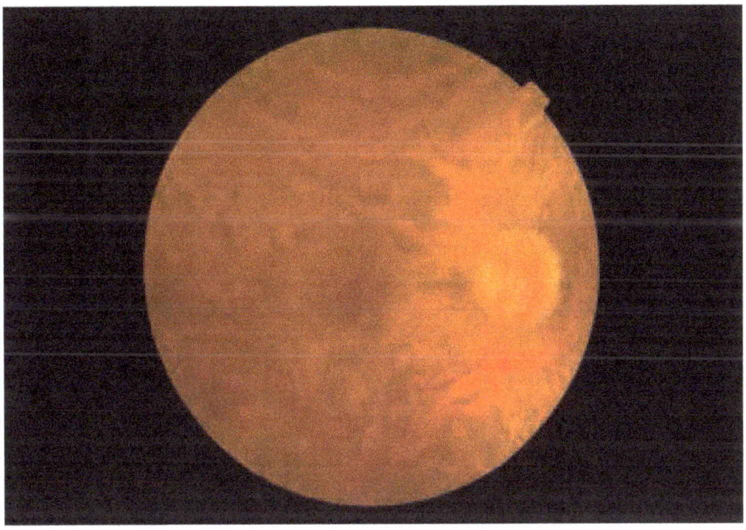

Figure 4. New vessels on disc and elsewhere inferotemporally

5. Classification

Diabetic retinopathy classification is based on who is classifying the disease. One approach has been for screening and one is based on grading severity in the context of ophthalmic signs. There are different screening systems in different parts of the developed world. In the UK, the English National Screening Criteria[122] is used to merit ophthalmological referral, seen in the table below. Two commonly used classification systems for classification in the context of ophthalmic signs are the Airlie House Classification [123] and the international (AAO) classification [124]. There are similarities and overlap in both. For the purpose of this chapter we will focus on the Airlie House classification.

The Airlie House classification was the original classification that has subsequently undergone modification in the Early Treatment of Diabetic Retinopathy Study (EDTRS)[125] aimed at grading retinopathy in the context of ophthalmic signs. EDTRS was first developed in 1997, but has undergone change and development for countries without significant screening and programmes and for the purpose of research. The sight threatening risk of diabetic retinopathy was incorporated into the later clinical grading system. Broadly this incorporates low risk non-proliferative retinopathy (3 substages), severe non-proliferative diabetic retinopathy, proliferative retinopathy and the presence of macula oedema.

Below is based on the Airlie House classification:

Mild Nonproliferative Diabetic Retinopathy (NPDR): At least one microaneurysm

Moderate NPDR: Severe retinal haemorrhages in at least one quadrant, cotton wool spots, venous beading or IRMA.

Severe NPDR: Severe retinal haemorrhages in four quadrants or venous beading in two quadrants; or extensive IRMA in one quadrant

Proliferative diabetic retinopathy: based on location and risk

Location: new vessels at disc (NVD) or elsewhere (NVE)

Risk: Low risk where neovascularisation of the optic disc is less than one-quarter to a third of the disc area with no vitreous haemorrhage.

High risk: mild NVD with vitreous haemorrhage.

Moderate to severe NVD (one quarter to a third disc areas)

New vessels elsewhere more than one half disc areas with vitreous haemorrhage.

ENSC Grade	Features
Retinopathy grade	
R0	No retinopathy
R1	Retinal microaneurysms, haemorrhages and or exudates not within the definition of maculopathy
R2	(Pre-proliferative) venous beading, venous loop or IRMA, dot or blot haemorrhages and cotton wool spots
R3	Proliferative: NVD, NVE or pre-retinal or vitreous haemorrhage, pre-retinal fibrosis and tractional retinal detachment
M0	No maculopathy
M1	Exudate within 1 disc diameter of fovea centre, or circinate exudates within the macula, or retinal thickening within 1 disc of fovea centre only if associated with vision of 6/12 or worse
P	Focal/grid laser to macula or peripheral scatter
U	Unobtainable

Table 2. The English National Screenin Committee Guidelines

Maculopathy

Focal: Well circumscribed areas of leakage with oedema and exudates, that may surround microaneurysms

Diffuse: Generalised leaking with oedema

Ischaemic: Reduced visual acuity with relatively normal clinical appearance but macula ischaemia on FFA.

Mixed: A combination of the above

Clinical significant macula oedema (CSMO)

- Retinal thickening at or within 500μm of the centre of the macula
- Hard exudates at or within 500μ of the centre of the macula if associated with adjacent retinal thickening
- Retinal thickening of > 1 disc area any part of which is within one disc diameter of the centre of the macula.

More recently the terms centre involving and non-centre involving macula oedema have been used.

6. Investigations

Diabetes Mellitus is a complex disease requiring a multidisciplinary approach. The systemic investigations requested for a patient identified with ocular manifestations of the disease may provide valuable information regarding other organ systems affected which are not yet clinically apparent. Some of the general investigations below may be requested by an ophthalmologist depending on the local health setting but require referral for result interpretation and subsequent management by diabetologist colleagues.

6.1. Systemic Investigations

6.1.1. HbA1C

The Diabetes Control and Complication Trial (DCCT) [126] and subsequent follow-up study, Epidemiology of Diabetes Interventions and Complications (EDIC), highlighted that the effect of good glycaemic control on progression of retinopathy is significant and persists for at least 10 years. Due to the 8-12 week turnover of erythrocytes the glycosylated haemoglobin molecule is a more useful marker of glucose control than a random blood glucose measurement.

6.1.2. Lipids

Recent studies [127] have identified the importance of cholesterol lowering medications to both treatment naïve and previously treated hypercholestrolaemic type 2 diabetics in reducing the risk of clinically significant macular edema (CSME), and diabetic retinopathy progression[127, 128]. Fasting lipids should therefore be requested in new patients.

6.1.3. Urea & electrolytes

Diabetic nephropathy is an important consequence of microvascular disease and all patients should be screened for any renal dysfunction.

6.1.4. Genetic markers

Various clinical studies have looked at retinopathy clusters in families with type 1 diabetes. Genetic studies have analysed risk genes for retinopathy [The Diabetes Control and Complications Trial Research Group, 1997][126]. No study has provided an evidence base for genetic testing in diabetic patients to predict the rate of retinopathy progression and therefore genetic testing is not currently recommended for routine practice.

6.1.5. Blood pressure

Patients should be referred to a physician for investigation of all modifiable risk factors including blood pressure and smoking cessation, both known to contribute to the rate of diabetic retinopathy progression. [Gaede *et al.* 2008][129]·

7. Imaging

7.1. Fundus Photography

Fundus photography provides a useful photographic record of the posterior pole and is useful in the Diabetic Screening Programme, but relies on 2-dimensional surrogate markers of macular thickening since it cannot quantify actual thickening.

7.2. Optical Coherence Tomography (OCT)

Optical Coherence Tomography is a non-invasive imaging technique which is non-contact and facilitates high resolution cross-sectional imaging of the anterior segment, vitreous, retina and optic nerve head. Rather than the sound waves of B-scan ultrasonography, OCT uses light interferometry (near-infrared) to interpret the interference patterns of wave superposition.

OCT is useful is very sensitive in detecting change in macula thickness and therefore useful in the diagnosis of diabetic macula oedema. It is also able to identify the loss of ganglion cells in the retina, which precedes vascular changes. Because OCT gives a quantitative measure of retinal thickness it is critical in monitoring retinal thickness in response to treatment e.g. Macula laser or Anti-VEGF agents.

Different tissue reflectivities are depicted by different colours; red denotes high reflectivity, green-yellow intermediate reflectivity and blue-black low reflectivity. In addition to numerical measures of retinal thickness a topographical map is created which is colour coded according to thickness.

7.3. Fundus Fluorescein Angiography (FFA)

Fundus Fluorescein Angiography involves the injection of an orange water-soluble dye; sodium fluorescein into the systemic circulation. It remains predominantly intravascular and is fluorescent; i.e. it emits light of a longer wavelength when stimulated by light of a lower wavelength. After intravenous injection, fundus photography is performed in a rapid sequence. Blue filtered light is absorbed by the molecule as it enters the retinal circulation and in turn emits yellow-green light.

The FFA image maps the retinal vasculature and the structural and functional integrity of the vessels.

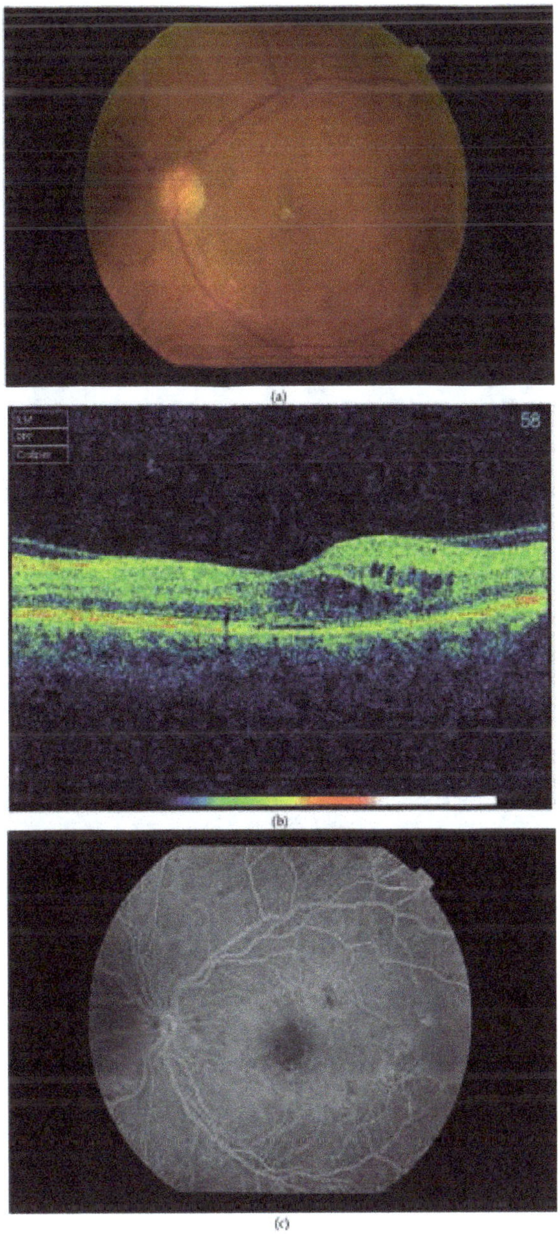

Figure 5. a. Fundus photograph of Diabetic Maculopathy (Circinate hard exudates, haemorrhages) **b.** Optical Coherence Tomography of Diabetic Maculopathy (Intraretinal cystic thickening) **c.** Fundus Fluorescein Angiogram of Diabetic Maculopathy

Normally 10-15 seconds elapse between dye injection and arrival of the dye in the short ciliary arteries. Choroidal circulation precedes retinal circulation by 1 second. Transit of dye through the retinal circulation takes approximately 15 to 20 seconds.

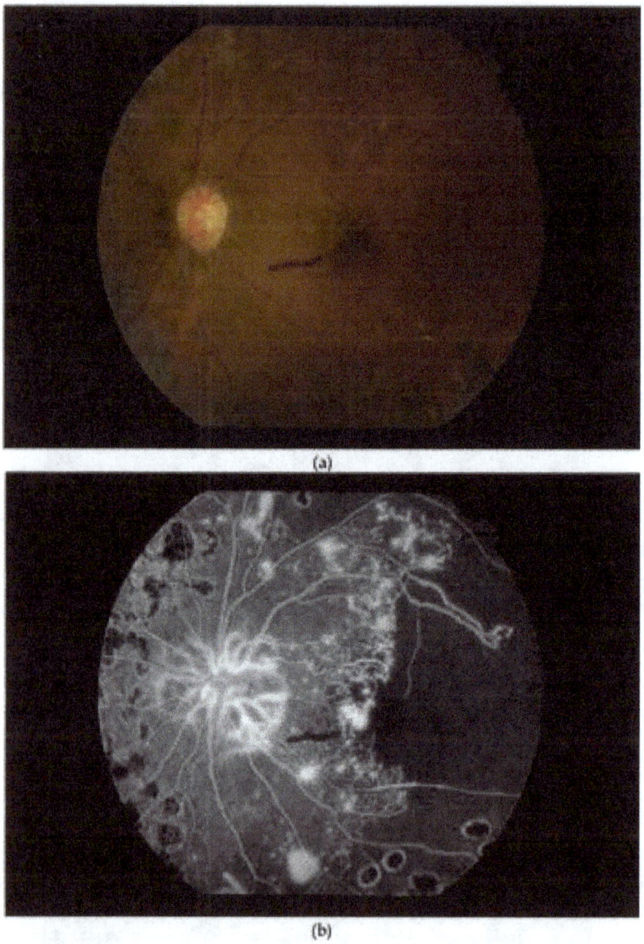

Figure 6. a. Fundus Photograph of New Vessel at Disc (NVD). Note PRP laser scars **b.** Fundus Fluorescein Angiogram of New Vessel at Disc (NVD) with evidence of peripheral ischaemia

The normal angiogram can be divided into five phases

1. **Choroidal phase**: The choroid is filled by the short ciliary arteries resulting in initial patching filling of lobules, quickly followed by a diffuse blush as dye leaks out of the choroidocapillaris.
2. **Arterial phase**: The central retinal artery fills about 1 second after choroidal filling
3. **Capillary phase**: The capillaries quickly fill following the arterial phase. The perifoveal capillary network is particularly prominent, as the underlying choroidal circulation is

masked by luteal pigment in the retina and melanin pigment in theretinal pigment epithelium (RPE). At the centre of this capillary ring is the foveal avascular zone 500um in diameter.

4. **Venous phase:** Early filling of the veins is from tributaries joining their margins, resulting in a tramline effect. Later the whole diameter of the veins is filled.

5. **Late (recirculation) phase:** 10 to 15 minutes later only a little dye remains within the blood circulation. Dye which has left the blood to ocular structures is particularly visible during this phase.

Below images are taken from clinical practice for common diabetic pathology (Images kindly provided by Mr Jignesh Patel, Essex County Hospital, Colchester).

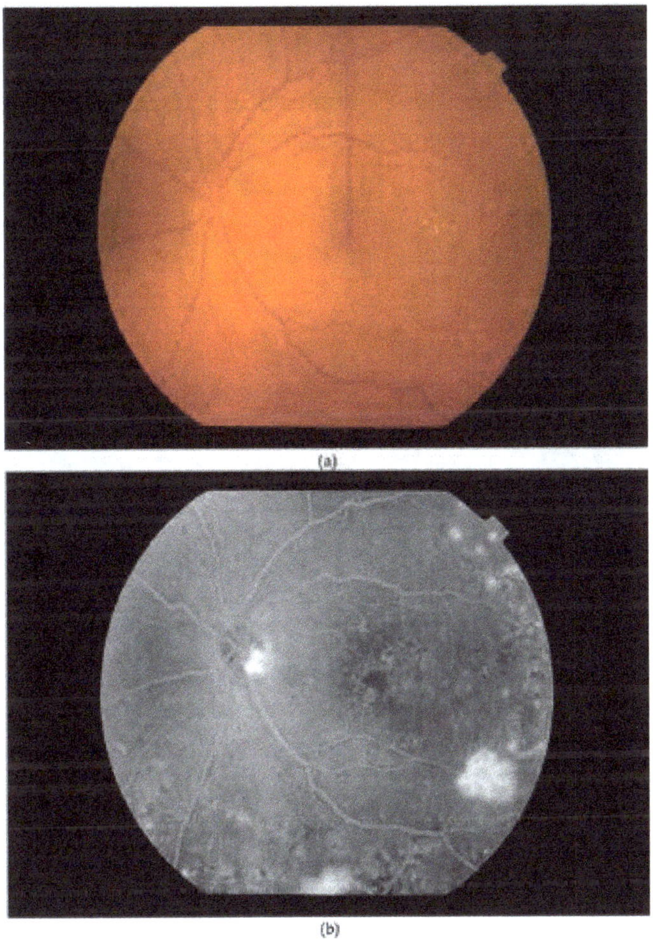

Figure 7. a. Fundus Photograph of New Vessels Elsewhere (NVE). **b.** Fundus Fluorescein Angiogram of New Vessels Elsewhere (NVE)

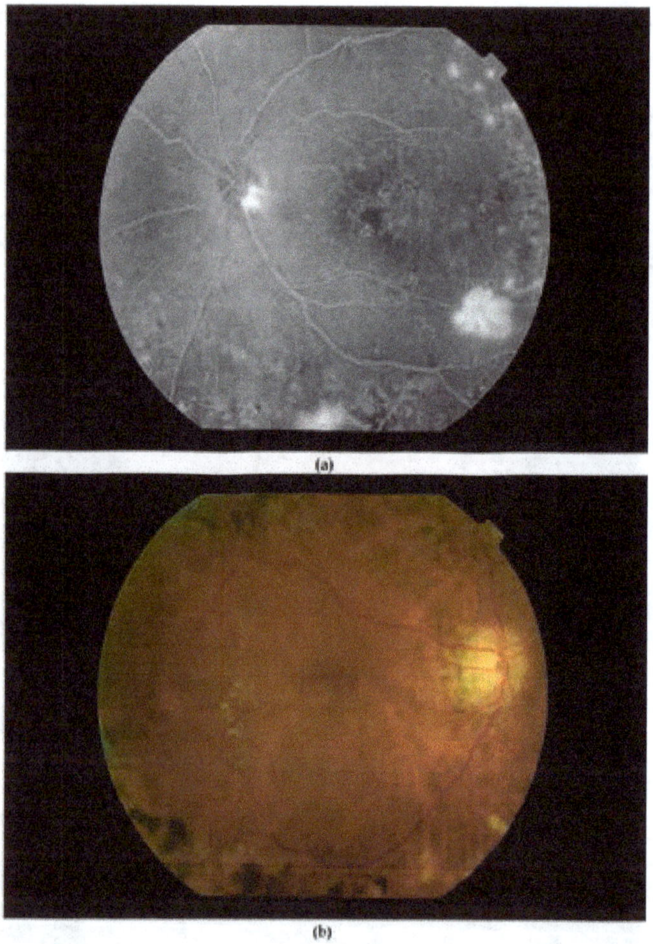

Figure 8. a. Fundus Photograph demonstrating PRP laser burns **b.** Fundus Fluorescein Angiogram of the above patient showing laser scars

8. Management of diabetic retinopathy

The management of diabetic retinopathy involves a multidisciplinary approach with involvement of the ophthalmologist, physician and dietician. The underlying diabetes and risk factors should be managed concurrently with the ocular complications of diabetes.

8.1. Medical management

8.1.1. Blood glucose control

Tight glycaemic control reduces the incidence and progression of diabetic retinopathy. The Diabetes Control and Complications Trial (DCCT)[131] showed that in type 1 diabetics effective glycaemic control reduced the incidence of diabetic retinopathy by 76% and progression of diabetic retinopathy by 54%. Similarly the United Kingdom Prospective Diabetes Study (UKPDS)[132] reported reduced microvascular complication, by 25% and the need for laser photocoagulation by 29% in type 2 diabetics.

8.1.2. Blood pressure control

The current British Hypertension Society guidelines define hypertension as systolic blood pressure ≥ 140mmHg and/ or diastolic blood pressure ≥ to 90mmHg [133]. In diabetes treatment targets should be systolic level <130 mm Hg and diastolic <80 mm Hg. Lower levels may be required for younger patients with Type 1 diabetes and microvascular complications. In this group of patients treatment with ACE inhibitors resulted in a 50% reduction in the progression of retinopathy and progression to proliferative diabetic retinopathy by 80% in the EURODIAB Controlled Trial of Lisinopril in Insulin Dependent Diabetes Mellitus (EUCLID) trial [134]. Type 2 diabetics in the UKPDS study showed that tight BP control prevented the progression of retinopathy. The beneficial effects of anti-hypertensive medication are immediate on commencing treatment, however the effects wear off as soon as control is lost. It is imperative therefore that blood pressure is measured at every clinical visit.

8.1.3. Lipid control

Observational studies suggest that dyslipideamia increases the risk of diabetic retinopathy particularly diabetic macula oedema[135, 136].

In the Fenofibrate Intervention and Event Lowering in Diabetes (FIELD) study [137], type 2 diabetic patients were treated with fenofibrate. Those patients treated with fenofibrate were less likely than controls to need laser treatment (5.2% vs 3.6%, $p<0.001$).

8.1.4. Cigarette smoking

In type 1 diabetes smoking increases the risk of diabetic retinopathy, nephropathy and neuropathy. Discontinuation of smoking is recommended for reducing the development of other complications of diabetes especially cardiovascular disease.

8.1.5. Management of macula oedema

Diabetic macula oedema is the most common cause for visual impairment particularly in type 2 diabetic patients. The management of clinically significant macula oedema depends on whether there is evidence of central macular thickening or vitreomacular traction. There are a wide variety of new treatments available currently some licensed and some unlicensed. A summary guideline as to the use of these treatments and their indications are summarized in Table 3.

Is the centre involved?	Visual Acuity	Phakic/ Pseudophakic	OCT- central retinal thickness	Treatment options
No		Either		Focal/Grid laser
Yes	Normal or "/>78 letters	Either		Focal/Grid laser/Observation if lesions too close to fovea
Yes	78-24 letters or symptomatic	Phakic	≥ 250 microns	Intravitreal anti- VEGF with or without laser. If unresponsive consider flucinolone implant.
Yes	78-24 letters	Pseudophakic	≥250 microns	Intravitreal anti- VEGF or intravitreal triamcinolone preservative free with or without laser. If unresponsive consider flucinolone implant.
Yes	<24 letters	Pseudophakic	≥250 microns	Observation especially if long standing or unrepsonsive to laser. Consider macula ischaemia. Otherwise consider anti-VEGF or intravitreal steroid
Yes		Either	Vitreomacular traction	Consider vitrectomy with or without adjunctive intravitreal anti-VEGF or steroid treatment

Management of diabetic maculopathy. Adapted from Royal College of Ophthalmologists. Diabetic Retinopathy Guidelines December 2012 (19)

Table 3. Table for management of CMO in Royal College of Ophthalmology

8.1.6. Laser photocoagulation

There is a strong evidence from the Early treatment of Diabetic retinopathy Study that focal and grid laser photocoagulation for clinically significant macula oedema reduces the chance of moderate vision loss (3 ETDRS lines) by 50%, (from 24% for the control group to 12% for the treatment group) at 3 years [19].

It is important to perform a fundus fluorescein angiography prior to treatment to delineate the area of leakage and identify areas of macula ischaemia. In focal maculopathy, focal laser treatment burns are applied directly to microaneurysms and and microvascular lesions in the centre of rings of exudates located 500-3000 microns from the centre of the macula. The spot size is 50-100 microns and exposure time 0.1 second with sufficient power to obtain gentle whitening or darkening of the microaneurysm. In macula grid laser treatment burns are applied to areas of diffuse retinal thickening more than 500 microns from the centre of the macula and 500 microns from the temporal margin of the optic disc. The spot size is 100 microns and exposure time 0.1 sec giving a very light intensity burn. Treatment should be lighter if significant macular ischaemia is present.

In addition to argon laser treatment two other forms of laser treatment frequency-doubled Nd:YAG laser and micropulse laser are available for the treatment of macula oedema which reduce the degree of retinal collateral thermal damage. The 'Pattern Scan Laser' (Pascal) uses frequency –doubled micropulse YAG in single shot mode or in a predetermined array of upto 56 shots applied in less than a second. This not only reduces the potential destructive retinal effect but allows the operator to apply multiple spots simultaneously with a single foot pedal depression.

Using a micropulse mode laser, energy is delivered with a train of repetitive short pulses, micropulse power as low as 10%-25% of the visible threshold power has been demonstrated to be sufficient to show RPE-confined photothermal effect.

8.1.7. Intravitreal anti-vascular endothelial growth factors (anti-VEGF) agents

Multiple studies have demonstrated the benefit of the anti-VEGF agents including pegaptanib, ranibizumab and bevacizumab for the treatment of central involving diabetic macula oedema. A large multicenter trial DRCRnet(The Diabetic Retinopathy Research Network Laser-Ranibizumab-Triamcinolone Study)[138] showed that intravitreal injection of 0.5mg ranibizumab initially given monthly for 3 months with prompt or deferred (≥ 24 weeks) macular laser had significantly superior visual and OCT outcomes to laser alone in eyes with diabetic macula oedema involving the fovea.

The READ-2 (Ranibizumab for oedema of macula in diabetes) [139], RESOLVE (Safety and Efficacy of Ranibizumab in diabetic macula oedema) [140], RESTORE (Ranibizumab monotherapy or combined with laser versus laser monotherapy for diabetic macula oedema) [141], and BOLT (Bevacizumab or Laser therapy)[142] studies have all demonstrated that centre-involving macula oedema should be considered for treatment with a VEGF inhibitor alone or in conjunction with focal laser.

Ranibizumab is now licensed for use in the European Union for the treatment of centre involving diabetic macula oedema and NICE have approved its use in patients with a central retinal thickness of ≥ 400 microns on OCT.

The Da VINCI trial (14) evaluated the safety and efficacy of intravitreal aflibercept for diabetic macula oedema. Four treatment regimes were studied versus laser positive results have been reported at 1 year with aflibercept. The maximum letters gain with aflibercept has been 13.1 letters vs 1.3 letters in the laser treated group. It is expected that this treatment will be licensed for Diabetic retinopathy in 2014.

8.1.8. Intraocular steroid

DRCRnet[138] study found that in pseudophakic eyes intravitreal triamcinolone injection followed by prompt laser may be as effective as ranibizumab at improving vision and reducing retinal thickening. However, there was a significant risk of an elevation of intraocular pressure. No corresponding visual benefit above laser was shown for phakic eyes, which also has had a substantially increased rate of cataract surgery by two years.

Flucinolone acetonide is a non-biodegradable intravitreal insert (Illuvein) with sustained release flucinolone and is licensed for use in the UK for chronic diabetic macula oedema unresponsive to other treatment options but it is not yet approved by NICE. Studies have shown that Illuvein can provide treatment benefit for three years-the best corrected visual acuity showed an improvement of 15 or more letters in 28.7% of the low dose group vs 16.2% in controls[144]. The longer acting nature is advantageous in that the patient would not require monthly injections as is the case with the anti-VEGFs. However there is a greater chance of development of cataract and raised intraocular pressure.

8.1.9. Pars plana vitrectomy

A vitrectomy with or without ILM peel may be indicated when macular oedema with or without ischaemia is associated with tangential traction from a thickened and taut posterior hyaloid. Often the oedema is unresponsive to laser and optical coherence tomography scanning may show vitreomacular traction.

8.2. Management of Proliferative Diabetic Retinopathy (PDR)

8.2.1. Pan retinal photocoagulation

This is indicated in the presence of new vessels at the optic disc, iris, angle or elsewhere with or without associated vitreous haemorrhage. Where possible PRP laser treatment should be initiated on the same day and maximum within 2 weeks.

PRP laser treatment should be applied as far peripheral as possible using the laser contact lens up to the ora serrata as the main areas of retinal ischaemia exist in the far peripheral retina. The laser settings depend on the type of lens that is used. With a Goldmann lens the spot size is set at 200-500 microns but with a panfundsocopic-type lens it is set at 100-300 microns. The burn duration should be set between 0.05-0.1 seconds and the power should be sufficient to produce only a light intensity burn.

Initial treatment involves 1500-2000 burns in a scatter pattern extending from the posterior fundus to cover the peripheral retina in one or more sessions. PRP completed in one session carries a higher risk of complications and therefore treatment should be staggered. The number of burns recommended is dependent on the stage of PDR ; early PDR 1200-1800 burns, in moderate PDR 2000-2500 burns and in severe PDR 3000 burns.

The Diabetic Retinopathy Study[145] found that the risk of severe visual loss (5/200) was reduced by 50% in the "high-risk" group treated with PRP. Patients with early proliferative diabetic retinopathy were evaluated in the ETDRS study. In this group PRP decreased the risk of patients developing high risk characteristics by 50%.

The main side effects of PRP laser treatment is the progression or development of diabetic macula oedema, vitreous haemorrhage, tractional retinal detachment, loss of night vision and constricted peripheral visual fields. Vision loss within 6 weeks of treatment has also been reported in 10-23% of patients compared with 6 % of controls.

8.2.2. VEGF inhibitors

VEGF is implicated in the development of retinal neovascularization. Intravitreal anti-VEGF is likely to have an increasing role in the treatment of proliferative diabetic retinopathy, probably as an adjunct to laser. Anti-VEGFS can also be used in the setting of proliferative diabetic retinopathy and vitreous haemorrhage to facilitate sufficient clearing of the haemorrhage and allow administration of PRP.

8.2.3. Vitrectomy

Indications for pars plana vitrectomy are listed below:

1. Severe persistent vitreous haemorrhage

The surgical goal is to remove the vitreous opacity through a 3 port pars plana vitrectomy. The posterior hyaloid face should be removed as this provides a scaffold for fibrovascular proliferation. The Diabetic Retinopathy Vitrectomy Study (DRVS)[146] 2 year results demonstrate that in eyes with central vitreous haemorrhage that reduced acuity to 50/200 or less for at least a month, vitrectomy carried out before 6 months resulted in an increase in the number of eyes achieving 20/40 or better acuity compared with eyes in which vitrectomy was deferred to a year. Patients with vitreous haemorrhage should be monitored weekly to ensure early detection of retinal detachment.

Type 2 diabetics are less likely to have severe proliferative retinopathy, however there is a growing trend to operate within 3 months as opposed to deferred surgery in both type 1 and type 2 diabetics.

2. Tractional retinal detachment

Tractional retinal detachment recently involving or imminently threatening the fovea is another common indication for surgery. Progressive traction produces a retinal break usually posterior to the equator and near an area of fibrous proliferation. These detachments progress quickly and usually result in a worse prognosis. Fibrovascular tissue proliferation and contraction attached to multiple retinal foci results in macular distortion (heterotropia) or tractional detachment.

3. Combined tractional/rhegmatogenous retinal detachments

These should be treated urgently even if the macula is not involved as subretinal fluid is likely to spread quickly and involve the macula.

4. Premacular subhyaloid haemorrhage

If dense and persistent should be considered for vitrectomy because if untreated the internal limiting membrane or posterior hyaloid face may serve as a scaffold for subsequent fibrovascular proliferation and consequent tractional macular detachment or macular epiretinal membrane formation.

5. Ghost Cell Glaucoma

Vitrectomy has also been shown in case series to be of benefit when there is ghost cell glaucoma [147]. Raised intraocular pressure may be caused by partially lysed red cells (erthyroclasts) particularly in eyes with a disrupted anterior hyaloid face after previous vitrectomy for vitreous haemorrhage or in aphakic eyes with vitreous haemorrhage.

8.2.4. Management of Rubeosis Iridis

This occurs in eyes with severe retinal ischaemia or persistent retinal detachment. New vessels on the iris should be treated with PRP laser to induce regression of these vessels.

Current practice for new vessels on the iris and at the angle includes full PRP and an intravitreal anti-VEGF injection to prevent the progression to neovascular glaucoma. Treatment for neovascular glaucoma include cycloablative procedures, trabeculectomy with anti-proliferatives and implantation of a drainage tube.

Eyes that have become blind from neovascular glaucoma should be kept comfortable with topical steroids and atropine.

9. Conclusion

The global pandemic of diabetes means that retinopathy and associated visual difficulties are an ongoing problem. Further research is needed into the impact of diabetes on the neurovascular unit to facilitate greater understanding of pathophysiology. Improved screening and outcomes of treatment in developed countries mean vision can be maintained for longer. Ideally however, socioeconomic barriers need to be overcome to facilitate translational research to all parts of the world, including poorer areas. Most importantly, education on risk factors and tight glycaemic control are paramount to help prevent visual problems occurring.

Author details

Vikas Tah[1,3], Sonia Mall[2], James Myerscough[4], Kamran Saha[3], Elizabeth Emsley[5], Andrew Swampillai[6], Ganeshan Ramsamy[1], Daren Hanumunthadu[3] and Mandeep Bindra[1]

1 Stoke Mandeville Hospital, UK

2 Oxford Eye Hospital, UK

3 Moorfields Eye Hospital, UK

4 Colchester Hospital University Foundation Trust, UK

5 Imperial College London, UK

6 Barts and The London, School of Medicine and Dentistry, UK

References

[1] Diabetes in the UK 2010: Key statistics on diabetes. Diabetes UK. 2010.

[2] American Diabetes Association. Diabetes Basics. Available from: http://www.diabetes.org/diabetes-basics/diabetes-statistics/ (accessed 27th July 2013)

[3] Quality and Outcomes Framework (QOF) 2009:England: http://www.ic.nhs.uk/statistics-and-data-collections/supporting-information/audits-andperformance/the-quality-and-outcomes-framework/qof-2008/09/data-tables/prevalence-data-tablesScotland:http://www.isdscotland.org/isd/servlet/FileBuffer?namedFile=QOF_Scot_200809_Boards_all_prevalence.xls&pContentDisposition-Type=attachment

[4] Figures based on PBS diabetes prevalence model phase 3: key findings, Yorkshire and Humber Public Health Observatory, May 2008. The PBS model estimates that by 2025 there will be 3.6 million people with diabetes in England and that the diabetes prevalence will be 6.48 per cent of the population in England. The total UK figures have been calculated by including forecasts for the population of Wales, Scotland and Northern Ireland which gives a total of 4.2 million people with diabetes by 2025.

[5] Figures based on PBS diabetes prevalence model phase 3: key findings, Yorkshire and Humber Public Health Observatory, May 2008. The PBS model estimates that by 2025 there will be 3.6 million people with diabetes in England and that the diabetes prevalence will be 6.48 per cent of the population in England. The total UK figures have been calculated by including forecasts for the population of Wales, Scotland and Northern Ireland which gives a total of 4.2 million people with diabetes by 2025.

[6] Department of Health (2007). About diabetes www.dh.gov.uk/en/Healthcare/NationalServiceFrameworks/Diabetes/DH_074762

[7] Stratton IM, Adler AI, Neil HAW et al (2000). Association of glycaemia with macrovascular and microvascular complications of Type 2 diabetes (UKPDS 35): prospective observational study. BMJ 321;405–412

[8] Stratton IM, Adler AI, Neil HAW et al (2000). Association of glycaemia with macrovascular and microvascular complications of Type 2 diabetes (UKPDS 35): prospective observational study. BMJ 321;405–412

[9] Harris MI, Klein R, Welborn TA et al (1992). Onset of NIDDM occurs at least 4-7 years before clinical diagnosis. Diabetes Care 15 (7); 815–819

[10] Stitt A, Lois N, Medina R, et al. Advances in our understanding of diabetic retinopathy. Clinical Science. 2013;125;1-17

[11] Hamilton AMP, Ulbig MW, Polkinghorne P (1996). Management of diabetic retinopathy, London:BMJ Publishing

[12] Williams R, Airey M, Baxter H. Epidemiology of diabetic retinopathy and macular oedema: A systematic review. Eye. 2004;18;963-83.

[13] Malone J, Morrison A, Pavan P, et al. Diabetic Control and Complications Trial: Prevalence and significance of retinopathy in subjects with type 1 diabetes of less than 5 years duration screened for the diabetes control and complications trial. Diabetes Care. 200;124;522-6.

[14] Kohner E, Aldington S, Stratton I. United Kingdom Prospective Diabetes Study, 30: Diabetic retinopathy at diagnosis of non-insulin-dependent diabetes mellitus and associated risk factors. Arch Ophthalmol. 1998;116;297-303.

[15] Klein R, Klein B, Moss S. Visual impairment in diabetes. Ophthalmology. 1984;91;1-9.

[16] Moss S, Klein R, Klein B. Ten-year incidence of visual loss in a diabetic population. Ophthalmology. 1994; 101(6); 1061-70.

[17] Forlenza G, Stewart M. Diabetic retinopathy in children. Pediatr Endocrinol Rev. 2012-13; 10(2);217-26.

[18] Photocoagulation treatment of proliferative diabetic retinopathy: the second report of Diabetic Retinopathy Study findings. Ophthalmology. 1978;85;82-105.

[19] Photocoagulation for diabetic macular oedema: Early Treatment Diabetic Retinopathy Study report number 1. Arch Ophthalmology. 1985;103;1796-806.

[20] Antonetti D, Klein R, Gardner T. Diabetic retinopathy. NEJM. 2012;366;1227-39.

[21] Klein R, Lee K, Gangnon R, et al. The 25-year incidence of visual impairment in type 1 diabetes mellitus: the Wisconsin Epidemiologic Study of Diabetic Retinopathy. Ophthalmology. 2010;117;63-70.

[22] Hovind P, Tarnow L, Rossing K, et al. Decreasing incidence of severe diabetic microangiopathy in type 1 diabetes. Diabetes care. 2003;26;1258-64.

[23] Nordwall M, Bojestig M, Arnqvist H, et al. Declining incidence of severe retinopathy and persisting decrease of nephropathy in an unselected population of Type 1 diabetes – the Linkoping Diabetes Complications Study. Diabetologia. 2004;47;1266-72.

[24] Kempen J, O'Colmain B, Leske M, et al. The prevalence of diabetic retinopathy among adults in the United States. Arch Ophthalmol. 2004;122;552-63.

[25] Sloan F, Belsky D, Ruiz D, et al. Changes in incidence of diabetes mellitus-related eye disease among US elderly persons 1994-2005. Arch Ophthalmol. 2008;126;1548-53.

[26] Klein R, Klein B. Are individuals with diabetes seeing better? A long term epidemiological perspective. Diabetes. 2010;59;1853-60.

[27] Wild S, Roglic G, Green A, et al. Global prevalence of diabetes: estimates for the year 2000 and projections for 2030. Diabetes Care. 2004;27;1047-53.

[28] Al-Rubeaan K. Type 2 diabetes mellitus red zone. Int J Diabetes Mellitus. 2010;2(1); 1-2.

[29] Rema M, Premkumar S, Anitha B, et al. Prevalence of diabetic retinopathy in urban India: the Chennai Urban Rural Epidemiology Study (CURES) eye study. Invest Ophthalmol Vis Sci. 2005;46;2328-33.

[30] Targher G, Bertolini L, Chonchol M, et al. Non-alcoholic fatty liver disease is independently associated with an increased prevalence of chronic kidney disease and retinopathy in type 1 diabetic patients. Diabetologia. 2010;53;1341-8.

[31] Nguyen T, Alibrahim E, Islam F, et al. Inflammatory, haemostatic and other novel biomarkers for diabetic retinopathy: the multi-ethnic study of atherosclerosis. Diabetes Care. 2009;32;1704-9.

[32] West S, Groves D, Lipinski H, et al. The prevalence of retinopathy in men with Type 2 diabetes and obstructive sleep apnoea. Diabet Med. 2010;27;423-30

[33] Arnold E, Rivera J, Thebault S, et al. High levels of serum prolactin protect against diabetic retinopathy by increasing ocular vasoinhibins. Diabetes. 2010;59;3192-7.

[34] Zietz B, Buechler C, Kobuch K, et al. Serum levels of adiponectin are associated with diabetic retinopathy and with adiponectin gene mutations in Caucasian patients with diabetes mellitus type 2. Exp Clin Endocrinol Diabetes. 2008;116;532-6.

[35] Nathan D, Zinman B, Cleary P et al. Modern day clinical course of type 1 diabetes mellitus after 30 years' duration: the Diabetes Control and Complications Trial/ Epidemiology of Diabetes Interventions and Complications and Pittsburgh Epidemiology of Diabetes Complications experience (1983-2005). Arch Intern Med. 2009;169; 1307-16.

[36] Matthews D, Stratton S, Aldington S, et al. Risks of progression of retinopathy and vision loss related to tight blood pressure control in type 2 diabetes mellitus: UKPDS 69. Archives of Ophthalmology. 2004; 122 (11); 1631-1640.

[37] White N, Cleary P, Dahms W, et al. Beneficial effects of intensive therapy of diabetes during adolescence: outcomes after the conclusion of the Diabetes Control and Complications Trial (DCCT). The Journal of Paediatrics. 139 (6); 804-812.

[38] Tarr J, Kaul K, Chopra M, et al. Pathophysiology of Diabetic Retinopathy. ISRN Ophthalmology. 2013;343560.

[39] Singh R, Ramasamy K, Abraham C, et al. Diabetic retinopathy: an update. Indian Journal of Ophthalmology. 2008;56(3);179-188.

[40] Gabbay K. Hyperglycaemia, polyol metabolism and complications of diabetes mellitus. Annual Review of Medicine. 1975;26;521-536.

[41] Gabbay K. The sorbitol pathway and the complications of diabetes. The New England Journal of Medicine. 1973;288(16);831-836.

[42] Szwergold B, Kappler F, Brown T. Identification of fructose 3-phosphate in the lens of diabetic rats. Science. 1990;247(4941);451-454.

[43] Barnett P, Gonzalez R, Chylack L, et al. The effect of oxidation on sorbitol pathway kinetics. Diabetes. 1986;35(4);426-432.

[44] Hohman T, Nishimura C, Robison E. Aldose reductase and polyol cultured pericytes of human retinal capillaries. Experimental Eye Research. 1989;48 (1);55-60.

[45] Chakrabarti S, Sima A, Nakajima T. Aldose reductase in the BB rat: isolation, immunological identification and localisation in the retina and peripheral nerve. Diabetologia. 1987;30(4);244-251.

[46] Cheung A, Fung M, Lo A, et al. Aldose reductase deficiency prevents diabetes-induced blood-retinal barrier breakdown, apoptosis and glial reactivation in the retina of db/db mice. Diabetes. 2005;54(11);3119-3125.

[47] Dagher Z, Park Y, Asnaghi V, et al. Studies of rat and human retinas predict a role for the polyol pathway in human diabetic retinopathy. Diabetes. 2004;53(9); 2404-2411.

[48] Kuwabara T, Cogan D. Retinal vascular patterns. VI. Mural cells of the retinal capillaries. Arch Ophthalmol. 1963; 69; 492-502.

[49] Roy S, Lorenzi M. Early biosynthetic changes in the diabetic-like retinopathy of galactose-fed rats. Diabetologia. 1996;39(6);735-738.

[50] Glover J, Jacot J, Basso M, et al. Retinal capillary dilation: early diabetic-like retinopathy in the galactose-fed rate model. Journal of Ocular Pharmacology and Therapeutics. 2000;16(2);167-172.

[51] 51. Hattori T, Matsubara A, Taniguchi K, et al. Aldose reductase inhibitor fidarestat attenuates leukocyte-endothelial interactions in experimental diabetic rat retina in vivo. Current Eye Research. 2010;35(2);146-154.

[52] Chung S, Chung S. Genetic analysis of aldose reductase in diabetic complications. Current Medicinal Chemistry. 2003;10(15);1375-1387.

[53] Hammes H, Martin S, Federlin K, et al. Aminoguanidine treatment inhibits the development of experimental diabetic retinopathy. Proceedings of the National Academy of Sciences of the United States of America. 1991;88(24);11555-11558.

[54] Peppa M, Uribarri J, Vlassara H. Advanced glycation end products and diabetes complications: what is new and what works. Clinical Diabetes. 2003;21(4)186-187.

[55] Zong H, Ward M, Stitt A. AGEs, RAGE and diabetic retinopathy. Current Diabetes Reports. 2011;11(4);244-252.

[56] Stitt A, Gardiner T, Anderson N, et al. The AGE inhibitor pyridoxamine inhibits development of retinopathy in experimental diabetes. Diabetes. 2002;51(9);2826-2832.

[57] Hammes H, Weiss A, Fuhrer D, et al. Acceleration of experimental diabetic retinopathy in the rat by omega-3 fatty acids. Diabetologia. 1996; 39(3); 251-255.

[58] Williamson J, Kilo C. Extracellular matrix changes in diabetes mellitus. In: Scarpelli D, Migahi D, editors. Comparative pathobiology of major age-related diseases. New York: Liss, 1984. Pp 269-88.

[59] Koya D, King G. Protein kinase C activation and the development of diabetic complications. Diabetes. 1998;47(6);859-866.

[60] Wang Q. PKD at the crossroads of DAG and PKC signaling. Trends in pharmacological sciences. 2006;27(6);317-323.

[61] Aiello L, Bursell S, Clermont A, et al. Vascular endothelial growth factor-induced retinal permeability is mediated by protein kinase C in vivo and suppressed by an orally effective beta-isoform-selective inhibitor. Diabetes. 1997;46(9);1473-1480.

[62] Aiello L, Clermont A, Arora V, et al. Inhibition of PKC beta by oral administration of ruboxistaurin is well tolerated and ameliorates diabetes-induced retinal haemodynamic abnormalities in patients. Investigative Ophthalmology and Visual Science.

[63] Joy S, Scates S, Bearelly S, et al. Ruboxistaurin, a protein kinase C Beta inhibitor, as an emerging treatment for diabetes microvascular complications. Annals of Pharmacotherapy. 2005;39(10);1693-1699.

[64] Clarke M, Dodson P. PKC inhibition and diabetic microvascular complications. Best practice and research: clinical endocrinology and metabolism. 2007;21(4);573-586.

[65] Kohner E. The retinal blood flow in diabetes. Diabete et Metabolisme. 1993;19(5); 401-404.

[66] Wilkinson-Berka J. Angiotensin and diabetic retinopathy. International Journal of Biochemistry and Cell Biology. 2006;38(5-6);757-765.

[67] Funatsu H, Yamashita H, Nakanishi Y, et al. Angiotensin II and vascular endothelial growth factor in the vitreous fluid of patients with proliferative diabetic retinopathy. British Journal of Ophthalmology. 2002;86(3);311-315.

[68] Sjolie A, Klein R, Porta M, et al. Effect of candesartan on progression and regression of retinopathy in type 2 diabetes (DIRECT-Protect 2): a randomised placebo-controlled trial. The Lancet. 2008;372(9647);1385-1393.

[69] Chaturvedi N, Porta M, Klein R, et al. Effect of candesartan on prevention (DIRECT-Prevent 1) and progression (DIRECT-Protect 1) of retinopathy in type 1 diabetes: randomised, placebo-controlled trials. The Lancet. 2008;372(9647);1394-1402.

[70] Mauer M, Ziman B, Gardiner R, et al. Renal and retinal effects of enalapril and losartan in type 1 diabetes. The New England Journal of Medicine. 2009;361(1);40-51.

[71] Otani A, Takagi H, Suzuma K,et al. Angiotensin II potentiates vascular endothelial growth-factor induced angiogenic activity in retinal microcapillary endothelial cells. Circulation Research. 1998;82(5);619-628.

[72] Schroder S, Palinksi W, Schmid-Schonbein G. Activated monocytes and granulocytes, capillary nonperfusion and neovascularization in diabetic retinopathy. American Journal of Pathology.

[73] Lutty G, Cao J, McLeod D. Relationship of polymorphonuclear leukocytes to capillary dropout in the human diabetic choroid. American Journal of Pathology. 1997; 151(3);707-714.

[74] Chibber R, Ben-Mahmud M, Coppini D, et al. Activity of the glycosylating enzyme, core 2 GlcNAc (Beta1,6) transferase, is higher in polymorphonuclear leukocytes from diabetic patients compared with age-matched control subjects: relevance to capillary occlusion in diabetic retinopathy. Diabetes. 2000;49(10);1724-1730.

[75] Chibber R, Ben-Mahmud B, Mann G, et al. Protein kinase C Beta2-dependent phosphorylation of core 2 GlcNAc-T promotes leukocyte-endothelial cell adhesion: a mechanism underlying capillary occlusion in diabetic retinopathy. Diabetes. 2003;52(6);1519-1527.

[76] Kaul K, Hodgkinson A, Tarr J, et al. Is inflammation a common retinal-renal-nerve pathogenic link in diabetes? Current Diabetes Reviews. 2010;6(5);294-303.

[77] Hernandez C, Segura R, Fonollosa A, et al. Interleukin-8, monocyte chemoattractant protein01 and IL-10 in the vitreous fluid of patients with proliferative diabetic retinopathy. Diabetic Medicine. 2005;22(6);719-225.

[78] Doganay S, Evereklioglu C, Er H, et al. Comparison of serum NO, TNF-alpha, IL-1beta, SIL-2R, IL-6 and IL-8 levels with grades of retinopathy in patients with diabetes mellitus. Eye. 2002; 16(2);163-170.

[79] Takami S, Yamashita S, Kihara S, et al. High concentration of glucose induces the expression of intercellular adhesion molecule-1 in human umbilical vein endothelial cells. Atherosclerosis. 1998;138(1);35-41.

[80] Larson E, Springer T. Structure and function of leukocyte integrins. Immunological Reviews. 1990;114;181-217.

[81] Sfikakis P, Grigoropoulos V, Emfietzoglou I, et al. Infliximab for diabetic macular edema refractory to laser photocoagulation: a randomized, double-blind, placebo-controlled, crossover, 32-week study. Diabetes Care. 2010;33(7);1523-1528.

[82] Baynes J. Role of oxidative stress in development of complications in diabetes. Diabetes. 1991;40(4);405-412.

[83] Cui Y, Xu X, Bi H, et al. Expression modification of uncoupling proteins and MnSOD in retinal endothelial cells and pericytes induced by high glucose: the role of reactive oxygen species in diabetic retinopathy. Experimental Eye Research. 2006; 83(4); 807-816.

[84] Kowluru R, Chan P. Oxidative stress and diabetic retinopathy. Experimental Diabesity Research. 2007;43603.

[85] 85. El-Remessy A, Bartoli M, Platt D, et al. Oxidative stress inactivates VEGF survival signaling in retinal endothelial cells via PI 3-kinase tyrosine nitration. Journal of Cell Science. 2005;118(1);243-252.

[86] Hartnett M, Stratton R, Browne R, et al. Serum markers of oxidative stress and severity of diabetic retinopathy. Diabetes Care. 2000;23(2);234-240.

[87] Brownlee M. The pathobiology of diabetic complications: a unifying mechanism. Diabetes. 2005;54(6);1615-1625.

[88] Grant M, Mames R, Fitzgerald C, et al. The efficacy of octreotide in the therapy of severe nonproliferative and early proliferative diabetic retinopathy: a randomised controlled study. Diabetes Care. 2000;23(4);504-509.

[89] Zimmerman B, Molnar G. Prolonged follow up in diabetic retinopathy treated by sectioning the pituitary stalk. Mayo Clinic Proceedings. 1977;52(4);233-237.

[90] Comer G, Ciulla T. Pharmacotherapy for diabetic retinopathy. Current Opinion in Ophthalmology. 2004;15(6);508-518.

[91] Ishida S, Usui T, Yamashiro K, et al. VEGF164 is proinflammatory in the diabetic retina. Investigative Ophthalmology and Visual Science. 2003;44(5);2155-2162.

[92] Zhang X, Wen L, Chen Y et al. Vascular endothelial growth factor upregulates the expression of intracellular adhesion molecule-1 in retinal endothelial cells via reac-

tive oxygen species, but not nitric oxide. Chinese Medical Journal. 2009;122(3); 338-343.

[93] Adamis A, Shima D, Yeo K, et al. Synthesis and secretion of vascular permeability factor/vascular endothelial growth factor by human retinal pigment epithelial cells. Biochemical and Biophysical Research Communications. 1993;193(2);631-638.

[94] Wirostko B, Wong T,Simo R. Vascular endothelial growth factor and diabetic complications. Progress in Retinal and Eye Research. 2008;27(6);608-621.

[95] Gao B, Clermont A, Rook S, et al. Extracellular carbonic anhydrase mediates haemorrhagic retinal and cerebral vascular permeability through prekallikrein activation. 2007;13(2);181-188.

[96] Weiwei Z, Hu R. Targeting carbonic anhydrase to treat diabetic retinopathy: emerging evidences and encouraging results. Biochemical and Biophysical Research Communications. 2009;390(3);368-371.

[97] Park S, Park J, Park S, et al. Apoptotic death of photoreceptors in the streptozotocin-induced diabetic rat retina. Diabetologia. 2003;46(9);1260-1268.

[98] West SD, Groves DC, Lipinski HJ, et al. The prevalence of retinopathy in men with Type 2 diabetes and obstructive sleep apnoea. Diabet Med 2010;27:423-430

[99] Tong Z, Yang Z, Patel S, et al. Promoter polymorphism of the erythropoietin gene in severe diabetic eye and kidney complications. Proc Natl Acad Sci U S A 2008;105:6998-7003

[100] Klein R, Klein BE, Moss SE, Davis MD, DeMets DL. The Wisconsin epidemiologic study of diabetic retinopathy. II. Prevalence and risk of diabetic retinopathy when age at diagnosis is less than 30 years. Arch. Ophthalmol 1984; 102(4), 520–526

[101] Roy MS. Diabetic retinopathy in African Americans with type 1 diabetes: The New Jersey 725: I. Methodology, population, frequency of retinopathy, and visual impairment. Arch Ophthalmol 2000;118:97–104

[102] Klein R, Klein BE, Moss SE, Davis MD, DeMets DL. The Wisconsin epidemiologic study of diabetic retinopathy. III.

[103] Harvey JN. The influence of sex and puberty on the progression of diabetic nephropathy and retinopathy. *Diabetologia* 2011;54(8), 1943–1945

[104] Klein BE, Moss SE, Klein R. Is menarche associated with diabetic retinopathy? *Diabetes Care 1990*; 13(10), 1034–1038

[105] EDIC research group. Retinopathy and nephropathy in type 1 diabetes patients four years after trial of intensive therapy. N Engl J Med. 2000;342:381–9

[106] The Diabetes Control and Complications Trial Research Group. The effect of intensive treatment of diabetes on the development and progression of long-term complications in insulin-dependent diabetes mellitus. N Engl J Med. 1993;329:977–86

[107] Hirsch IB, Brownlee M. Beyond hemoglobin A1c — need for additional markers of risk for diabetic microvascular complications. JAMA 2010;303:2291-2

[108] Kern PA. Lipid disorders in diabetes mellitus. Mt Sinai J Med 1987-54: 245-252.

[109] Ferris III FL, Chew KY, Hoogwerf HJ. Serum lipids and diabetic retinopathy. Early treatment diabetic retinopathy study research group. Diabetes Care 1996; 19: 1291

[110] Chew EY. Diabetic retinopathy and lipid abnormalities. Curr Opin Ophtthal. 1997; 8: 59-62

[111] Hypertension in Diabetes Study (HDS). II. Increased risk of cardiovascular complications in hypertensive type 2 diabetic patients. J Hypertens 1993;11:319-25

[112] Patel V, Rassam S, Newsom R, Wiek J, Kohner EM. Retinal blood flow in diabetic retinopathy. BMJ. 1992;305678-683

[113] Rassam SMB, Patel V, Kohner EM. The effect of experimental hypertension on retinal autoregulation in humans: a mechanism for the progression of diabetic retinopathy. Exp Physiol. 1995;8053-68

[114] Hogeboom van Buggenum IM, Polak BC, Reichert-Thoen JW, et al. Angiotensin converting enzyme inhibiting therapy is associated with lower vitreous vascular endothelial growth factor concentrations in patients with proliferative diabetic retinopathy. Diabetologia. 2002;45:203-209

[115] UK Prospective Diabetes Study Group: Efficacy of atenolol and captopril in reducing risk of macrovascular and microvascular complications in Type 2 diabetes. UKPDS 39. Br Med J 1998;317:713-20.

[116] The Diabetes Control, Complications Trial Research Group. Effect of pregnancy on microvascular complications in the Diabetes Control and Complications Trial. Diabetes Care 2000; 23: 1084–1091

[117] Klein BE, Moss SE, Klein R. Effect of pregnancy on progression of diabetic retinopathy. Diabetes Care 1990; 13: 34–40

[118] Axer-Siegel R, Hod M, Fink-Cohen S, Kramer M, Weinberger D, Schindel B, Yassur Y. Diabetic retinopathy during pregnancy. Ophthalmology 1996; 103(11): 1815-1819

[119] Phelps RL, Sakol P, Metzger BE, Jampol LM, Frienkel N. Changes in diabetic retinopathy during pregnancy. Correlations with regulation of hyperglycaemia. Arch Ophthalmol 1986; 104: 1806–1810

[120] Diabetes in Early Pregnancy Study. Metabolic control and progression of retinopathy. Diabetes Care 1995; 18: 631–637

[121] Chew EY, Mills JL, Metzger BE, Remaley NA, Jovanovich-Peterson L, Knopp RH. Metabolic control and the progression of retinopathy. The diabetes in Early Pregnancy Study. Diabetes Care 1995; 18: 631–637

[122] Harding, S., R. Greenwood, S. Aldington, J. Gibson, D. Owens, R. Taylor, E. Kohner, P. Scanlon, and G. Leese. 2003. Grading and disease management in national screening for diabetic retinopathy in England and Wales. Diabet Med 20:965.

[123] Diabetic Retinopathy Study Research Group. Report 7. A modification of the Airlie House classification of diabetic retinopathy. Invest Ophthalmol Vis Sci 1981;21:210–26.

[124] Wilkinson, C. P., F. L. Ferris, 3rd, R. E. Klein, P. P. Lee, C. D. Agardh, M. Davis, D. Dills, A. Kampik, R. Pararajasegaram, and J. T. Verdaguer. 2003. Proposed international clinical diabetic retinopathy and diabetic macular edema disease severity scales. Ophthalmology 110:1677.

[125] Grading diabetic retinopathy from stereoscopic colour fundus photographs--an extension of the modified Airlie House classification. ETDRS report number 10. Early Treatment Diabetic Retinopathy Study Research Group. Ophthalmology 1991. 98:786.

[126] The Diabetes Control and Complications Trial Research Group (1997) Clustering of long-term complications in families with diabetes in the diabetes control and complications trial. The Diabetes Control and Complications Trial Research Group. Diabetes 46: 1829–1839.

[127] Chew, E., Klein, M., Ferris, F., III, Remaley, N., Murphy, R., Chantry, K. et al. (1996) Association of elevated serum lipid levels with retinal hard exudate in diabetic retinopathy. early treatment diabetic retinopathy study (ETDRS) report 22. Arch Ophthalmol 114: 1079–1084

[128] Keech, A., Mitchell, P., Summanen, P., O'Day, J., Davis, T., Moffitt, M. et al. (2007) Effect of fenofibrate on the need for laser treatment for diabetic retinopathy (FIELD study): a randomised controlled trial. Lancet 370: 1687–1697

[129] Gaede, P., Lund-Andersen, H., Parving, H. and Pedersen, O. (2008) Effect of a multifactorial intervention on mortality in type 2 diabetes. N Engl J Med 358: 580–591.

[130] Images courtesy of Mr Jignesh Patel, Essex County Hospital, Colchester.

[131] Diabetes Control and Complications Trial/Epidemiology of Diabetes Interventions and Complications Research Group. Retinopathy and nephropathy in patients with type 1 diabetes mellitus four years after a trial of intensive therapy. N Eng J Med. 2000;342:381-9

[132] UK Prospective Diabetes Study (UKPDS) Group. Intensive blood-glucose control with sulphonylureas or insulin compared with conventional treatment and risk of complications in patients with type 2 diabetes (UKPDS 33). Lancet.1998;352:837-53.

[133] Guidelines from the British Hypertensive Society. BMJ. 2004;328:593-4.

[134] Chaturvedi N, Sjolie AK, Stephenson JM et al; EUCLID Study Group. Effect of lisinopril on progression of retinopathy in normotensive people with type 1 diabetes. Lancet. 1998;351 (9095):28-31

[135] Van Leiden HA, Dekker HA, Moll AC, et al. Blood pressure, lipids, and obesity are associated with retinopathy: the Hoorn study. Diabetes Care. 2002;25:1320-5.

[136] Klein R, Sharrett AR, Klein BE, et al. The association of atherosclerosis, vascular risk factors, and retinopathy in adults with diabetes: the atherosclerosis risk in communities study. Ophthalmology.2002;109:1225-34

[137] Keech A, Simes RJ, Barter P, et al. Effects of long term fenofibrate therapy on cardiovascular events in 9795 people with type 2 diabetes mellitus (the FIELD study): randomized controlled trial. Lancet. 2005; 366:1849-61

[138] Diabetic Retinopathy Clinical Research Network. A randomized trial comparing intravitreal triamcinolone acetonide and focal/grid photocoagulation for diabetic macular oedema. Ophthalmology. 2008;115:1447-59.

[139] Nguyen QD, Shah SM, Khwaja AA, et al. Two year outcomes of ranibizumab for oedema of the macula in diabetes (READ-2) study. Ophthalmology. 2010;117:2146-51.

[140] Massin P, Bandello F, Garweg JG, et al. Safety and efficacy of ranibizumab in diabetic macula oedema (RESOLVE Study): a 12 month, randomized, controlled, double-masked multicenter phase II study. Diabetes Care. 2010;33:2399-405.

[141] Mitchell P, Bandello F, Schmidt-Erfurth U et al. The RESTORE study: ranibizumab monotherapy or combined with laser versus laser monotherapy for diabetic macular edema. Ophthalmology. 2011;118:615-25.

[142] Michaelides M, Kaines A, Hamilton RD, Fraser-Bell S, et al. A prospective randomized trial of intravitreal bevacizumab or laser therapy in the management of diabetic macula edema (BOLT study) 12-month data: report 2. Ophthalmology. 2010;117:1078-86.

[143] Do DV, Nguyen QD, Boyer D, Schmidt-Erfurth U, Brown DM, Vitti R, Berliner AJ, Gao B, Zeitz O, Ruckert R, Schmelter T, Sandbrink R, Heier JS; DAVINCI Study Group. One-Year Outcomes of the DA VINCI Study Group of VEGF Trap-Eye in Eyes with Diabetic Macula Edema. Ophthalmology 2012. April 24 epub ahead of print.

[144] Campochiaro PA, Brown DM, Pearson A, et al. FAME Study Group Susutained Delivery Fluocinolone Acetonide Vitreous Inserts Provide Benefit for at Least 3 years in Patients with Diabetic Macula Edema, Ophthalmology 2012 Jun 21 (epub ahead of print)

[145] The Diabetic Retinopathy Research Group. Indications for photocoagulation treatment of diabetic retinopathy: Diabetic Retinopathy Study No.14 Int Ophthal Clin 1987;27:239-252.

[146] Diabetic Retinopathy Vitrectomy Study Research Group. Early Vitrectomy for severe vitreous haemorrhage in diabetic retinopathy. Two year results of a randomized trial. DRVS report No 2. Archives of Ophthalmology. 1985103:1644

[147] Brucker AJ, Michels RG, Green WR. Pars plana vitrectomy in the management of blood-induced glaucoma with vitreous haemorrhage. Ann Ophthalmol. 1978;10:1427-37

[148] Royal College of Ophthalmologists. Diabetic Retinopathy Guidelines December 2012 http://www.rcophth.ac.uk/page.asp?section=451&sectionTitle=Clinical+Guidelines

5

Low Vision Rehabilitation

Bennett McAllister and Rebecca Kammer

1. Introduction

Low vision rehabilitation has developed along two approaches based on either the education/ vocational system or the medical model. In 1999, Massof and Lidoff [1] reviewed the issues in vision rehabilitation from a public policy, service delivery, and funding perspective. They delineate the evolution of services for persons with visual impairment as primarily originating within the education and vocational rehabilitation systems. The end goals from these perspectives would be educational achievement or vocational training and placement. Simultaneously, though, a medical model of low vision rehabilitation also existed within the United States' Veteran's Administration as it historically has provided military veterans comprehensive, in-patient rehabilitation services including visual aids or adaptive devices, instruction in living skills, communication, orientation & mobility (O&M) and more. The objective of the medical model of low vision rehabilitation is to restore function for improveddaily living skills. Although the strategies for rehabilitation within the education model and the medical model may be similar, the framework of this chapter is primarily based on principles of the medical model while borrowing valuable insight from the educational model.

Outside of the Veterans Administration but within health care professionals, some version of low vision rehabilitation has developed over the last several decades from a specialty or area of emphasis practiced by a few scattered experts in optometry, ophthalmology, and most recently nursing and occupational therapy. Entry-level skills in low vision rehabilitation have become a required competency for all optometry graduates [2]. It is also a requirement of all U.S. ophthalmology residencies to expose students to low vision rehabilitation.. Even so, low vision rehabilitation remains a field that is difficult to define precisely in that it still faces barriers within reimbursement structures and funding mechanisms [1].

In 2006, some progress in funding models was made as rehabilitation codes were designated by Medicare as applicable to vision rehabilitation. Occupational therapists with their training in aging and activities of daily living began offering low vision rehabilitation under the order or referral of a physician. Under Medicare definitions, this physician role in most cases is fulfilled by the low vision optometrist or ophthalmologist. Together with occupational therapy, a rehabilitation model similar to physical therapy rehabilitation models has emerged, however, the consensus and uniformity of low vision rehabilitation service provision in the U.S. remains inconsistent. In 2009, Cynthia Owsley [3] performed a large census of non-Veterans Affairs entities that performed low vision rehabilitation in the United States in an effort to describe the characteristics of services, types of providers and profile of patients. The result was the first large scale picture on the state of low vision rehabilitation. Among several findings were that 74.1% of patients had central vision loss with its attendant reading (85.9%) and driving (44.9%) problems. 67.1% were diagnosed with age related macular degeneration (AMD). Notably, the patient complaints were function related. This chapter presents an overview of the low vision rehabilitation field from a functional care perspective with the goal of enhancing the patient's quality of life. The emphasis is on a comprehensive, inclusive and interprofessional approach to the treatment and management of the whole patient related to their visual impairment and their specific functional goals.

2. Definitions and model

Every doctor who prescribes minus lenses to allow a myope to see distance objects, or vision therapy to relieve symptoms of convergence insufficiency or cataract surgery to give clearer vision is practicing vision rehabilitation even if not using the term. Indeed, most primary ophthalmic and optometric treatments are designed to restore visual system efficiency and patient functioning, and can surely be considered forms of vision rehabilitation in the broadest sense. Low Vision Rehabilitation, however, emphasizes care for people who have degraded visual function such as visual acuity, visual fields or contrast sensitivity to the point that restoration of previous visual abilities with standard optical corrective techniques like glasses and contact lenses or surgical procedures is no longer possible. The World Health Organization (WHO) provides two definitions for low vision:

1. Low vision is visual acuity less than 6/18 and equal to or better than 3/60 in the better eye with best correction.
2. A person with low vision is one who has impairment of visual functioning even after treatment and/or standard refractive correction, and has a visual acuity of less than 6/18 to light perception, or a visual field less than 10 degrees from the point of fixation, but who uses, or is potentially able to use, vision for the planning and/or execution of a task for which vision is essential.

These definitions are primarily based on measurement of visual abilities rather than the loss of function secondary to the loss of vision. This difference is crucial to the vision rehabilitation of the individual. What is important to one person may be inconsequential to another and treatments based on only visual acuity or visual field may prove unsatisfying for the patient. Therefore, our focus will be on the functional loss of independence when performing critical and desired activities of daily life (ADL). For our purposes in this chapter we will maintain the World Health Organization definitions and propose an additional definition:

3. Low Vision is *a loss of visual function (i.e.* Visual acuity, visual fields and/or contrast sensitivity) caused by an organic or non-organic mechanism resulting in a loss of functional ability and quality of life

Our emphasis in this chapter will be on people who developed as fully sighted then suffered an event or series of events that negatively impacted their visual systems. While it is true that infants with Retinopathy of Prematurity, inborn errors in metabolism, trauma, or other sight affecting conditions can be, and are, considered in the low vision field, and the principles in this chapter are applicable to them, the core view for this chapter will include rehabilitation approaches for those who have acquired vision loss in adulthood, rather than on congenital vision loss. With most visual impairment caused by conditions related to aging or present in aging adults, acquired vision loss in older adults presents the most challenge and burden from a social and economic perspective [4].

Low vision rehabilitation is presented as a three-part paradigm to provide a framework for the physician's evaluation and guided rehabilitation process within the medical model to the linking of services available outside of that model but within the valuable educational and vocational system.

Vision Rehabilitation secondary to our above definition is approached herein as a three part paradigm:

1. *Cause* Visual abilities loss and their measures
2. *Effect* How a person functions given their visual status
3. *Impact* How vision loss impacts quality of life (QOL) and the amelioration of Impact

Cause refers to the loss of visual ability in the key areas of visual acuity, visual fields and contrast sensitivity and how such losses operate to interfere with optimal eye and vision system performance.

Whereas *Cause* implies a vision dysfunction, *Effect* is related to the level of functional visual ability and performance independence given the associated *Cause. Effect* is addressed with standard health history questioning, symptom survey measures of functional independence and observational evaluation of the patient performing a task or series of tasks.

Lastly but quite important, we consider *Impact,* or how the loss of visual function contributes to the degradation of the person's quality of life. This is viewed from a patient reported, subjective evaluation of life status but it is addressed through referral and partnership with a number of providers that may be within or outside the medical system. Whereas the first two, *Cause* and *Effect,* can be addressed within the evaluation process of physician and therapist, the concept of *Impact* can be addressed in a broad fashion with appropriate referrals and education about resources. *Cause, Effect* and *Impact,* will be considered herein as overlapping and interconnected in order to effectively practice comprehensive, inclusive and interprofessional low vision rehabilitation.

It should be noted that health care has become increasingly divided into specialties in spite of a number of initiatives to integrate care across and among various disciplines. The sheer volume of knowledge necessary to become expert in just the various specialties of the eye and visual system, let alone the whole human body, strongly mitigate against the interprofessional efforts of universities, governments and non-government groups. As each provider's specific view of the patient becomes more and more limited to the aspect unique of their specialty, the overall view of the wellbeing of the patient can become more at risk of being diminished or lost. While the results of specialty treatments are separately efficacious to the parts they address, there is a danger in viewing the patient as an assemblage of parts. Many patients with low vision report hearing, "nothing more can be done" from the authority they trust when the authority means "I cannot do any more". The critical missing part of the conversation is: "but there may be someone who can." [5]

3. Chain of vision

One approach to moderating this potential point of patient vulnerability is by addressing it early in the exam process with the analogy that vision is like a chain. Each link in the chain is necessary for full visual functioning but none is sufficient alone. Therefore, repairing a single link does not make one see if there is more than one issue, but rather removes one barrier to vision. All link weaknesses must be ameliorated and all links must be whole for the chain of vision to be strong.

Chain Link One:	Light
Chain Link Two :	Clarity of Ocular Media
Chain Link Three:	Optical Focus
Chain Link Four:	Receptor Elements
Chain Link Five:	Optic nerve and Pathways
Chain Link Six:	Neural processing and brain associations

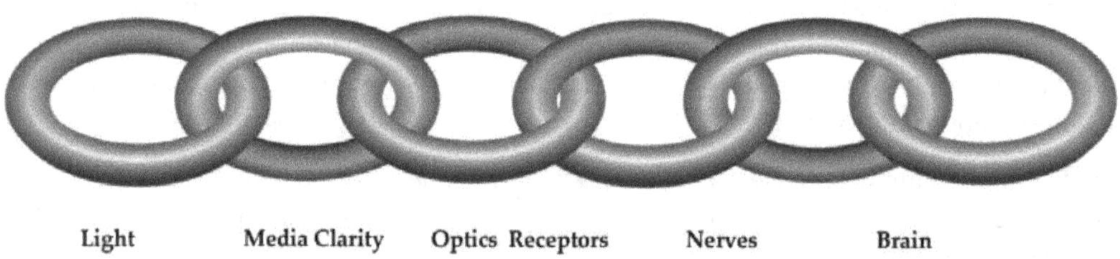

Figure 1. Chain of Vision

The first link is a sufficient amount of **light** to illuminate the object of regard and mitigation of glare.

The second link is **clear media** which can be compromised by cloudy corneas or lenses.

Third is the sharp **optical focus** of the image. This link is the only one impacted by glasses, contact lenses or refractive surgery.

Fourth are the **receptor elements** of the eye, or the retina which takes the "picture". Age related macular degeneration and diabetic retinopathy are primary diseases affecting this chain link.

Fifth we have transmission to the brain via the **optic nerve** and related pathways which can be compromised by atrophies, vascular accidents and trauma.

The sixth link is in the **brain** where **neural processing** takes place and associations occur. Stroke, aneurysms and accidents interfere with the chain of vision in this link.

While the Chain of Vision analogy sounds simplistic at first glance, it has proven memorable to patients who commonly believe it requires only glasses or surgery to make them see. Taking a few moments to introduce this model of Chain of Vision can yield multiple benefits down-stream. Once the patient realizes all the links must work to see and once the specialist acts on the reality that their specialized treatment for one link is necessary but potentially insufficient for restoration of visual ability, we can work toward improving the patient's quality of life using the tools and techniques of the Low Vision Rehabilitation field.

Caution:

When considering the *Cause* of loss of vision ability, it is important to remember that the patient is not to be equated with their condition [6]. Regrettably, language frequently betrays a, perhaps unintended though nevertheless real, diminishment of our patients into a single category of disease through our labels. The adjective becomes the noun and the person becomes the condition. It is easy to think of a person as a "diabetic" or "albino" or "strabismic" but in so labeling them, we belittle, in a real way, the totality of the individual in our substitution of their wholeness into a single attribute. A person with diabetes or a person with albinism or a person with strabismus is first and foremost a person. A whole, complete person who has all the hopes, traits, abilities, talents, relationships and fears comparable to any other person. This clarity of differentiation is not trivial for many of our patients as it is language that shapes perception of reality and influences attitudes that direct care and treatment.

4. Cause

As Cause refers to the etiology and assessment of vision loss, the measure of that dysfunction on the patient's function will guide the low vision rehabilitation practitioner's approach to understanding the *Effect* and to ameliorate the *Impact* on the patient's quality of life. Although there are many visual capacities explored in a comprehensive low vision rehabilitation exam, this chapter will highlight the three key measurable attributes of (1) visual acuity, (2) visual fields and (3) contrast sensitivity. Visual acuity (VA), or sharpness of vision, is the primary vision attribute measured in assessing visual ability as it directly affects reading and driving. Visual fields and contrast sensitivity are reviewed later in this chapter as they have been demonstrated to correlate with particular patient complaints and functioning such as reading ability, facial recognition, mobility and fall risk.

The two most common causes of low vision in the U.S. are age related macular degeneration and diabetic retinopathy affect all three of the above visual functions [7-9]. Most commonly found in people over age 65, age related macular degeneration primarily disrupts visual acuity and central visual fields. The leading cause of vision loss for those under age 65 is diabetic retinopathy which similarly yields reduced visual acuity but generally with greater contrast sensitivity loss and varying amounts of visual field loss. Though visual acuity is typically easy to measure, the standard in-office charts have been designed for the fully sighted person and the design assumptions underlying them can lead to invalid outcomes when used to measure visual acuity in people with low vision.

4.1. *Cause* — Visual acuity

There are several types of visual acuity. Therefore, it might be more appropriate to speak of "the visual acuities" rather than just the singular "visual acuity" and review them sequentially to develop a common foundation that provides us good confidence in the validity of our clinical results. Measurements in one category do not necessarily correlate with those of another. Indeed, as there can be significant variances between and among the categories, it is important to identify the type of acuity one is assessing and not compare across psychometric boundaries. We will then examine these systems used to measure and record VA and investigate how the proper documentation can generate useful extrapolations regarding patient performance and treatment choices.

The first type of VA is **Detection Acuity**. This is the "ah-ha" acuity often expressed by subjects with the expression, "look, something is there!" Detection acuity is useful for safe ambulation, scanning for new information sources in the environment, and defense against approaching dangers. It is not, however, much use in the gathering of form details such as reading, driving or facial recognition.

The second category of VA on our list is **Resolution Acuity**, or the ability to differentiate (resolve) a gap or change in an object or image. This allows an observer to tell a letter "C" from an "O" and forms the basis for the Landolt C acuity charts. The patient is to tell which direction the opening is pointing. Multiple presentations of the Landolt C in various orientations quickly yield a high level of confidence in the final result if the patient gets them all correct. Resolution is useful when an observer knows something is there (detection) but cannot recognize any elements. Extracting some details from the image can generate knowledge of space, distance and, in unfamiliar areas, safety. Resolution acuity does not, however, allow the observer to gather detailed or coded (e.g. alphabet) information.

Vernier Acuity is generally of more interest to vision scientists than to the clinician. Still, it has found utility in geographic areas where it is important to triage patients with severe cataracts when there are not enough ophthalmic surgeons to meet the need. Screening with vernier acuity can help determine who has macular function sufficient to benefit from cataract removal.

Recognition Acuity is the standard of most distance visual acuity test charts. Being able to not only know something is there (detection) and that there are gaps or a space in the image

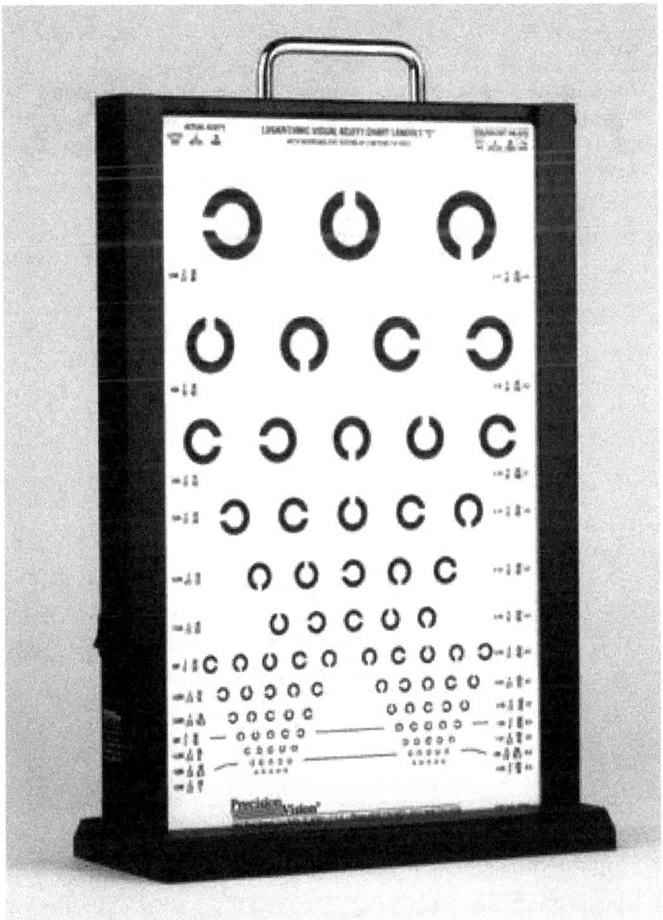

Figure 2. Landolt C Resolution Acuity Chart

(resolution), but to identify it with visual cues is the key to reading printed materials and language. This is the core issue for people with the central vision impairment caused by age related macular degeneration or diabetic retinopathy. Poor recognition acuity is the primary motivator for people with macular issues to present for a low vision rehabilitation evaluation. Inability to recognize faces and difficulty reading disempowers the individual leading to dependencies in the demands of modern daily life and, too frequently, less than optimal quality of life. The concept of recognition acuity, unfortunately, is so comfortably familiar to clinicians that its real meaning can become muddled when it is inappropriately used. Therefore, we need a psychometric standard for our results to have useful meaning in low vision rehabilitation.

The first chart incorporating the most significant psychometric principles was the Bailey-Lovie chart, first introduced in the late 1970s [10]. It was developed to address all the significant factors in the measurement of recognition acuity including equivalent readability of the letters, stroke height of letters, equal contour interaction both within and between rows of letters,

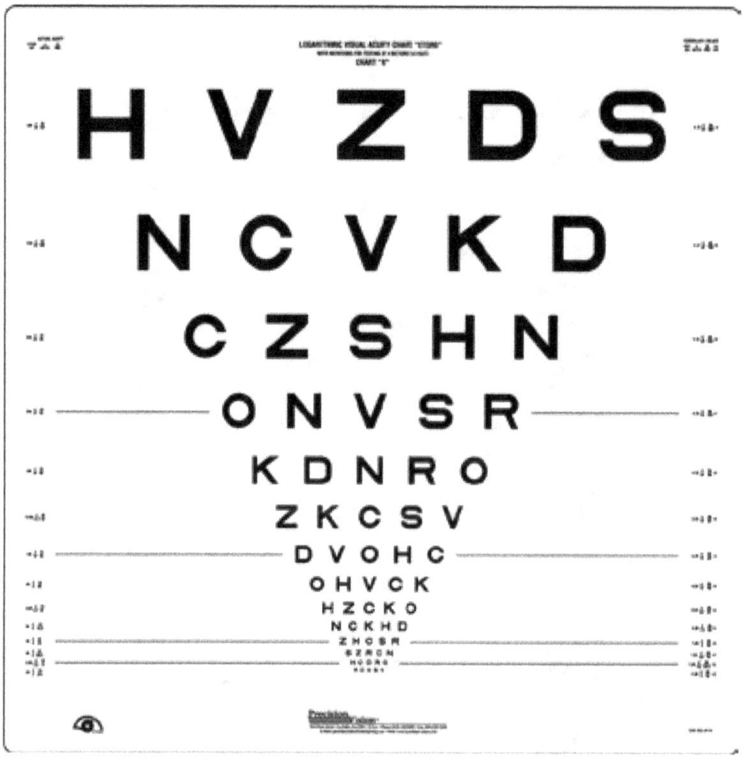

Figure 3. Recognition Acuity Chart ETDRS

equal numbers of single letters per row and logarithmic progression of test task within and between rows. This last aspect takes advantage of Weber's Law and yields valuable predictive power in choosing lenses, working distance, magnification and telescopes for patients' needs. In the early 1980s, the Early Treatment of Diabetic Retinopathy Study (ETDRS) test chart was developed, largely from the Bailey-Lovie design and has been the standard for Recognition visual acuity ever since. The standardizing of test task equivalence yielded by both these charts gives a high level of confidence in the validity and repeatability of measurements, allowing more accurate and consistent collection of data and a solid basis for comparison of past and future visual performance when tracking the course of the patient's condition and the success or lack thereof in treatment.

Recording recognition visual acuity is optimally done with the Snellen fraction, writing the numerator as the test distance, preferably in the logarithmic progression of distances and letter size read at threshold as the denominator, also in the logarithmic sequence of Just-Noticeable-Differences (JND) (both discussed more fully in the *Cause*-LogMAR section below) while always keeping the units in the same system (English or Metric). When visual acuity is always and only recorded as a fraction with actual test distance over actual letter size measured, all the pertinent visual acuity information is captured and available for use by the clinician.

Refraction is an aspect of visual acuity that requires addressing even if it is too large a topic to explore completely in our chapter context. The phoropter is the instrument developed for refraction of fully sighted patients and serves that purpose very well. It uses small steps of dioptric power to determine the patient's ametropia because the Just-Noticeable-Difference of fully sighted patients is roughly only a quarter of a diopter (0.25D) as found in the phoropter. Partially sighted patients, however, have variable Just-Noticeable-Differences depending on their level of acuity or sensitivity and therefore need an approach based on differential lens steps to accommodate the presenting Just-Noticeable-Difference. This is achieved by the use of a trial frame and trial lens set with techniques adapted to the sensitivity of the partially sighted patient. The whole range of visual acuities and Just-Noticeable-Difference variances can be addressed using the principles of LogMAR progression steps of significance.

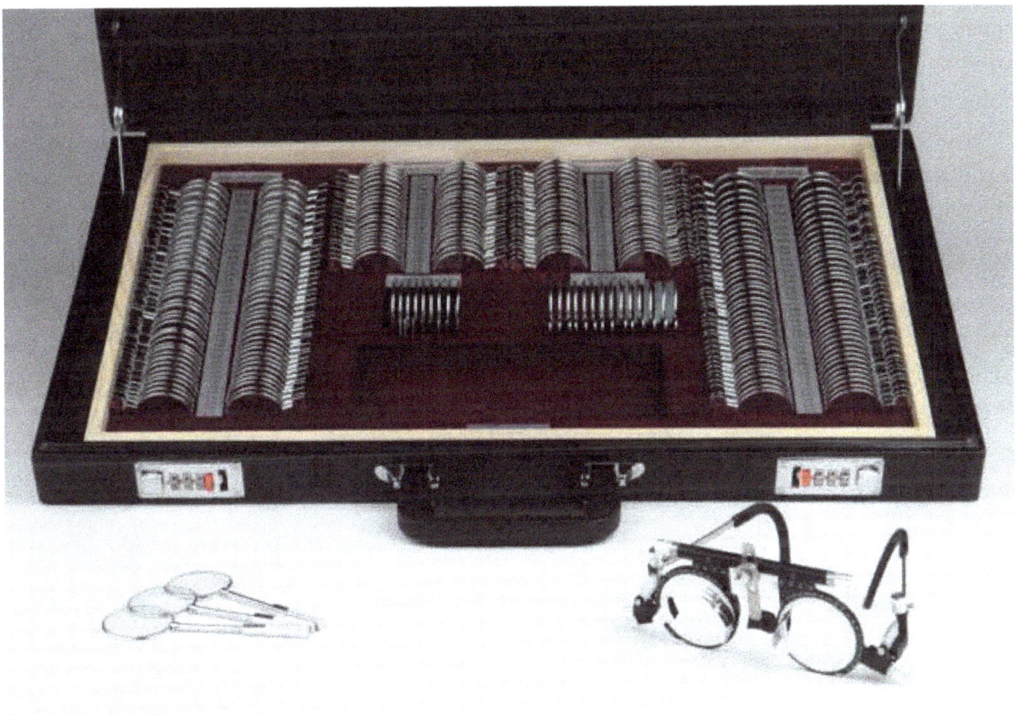

Figure 4. Trial Lens Set with Trial Frame and hand held Jackson Flip Cross Lenses

4.2. *Cause* — LogMAR

Weber's Law – The change in stimulus which is necessary to evoke a just-noticeable-difference (JND) in sensation bears a constant ratio to the original stimulus from which it was derived.

This broad law of human stimulus perception is deceptively simple in its presentation yet potentially powerful for predicting patient performance with induced changes in stimulus. While Weber's law is not immutable, especially with stimuli at the extremes of the spectrum, it does provide guidance with stimuli changes that are manifest in the activities of daily life. When considering formed image stimuli measurable by recognition acuity charts, the constant ratio, or logarithmic progression, of Just-Noticeable-Differences is remarkably consistent and reliable over the range of standard measures. Given this characteristic of Just-Noticeable-Differences being a constant ratio, and charts designed with the principles of psychometric integrity and test task equivalence, we have the foundation for using acuity measurements to predict visual performance when we introduce reading lens changes, working distance adjustments or telescopic power variations to the patient, other factors being equal. All that is missing for us to lever the potential power of Weber's Law in predicting patient performance is a starting "original stimulus." Fortunately, we have Robert Hooke, sometimes known as "England's DaVinci." We can thank him for developing an employment test aimed at potential astronomy assistants. Hooke had the assistant candidates count the stars in the Big Dipper. Since one "star" is really two stars (Alcor and Mizar) separated visually by approximately one minute of arc, he declared those that passed had good vision and the stage was set for one minute of arc to be the standard of visual acuity. However apocryphal the story might be, we have our "original stimulus" or minimum angle of resolution (MAR) from which to begin our logarithmic progression for charts, working distances, dioptric lens powers and telescopic magnification: one minute of arc.

Work in the late nineteenth century demonstrated the constant ratio for detecting visual change as 0.1 $\log_{10}$ units. From our starting point of a minimum angle of resolution of one minute of arc, and a Weber's Law constant of 0.1 log units we can build a table of significance for visual acuity:

LogMAR	MAR (′)	VA (English)	VA (Metric)
0.0	1.0	20/20	6/6
0.1	1.25	20/25	6/8
0.2	1.6	20/32	6/10
0.3	2.0	20/40	6/12.5
0.4	2.5	20/50	6/16
0.5	3.2	20/63	6/20
0.6	4.0	20/80	6/25
0.7	5.0	20/100	6/32
0.8	6.3	20/125	6/40
0.9	8.0	20/160	6/50
1.0	10.0	20/200	6/60

Table 1. MAR, LogMAR and Visual Acuity

This chart design enables thinking of the steps between the lines as "steps of significance". These steps can be Diopters (D), working distance, letter size when working at near, or telescopic magnification for distance. At near, a change in one step for diopters necessitates a change in one step of distance, resulting (all other variables being equal) of one step in letter size. As diopters add increases by a step, working distance decreases by a step as does letter size. In the above table, the MAR column can be thought of as the "Steps" column.

Steps	Diopters Add (D)	Working Distance (cm)	Letter Size (M)
Start	2.50	40	2.0
1	3.25	32	1.6
2	4.00	25	1.25
3	5.00	20	1.0
4	6.25	16	0.8
5	8.00	12.5	0.63
6	10.00	10	0.5

Table 2. LogMAR Reading Example

When working with telescopic powers, one always begins with best distance refraction and working distance is always infinity. Since the eye by definition has a magnification at distance of "1", all step changes start from there.

Steps	Telescope Power	Acuity
Start	1.0	20/200
1	1.25	20/160
2	1.6	20/125
3	2.0	20/100
4	2.5	20/80
5	3.25	20/63
6	4.0	20/50
7	5.0	20/40
8	6.3	20/32
9	8.0	20/25

Table 3. LogMAR telescope example

One can see the utility in charts built with LogMAR, but before using these steps of significance for treatment choices in the *Impact* section, it is important to examine near visual acuity and reading ability.

4.3. *Cause* — Reading

Near visual acuity and reading ability are different tasks yet sometimes conflated inappropriately thereby becoming a source of frustration for the doctor and patient when expectations of reading ability in the patient's life and near acuity measures from the doctor's office do not align.

Charts properly designed for near visual acuity give results strongly correlated with distance acuity. The rules of building significance for distance ETDRS charts apply for the near charts allowing maximum degrees of freedom in choosing working distance, add powers and magnification. Image 5 shows a single digit near visual acuity chart with a 40cm string that can be used to control working distance. The string can also be folded in half for a 20cm working distance but any distance on the LogMAR scale can reasonably be used.

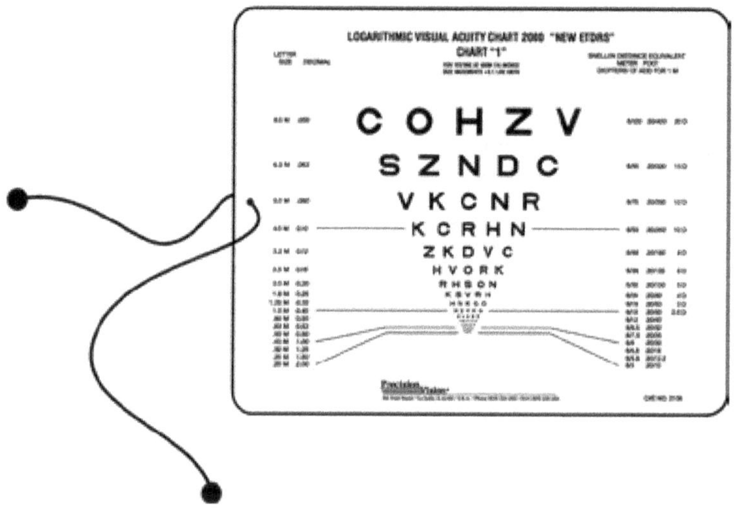

Figure 5. Single Digit near chart

Near Visual Acuity has four common systems of recording, only one of which has the psychometric integrity necessary for our purposes. (1) Reduced Snellen does not capture either letter size or working distance. (2) Point system (n-units) captures image size but not working distance in a useable format. (3) Jaeger or "J" size is not standardized among chart manufacturers and does not record working distance in a meaningful way. Only (4) M-Units recorded as a Snellen fraction of distance in meters over M size provides information in a fashion which can be used in calculating dioptric lens powers and working distances for low vision rehabilitation work.

Example of Recorded M-Unit acuity: 0.4/1.0M means at 40 cm, the patient was able to recognize a 1.0M letter

Once the near single digit visual acuity is determined and recorded in M-Unit fashion, variations in working distance and dioptric lens power can be manipulated to meet patient acuity goals using LogMAR principles discussed previously.

Reading for information, however, is a complex activity of which near Visual Acuity is only one part. Therefore, a reading task requires a more complete description than just acuity. One method that accounts for reading's complexity is the MN Read cards system which incorporates three factors affecting reading performance: (1) Reading Acuity, (2) Maximum Reading Speed and (3) Critical Print Size.

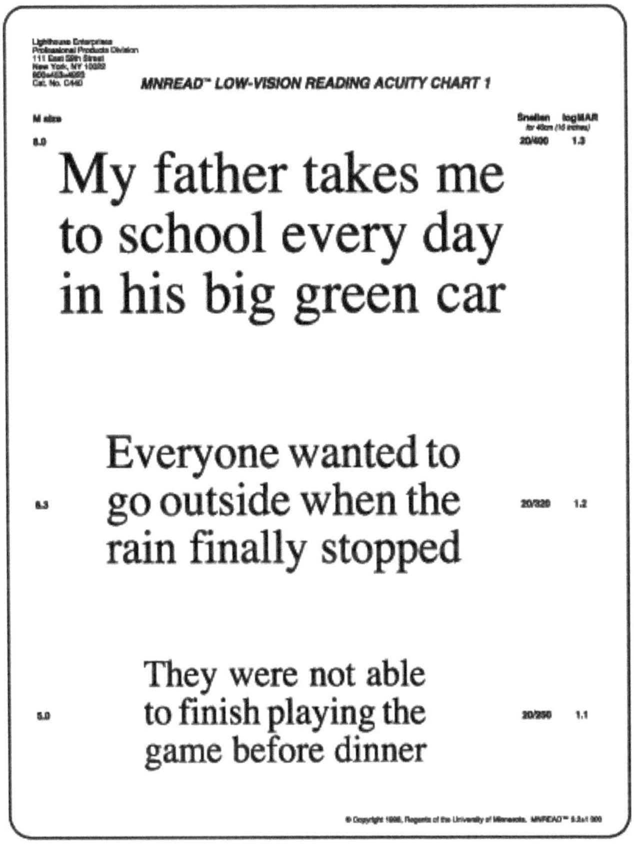
MNREAD™ LOW-VISION READING ACUITY CHART 1
My father takes me
to school every day
in his big green car
Everyone wanted to
go outside when the
rain finally stopped
They were not able
to finish playing the
game before dinner

Figure 6. MN Read Near Card

Reading acuity (1) is the smallest resolvable print size, similar to near visual acuity. Maximum Reading Speed (2) is the top rate at which a patient can read contextual words for information. Critical Print Size (3) is the smallest print size that the patient can read at maximum reading speed. Combining these three reading components allows a more thorough understanding of reading in patients with low vision. Additionally, it demonstrates to the patient how their reading is affected by the three factors and that it can be improved with changes in add, working distance and letter size.

A reading test developed primarily for the patient with the central field defects (scotomas) that are commonly found in age related macular degeneration is the Smith-Kettlewell Reading test (SK Read) by Don Fletcher. The test is different from the MN read as it uses words that when combined into a block of a particular size print, the block contains no contextual meaning. This means that reading errors caused by central field defects or scotomas and the corresponding preferred retinal locus (PRL) will be apparent as the patient cannot use context to guess words. Both the reading speed and number of errors are recorded which results in a reading error rate per block of text. The test instructions provide guidance for interpreting the locations of the errors as related to the location of the patient's scotoma relative to fixation. The test can also be used to educate the patient on the impact of central scotomas on reading so that when both magnification and fixation training are included in the final rehabilitation plan, the patient is aware of the complexities of their reading facility and the rehabilitation process.

4.4. *Cause* — Visual field

The low vision rehabilitation domain has traditionally divided visual field impairments into the two general areas of centralfields and peripheral fields. The type of loss in either area affects patient function in different ways. Peripheral field losses such as overall constriction and hemianopsias can affect mobility and activities of daily life but are a small percentage of total scotomas compared to acquired central field loss as found in age related macular degeneration. Therefore, the emphasis in low vision rehabilitation is properly on central and paracentral loss.

Although it has been well understood that scotomas or visual field defects occur in the progression of many visually debilitating conditions, the understanding of how to best measure the central and paracentral scotoma and relate that measurement to patient visual abilities and low rehabilitation strategies is a newer concept. Traditionally, a central automated visual field or an Amsler grid was considered the test of choice for evaluating the central visual field but both of these tests are problematic when applied to rehabilitation of a patient.

As early as 1987, Timberlake, Peli, and Augliere [12] used a Scanning LASER Ophthalmoscope (SLO) and derived the term preferred retinal locus (PRL) to describe a "single, idiosyncratic retinal area, immediately adjacent to the scotoma, for fixating, inspecting acuity targets, and scanning simple, nonsense-syllable text". They also determined the preferred retinal locus may not be the ideal location for reading text nor was it always situated as close to the fovea as possible. In 1999, Schuchard, Naseer and de Castro determined both that the location of the preferred retinal locus affects visual performance of the patient and the location may shift over the progression of the disease-true especially of patients with a ring scotoma [13]. Additional studies have suggested that the development of a preferred retinal locus occurs within 6 months of visual loss and that multiple fixation locations can be used depending on the visual task.

There are varying opinions about how the location of the scotoma relative to the preferred retinal locus impact reading rates and about how to best train patients to use their preferred retinal locus or to even use a new better positioned trained retinal locus (TRL). For example, Deruaz (2006) [14] asserted that reading requires two conditions (1) detailed discrimination and (2) global viewing (i.e. seeing the whole length or words). A natural preferred retinal locus may only provide detailed discrimination but might be in a location that prevents the second important reading criteria, global viewing (2006). Nillson (2003) [15] and Deruaz (2006) have successfully selected a new location for the patient, a trained retinal locus (TRL), typically above or below the scotoma for hopes of improving function. Although they achieved short term success in the use of a trained retinal locus or a combination of preferred retinal locus and trained retinal locus for reading, it is unclear how the patient may utilize the trained retinal locus alone or in combination with their preferred retinal locus for activities of daily life in the long term or for improved vision related quality of life (VRQOL).

Another rehabilitation approach, training with the existing preferred retinal locus for fixation stability, has been demonstrated to successfully improve reading speed. Most recent literature on scotomas and function support the use of strategies aimed at improving fixation stability with the natural preferred retinal locus strategies [16, 17].

Many clinicians, instead of using any type of perimetry with age related macular degeneration patients, employ techniques such as asking the patient to identify parts of the doctor's face that may be missing or numbers on a clock face that may be absent or difficult to view. These techniques suffer from subjectivity and poor quantification. The patient is an unreliable source to describe the presence of binocular scotomas and the "missing areas" that result. Fletcher found that out of 153 patients with age related macular degeneration who were asked if they were able to see or notice their blind spots, 56% were totally unaware of their presence, and of those patients who did notice something missing they were only able to vaguely describe how objects disappeared. Microperimetry and determination of the patients most commonly used preferred retinal locus is invaluable for modern rehabilitation methods that incorporate training strategies teaching steady eye fixation. [18]

According to Markowitz (2013), the three parameters of macular function that should be assessed during a low vision rehabilitation evaluation are (1) scotoma characteristics, (2) preferred retinal loci and (3) oculomotor control [19]. This can be done through the use of microperimeter or scanning LASER ophthalmoscope to view the fundus while simultaneous projecting viewing targets directly on areas of the retina. Although microperimetry is used extensively in research settings and in a few comprehensive low vision clinics, the cost and time to perform such testing limits their current use in low vision rehabilitation clinics. Until more widespread adoption of microperimetry in low vision clinics occurs, less expensive and time intensive strategies have been recommended such tests as the California Central Visual Field Test (CCVFT) by Fletcher, Cole, and Kammer [20]. The California Central Visual Field Test utilizes three different modified LASER pointers with varying output and beam diameters as visual stimulation. The fixation target is in the center of series of rings printed on letter size paper. The test is positioned at a near distance that allows for simple determination of size of the scotoma in degrees with simultaneous recording of scotoma boundaries directly on the test. The test is similar to a tangent screen in the utilization of both static and kinetic target presentations and does require the clinician to simultaneously observe both the patient's fixation and record the boundaries of the scotoma.

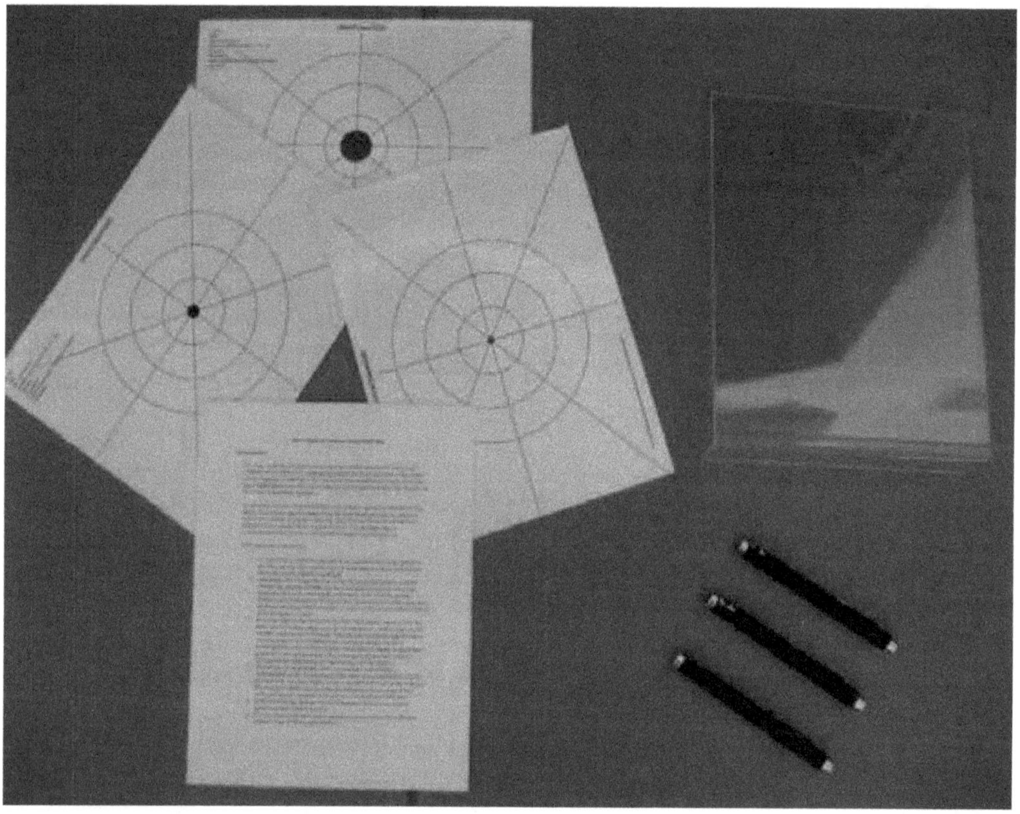

Figure 7. California Central Visual Field Test (CCVFT)

4.5. *Cause* — Contrast sensitivity

Contrast Sensitivity Function is the third important attribute of visual ability quantified in a low vision rehabilitation exam. The term "Contrast" refers to the difference between the highest and lowest brightness levels of a target. A person's ability to detect the minimum difference in contrast for a particular size image is designated "Contrast Sensitivity" and the plot of Contrast Sensitivity to object (letter) size is called the "Contrast Sensitivity Function". Contrast Sensitivity is affected primarily by optics, retinal function and neural processing. Since the most common conditions that cause visual impairment are age related macular degeneration and diabetic retinopathy, poor retinal function is the predominant cause of contrast sensitivity loss in this population.

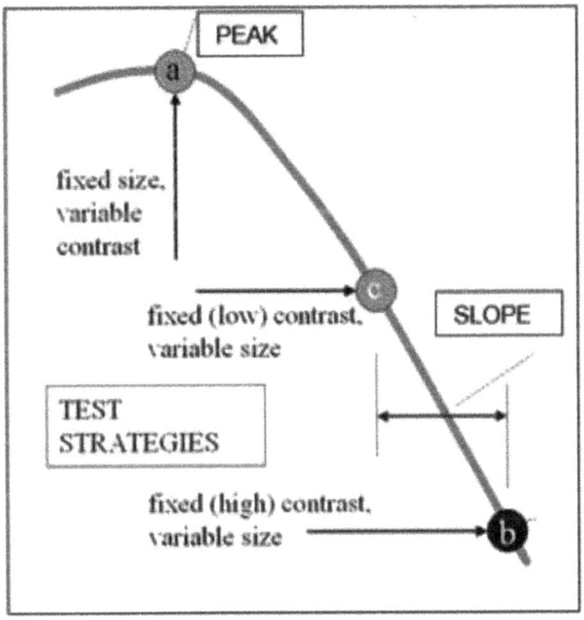

Figure 8. Contrast Sensitivity Curve

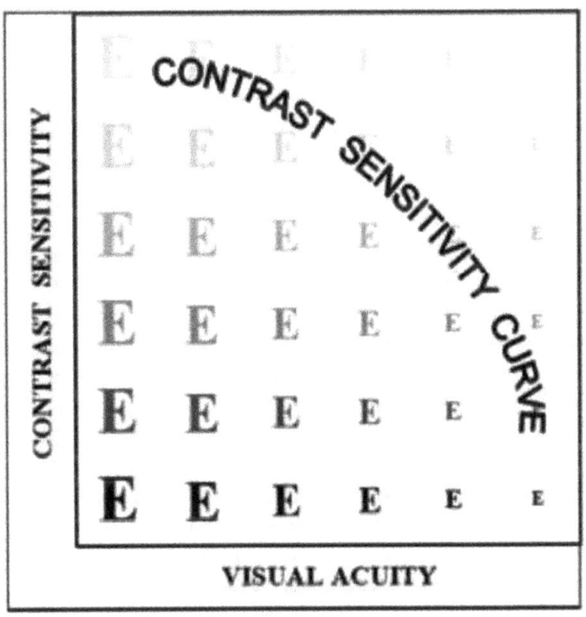

Figure 9. Contrast Sensitivity Curve Illustration

Threshold visual acuity is actually measured on a CSF graph being, in essence, the single point farthest to the right.

Reasonably, therefore, Contrast Sensitivity Function has not been shown to add any prescriptive value beyond standard visual acuity in measures of reading function when using high contrast materials. Activities of daily living such as walking, cooking, and grooming, however, often consist of visual cues with less than optimum contrast that present as various sizes and can cause functional visual difficulties for patients with low vision. In particular, mobility speed and safety are correlated with Contrast Sensitivity Function [21].

In examining the CSF, where visual acuity is along the X-axis and contrast sensitivity along the Y-axis, we find the peak contrast sensitivity for fully sighted people at mid-sized objects. As objects get smaller or larger, contrast sensitivity performance drops off. The CSF curve deviates differentially when retinal function is negatively affected by a condition or disease. Typical contrast measurements might be obtained with high contrast, small letter objects even while the ability to detect larger, lower contrast objects declines. This would be manifest by the ability to read standard vision charts well but subjective patient reports of significant issues in mobility such as not being able to see a curb or step. Functionally, this can lead to increased fall risk. When only considering visual acuity, these functional complaints seem to be out of proportion to the measured acuity, and indeed they are. Only when Contrast Sensitivity Function is considered are the subjective complaints accounted for.

There are several tests to evaluate CSF including sine wave gratings of variable contrast and size, Pelli-Robson or MARS letter triplets of varying contrast, and ETDRS or Text charts at distance or near with varying levels of contrast between presented charts. Each test has its own scoring which makes cross test extrapolation less than satisfactory, but each type of testing yields results that characterize patient complaints unaccounted for by acuity and visual field tests. Loss of Contrast in the higher spatial frequencies (small letters) usually signifies threshold visual acuity loss, while Contrast loss in lower spatial frequencies (large letters) could indicate poor ability to detect large, low contrast items in a path and lead to increased trip hazard and fall risk. Since visual acuity can be a good predictor of higher spatial frequency losses, particular attention regarding CSF should be paid to loss of contrast in lower spatial frequencies. In the past, contrast sensitivity testing was often left to the vision researchers and less commonly addressed in clinical vision examinations. This could be due to the complexity and the time required to complete and interpret testing. New types of charts that enable a quick screening of CSF loss such as the Mixed Contrast Chart by Gus Colenbrander [22] could be used to identify significant defects as well as educate patients and caregivers about the impact of loss.

Losses in the lower spatial frequencies are not generally improved by optical devices, but the attendant functional losses can be ameliorated with techniques and training by qualified professionals such as Orientation and Mobility (O&M) instructors and Occupational Therapists (OT).

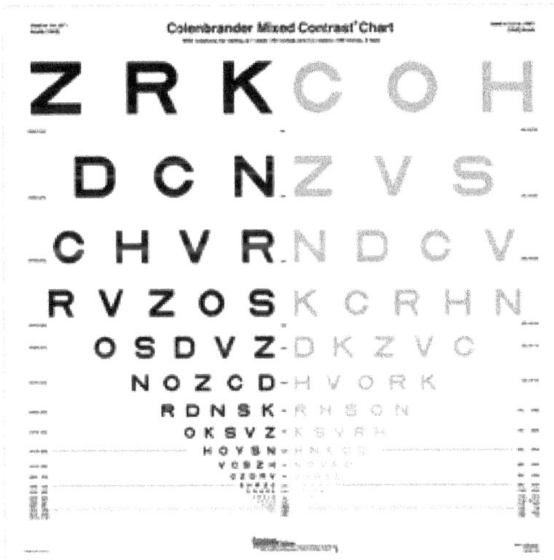

Figure 10. Colenbrander Mixed Contrast Chart

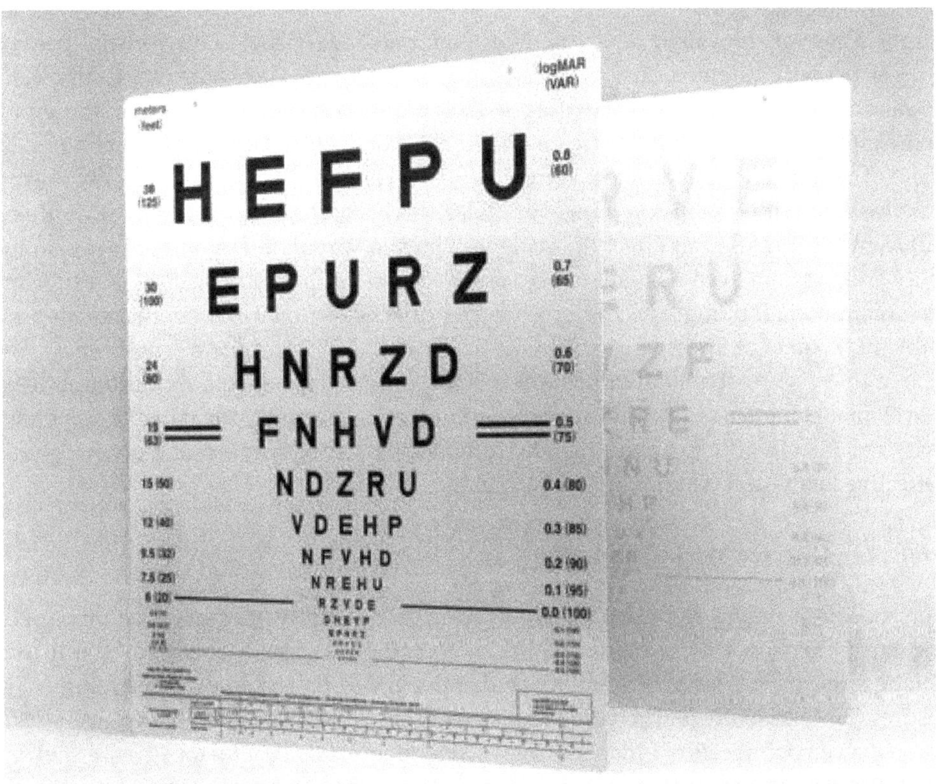

Figure 11. ETDRS Two Contrast Charts

4.6. *Cause* — Lighting

Lighting is more problematic to quantify than visual acuity, visual fields and contrast sensitivity function, and although it is not a measure of visual dysfunction directly, understanding how it may change the assessment of the other deficits is important. Lighting or illumination is a potentially key factor in ameliorating the *Effect* of the visual condition on function and its *Impact* on quality of life. For patients with significant contrast sensitivity loss, illumination can improve function and effectively decrease the amount of magnification needed to achieve the patients reading goals [23]. In addition, Schuchard and Lei discovered that in patients with relative central scotomas, some patients use different preferred retinal loci locations in high illumination settings for different visual and reading tasks [24]. Compounding contrast sensitivity loss with central scotomas can result in reading impairment to a much greater degree than would predicted by single optotype acuity testing under optimum office conditions. Therefore, evaluating the patient's response to lighting during the low vision rehabilitation exam process is necessary if both contrast sensitivity and the central visual field have been found to be compromised during standard testing of visual acuity, visual field and contrast sensitivity testing.

4.7. *Effect* — Functional sequelae of cause

Once the *Cause* of the vision deficit is determined and the visual acuity, visual fields and contrast sensitivity parameters measured, it is important to define how the visual deficit affects the patient's function regarding activities of daily life. This is done initially with the standard vision exam history. In a primary care exam, the standard measures of Chief Complaint, Review of Systems (ROS) and Past, Family & Social History (PFSH) are generally adequate. For the patient with low vision, however, these three standard history categories are often insufficient. Vision loss can affect the patient in such a way that they adapt by avoiding an activity and may not even recognize they can no longer perform it or that they even want to. Once accommodation is made, the specific loss of function may not be elicited in a Chief Complaint, Review of Systems, Past Family and Social History profile of questioning. Therefore, in a low vision rehabilitation history it is important to probe in a more comprehensive and systematic manner. Symptom surveys of independence and third party observations of activities of daily living can provide a more complete picture of the *Effect* and give us guidance for effective low vision rehabilitation treatment.

4.8. *Effect* — Directed symptom survey

Vision specific questions alone do not always address the totality of *Effect* on activities of daily living for the person with a vision loss. A more complete system needs to be utilized for evaluating the patient's level of ability and independence. The Functional Independence Measures (FIM) structure meets these requirements [25, 26]. FIM separately evaluates thirteen tasks on a seven point scale of Independence – Dependence. It is a useful tool to ascertain where a patient is having difficulty performing common activities of daily living, identify those activities a patient has given up on or is avoiding, and to direct the rehabilitation team's ongoing efforts. Functional independence measures can also be used to monitor progress of the patient's treatment regimen and evaluate care goals. While functional independence measure scaling is necessarily subjective, it is rubric driven around specified criteria to improve validity. Limiting the number of questions and the number of associated scaled responses to each question allows us to glean valuable information regarding activities of daily life objectives in a short time.

The following is a list of thirteen categories for the functional tasks that have been selected to be each graded using a seven point scale of perceived independence/dependence.

1. Cooking
2. Cleaning
3. Grooming
4. Finances
5. Self-Care
6. Ambulating Home
7. Ambulating Out
8. Reading Sustained
9. Reading Spot
10. Other Near Tasks
11. Intermediate Tasks
12. Distance Tasks
13. Technology

These thirteen functional task categories are reasonably self-explanatory and understandable for the patient who ranks each task on a seven point scale with a score of seven being completely independent and a score of one being total dependence. A measure of independence with no helper is only possible at the level of six or seven. Dependence levels are ranked from five to one with subscales for modified dependence and complete dependence. Details for scaling independence are described in Table 4.

After the level of Dependency is established for each of the thirteen categories, we can direct our rehabilitation efforts more rationally in mitigating the *Effect* of the vision deficit on the patient's life. For example, a patient with scores of six and seven in all categories except Sustained Reading needs little attention to distance rehabilitation devices or activities of daily living training. Rather, we should concentrate on reading devices, training and techniques. Similarly, a patient with scores of six and seven in all categories except Ambulating Out will need a referral to the Orientation and Mobility (O&M) member of the rehabilitation team, not new magnifiers. Processing functioning scores at the entrance testing level of our low vision rehabilitation evaluation not only directs the doctor toward the most efficacious avenue to proceed in the exam, but makes the patient aware there might be possibilities for them in

INDEPENDENT Another person is not required for the activity (NO HELPER).	
	7 Complete Independence - All of the tasks described as making up the activity are typically performed safely without modification, assistive devices (other than standard glasses or contact lenses) and within a reasonable time frame.
	6 Modified Independence - Activity requires any one or more of the following: An assistive device beyond standard glasses or contact lenses, more than reasonable time, or there are safety (risk) considerations.
DEPENDENT Another person is required for either supervision or physical assistance in order for the activity to be performed, or it is not performed (REQUIRES HELPER).	
	MODIFIED DEPENDENCE - The subject expends 50% or more of the needed effort to perform the task. The levels of assistance required are:
	5 Supervision or Setup - Subject requires no more help than standby, cueing or coaxing, without physical contact. Or, helper sets up needed items.
	4 Minimal Contact Assistance - With physical contact the subject requires no more help than touching, and subject expends 75% or more of the effort.
	3 Moderate Assistance - Subject requires more help than touching, or expends between 50% and 75% of the effort required to perform the task.
	COMPLETE DEPENDENCE - The subject expends less than 50% of the effort, maximal or total assistance is required, or the activity is not performed. The levels of assistance required are:
	2 Maximal Assistance - Subject expends between 25% and 50% of effort for task
	1 Total Assistance - Subject expends less than 25% of the effort.

Table 4. FIM Independence Rubric

categories on which they had given up or are avoiding. This sets functional scoring apart from standard history taking of Chief Complaint, Review of Systems and Past, Family and Social History and opens up options for addressing aspects in the life of the patient with low vision that are never manifest in fully sighted patients and hence have never become a part of standard history taking in a primary care vision exam. Asking the patient their Chief Complaint or reason for presenting is necessary yet many times inadequate for those with vision impairment. Directed probing at the beginning of the low vision rehabilitation evaluation rationalizes the process for the doctor, opens up the patient to possibilities they might not have considered and prepares the patient for thinking beyond just glasses and magnifiers. As the *Effect* on the low vision patient is qualitatively different from the fully sighted patient, so must the history be.

4.9. *Impact* — Quality of life

Impact in our paradigm of low vision rehabilitation refers to how the how the loss of vision and vision related function (*Cause* and *Effect*) contribute to the degradation of the individual's quality of life. Whereas *Cause* and *Effect* can be addressed within the evaluation process of physician and therapist, the concept of *Impact* may need to be additionally addressed in a broader fashion beyond low vision rehabilitation optical devices with appropriate referrals and education about resources.

Quality of life is a common phrase, but as a precisely definable concept remains elusive. The various conceptualizations of quality of life do, however, generally tend to include objective and subjective measures in a multi-dimensional manner while recognizing individual, societal and economic values. Though details do vary between the various instruments of quality of life measures, the categories essentially overlap and usually include aspects of a person's physical, material, social and emotional well-being. Therefore, rather than a blueprint of precision, quality of life definitions and measurement tools present a more general framework of reference. They are not typically used clinically on every low vision rehabilitation patient due to the time limitations for their administration, but have been used to validate the efficacy of treatment models.

Patient Reported Outcomes (PRO) are being increasingly used by third party and government regulators to assess care quality from the viewpoint of the patient and society. Among these are a number of quality of life surveys that seek to validate treatment efficacy. Khadka, McAlinden, and Pesudovs [27] conducted a comprehensive survey of the field in 2013 and found 121 vision related patient reported outcomes with 48 meeting the quality inclusion criteria for question unidimensionality and interval-level measurement. Of those, only six were related to low vision rehabilitation and one, the Veteran Affairs Low-Vision Functioning Questionnaire was considered highest quality. This patient reported outcome structure was validated in the Veteran Affairs Low Vision Intervention Trial (LOVIT) which reported significant improvement in every facet of visual function outcomes for patients who received low vision rehabilitation treatment. Even so, with 48 questions, it involved a significant time commitment to administer. While the outcomes of low vision rehabilitation have been shown to be positive, the studies point to time constraints as one of the main difficulties in performing current quality of life surveys on every patient. In addition, the current state of quality of life surveys is limited by the fixed question format which does not provide for adaptive questions based on preceding answers, thus limiting the comprehensiveness and individuality of the results.

The World Health Organization [28] broadly defines quality of life as "an individual's perception of their position in life in the context of the culture and value systems in which they live and in relation to their goals, expectations, standards and concerns. It is a broad ranging concept affected in a complex way by the person's physical health, psychological state, personal beliefs, social relationships and their relationship to salient features of their environment."

The Center for Disease Control [29] subsequently added the concept of health related quality of life (HRQOL) in order to parse out those aspects of overall quality of life pertaining particularly to health. Defining, measuring and tracking health related quality of life is intended to be used to improve public health decision-making and allocation of resources.

Vision Related Quality of Life (VRQOL) [30] is a term referring to those parts of quality of life affected by vision. Instruments have been developed that seek to provide guidance in making economic health evaluations of eye care and rehabilitation programs. These instruments have currently not received widespread clinical acceptance.

A factor impacting quality of life that is commonly seen in low vision rehabilitation practice is that of depression. Renaud and Bedard (2013) completed a review of the literature of studies linking the relationship between quality of life and depression in elders with visual impairment and, as is expected, their findings indicate that better quality of life is strongly related to less severe depressive symptoms. The complexity of psychological evaluation makes it difficult to deconstruct out the exact link with vision loss in seniors, but Eramudugolla, Wood and Anstey [31] showed a significant association between objective indices of visual impairment (visual acuity, contrast sensitivity, visual fields) and functional vision with depressive and anxiety symptoms. This would lead us to encourage primary care practitioners to consider deeper evaluation of depression and anxiety in adults with age related eye disease. Several studies have demonstrated a lack of appropriate screening methods among practitioners while also calling for methods to train low vision rehabilitation practitioners in screening and referral methods [32, 33]. Some leaders have been successful in developing a training program to assist health professionals and rehabilitation professionals in detection but the program has not been adopted in widespread use in the U.S [34].

Another impacting phenomenon for people with low vision is Charles Bonnet Syndrome (CBS). This involves visual hallucinations that many people with binocular vision loss experience, many times, on a regular basis. Some scholars suggest that 30% of persons with ARMD and binocular vision loss experience these [35]. Commonly described as colorful and sometimes dynamic scenes, they do not usually induce an unpleasant experience. The symptoms may decrease over time but in some patients it is an ongoing phenomenon. The exact process causing the hallucinations is unknown but thought by some to be similar to the mechanisms of "phantom limb syndrome". Others based their theories on functional MRI studies suggesting Charles Bonnet Syndrome results from increased function in certain pathways other than those caused by external visual stimulus [36]. Regardless of the cause, doctors may reassure patients of the benign nature of these hallucinations and that they are unrelated to cognitive decline.

5. Interventions and management

5.1. *Impact* — Vision enhancement — Optical

Vision enhancement by optical and electronic devices have been a mainstay of low vision rehabilitation but modern low vision approaches and advancement in knowledge have supported the evolution of prescribing to include more factors for enabling patients to use the devices and incorporate them in daily life. For example, rather than prescribing optical or electronic devices after an evaluation with a low vision physician, many rehabilitation teams provide basic tools but incorporate rehabilitation methods such as teaching stable fixation with a preferred retinal locus (PRL) in patients with age related macular degeneration prior to prescribing final devices. This allows for an evaluation of activities of daily life, lifestyle, and cognitive dimensions alongside the low vision physician that supports an integration of the devices by the rehabilitation therapist into daily life. Rehabilitation then becomes an ongoing process where the patient is encouraged to develop lifestyle adaptations over the course of rehabilitation. After several sessions with the therapist, the low vision physician would re-evaluate the patient's progress and prescribe additional devices as needed. In the U.S. a growing trend is for the low vision physician (optometrist or ophthalmologist) to refer to a low vision experienced occupational therapist (OT) who can be supported within the medical model by the Center for Medicare and Medicaid Services (CMS). [37].

Optical vision enhancement devices encompass high dioptric add powers, single vision near point glasses, magnifiers of various types (hand held, stand, illuminated) and telescopes. Unfortunately for our model of psychometric integrity, these devices can be variously labeled with non-standard power and/or magnification descriptors leading to confusion and frustration when attempting to compare patient performance and response. Magnification nomenclature is not homogeneous between companies that manufacture low vision rehabilitation devices and, in addition, are based on different assumptions of working distance. The assumptions are limiting and the various magnification formulae confusing.

The power of lenses and lens systems is most correctly defined with diopters and Equivalent Power (F_e) is the standard by which they are most properly described. Eyeglasses for the fully sighted are generally such low power that thin lens formulae give good approximations of Equivalent power (F_e). Therefore, office lensometers which measure back vertex power (F_v) give results which can be considered correspondent with F_e when used for the most common eyeglass powers. As lens powers increase to the ranges often used in low vision rehabilitation, the thin lens calculations generate measurement errors that become significant. Using F_e rationalizes observed lens effects on performance and makes treatment decisions on lens more systematic and rational. Consequently, describing the power of low vision rehabilitation optical devices with F_e is desirable.

The logarithmic progression of steps of significance in the ETDRS chart design in combination with the standardization of F_e for describing the power of low vision rehabilitation optical devices means predictions of patient near point performance can be made with good levels of confidence. Since each step on the LogMAR scale is a Just Noticeable Difference (JND), the steps can be thought of as either dioptric power steps, working distance steps or M-Unit size steps. Following is a four stage procedure that leads to performance predictions with changes in working distance, letter size and lens power for near acuity:

Stage 1-Measure and Record Visual Acuity in M-Units

Stage 2-Set letter size Goal for Performance Improvement

Stage 3-Count steps from Measurement to Goal

Stage 4-Implement counted steps for both working distance and F_e

0.4	0.5	0.63	0.8	1.0	1.25	1.6	2.0	2.5	3.2	4.0	5.0	6.3	8.0	10.0	12.5	16.0	20.0

Table 5. LogMAR steps of significance in JND increments of Diopters, Working Distance and M-Units

Once the Equivalent power needed to attain the patient's goal has been determined, the manner of delivery is chosen. Given that the important factor is the angular subtense of the image on the retina, the dioptric power can be supplied to the patient by single vision glasses, bifocal add, hand held magnifier, stand magnifier or telescope. In choosing between the various power delivery methods, factors other than diopters come into play. These factors include the particular task logistics, the ability of the patient to hold magnifiers steady, spot vs. sustained reading and others.

Low vision rehabilitation single vision glasses and bifocals delivery equivalent power to the eye by traditional means but with much higher dioptric power. The advantage to the patient is both hands are free to manipulate books and objects. The disadvantage is the close working distance. Since the working distance is the reciprocal in meters of the dioptric power and powers over+4.00D make binocular fusion problematic with high convergence demands, low vision rehabilitation glasses tend to be reserved for monocular use. This is in keeping with the common asymmetry in visual acuity found in patients with age related macular degeneration and diabetic retinopathy. Monocular spectacle powers in low vision rehabilitation glasses are prescribed in powers as high as+48.00D

Hand held magnifiers are the traditional means of delivering power for spot reading mail, prices in stores and other time limited near visual tasks. They can be lens power alone with a handle or in combination with illumination. Their advantage is easy portability and general inexpensiveness. The chief disadvantage is the necessity to reserve one hand for manipulation of the device while attempting to hold the object of regard with the other. This makes sustained reading difficult.

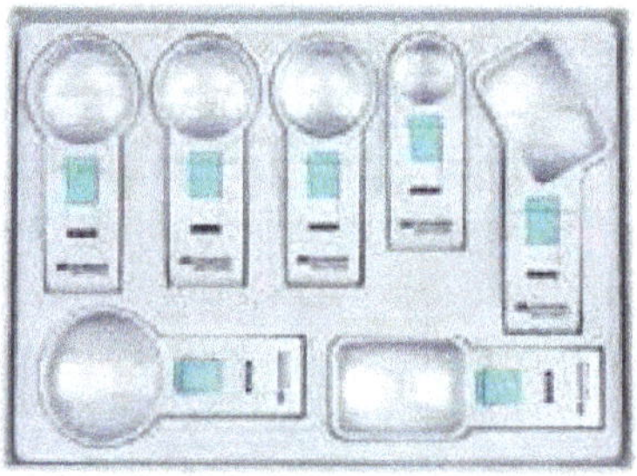

Figure 12. Hand Held Magnifier Set

Stand magnifiers were developed from hand held magnifiers in order to provide an optimal lens placement from the object of regard. While helping to alleviate the issue of managing lens to object distance, stand devices are bulkier and less portable. They can be found with handles and illumination, no handles with open plastic stands or in domes. In any form, spot reading is the primary task for which they are used.

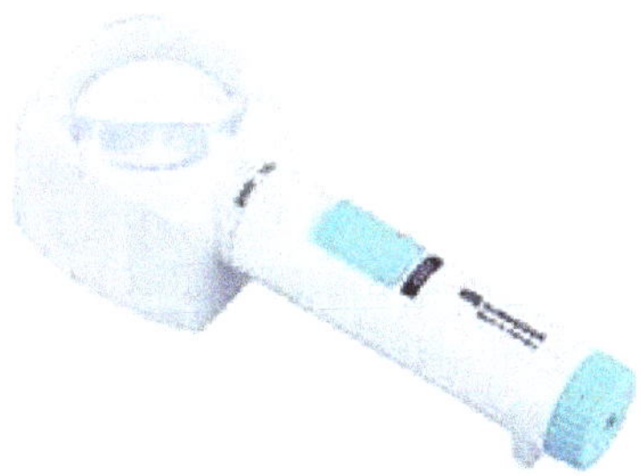

Figure 13. Stand Magnifier with Illumination

Telescopes have traditionally been prescribed for distance tasks such as reading street signs, taking notes from the board or spotting for mobility. New, closer focusing monocular or binocular telescopes allow television watching, computer viewing and even near point reading with extended length or reading caps on the telescope's objective lens. Telescopes can be hand held for spot use as needed or spectacle mounted for more continuous use. The tradeoff for improving distance visual acuity with any telescope is visual field restriction.

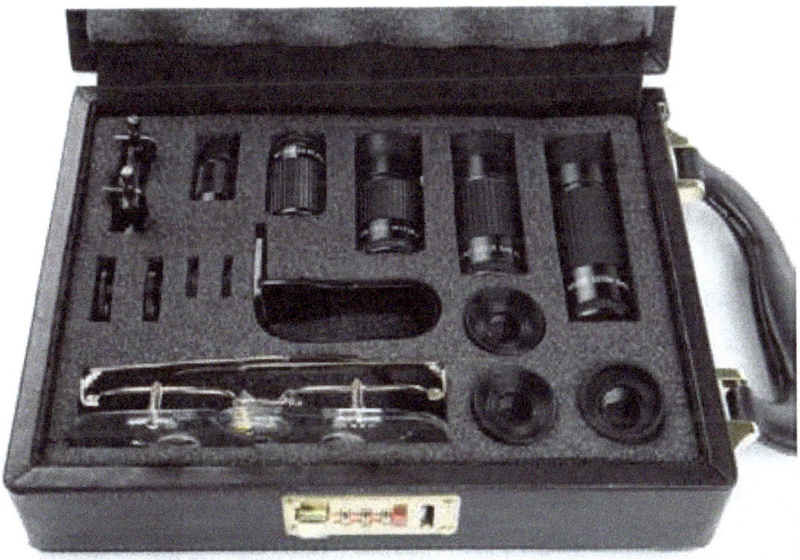

Figure 14. Telescope Set

Although all low vision optical and electronic magnification devices have until recently been extraocular, three intraocular devices have recently been developed; (1) the Implantable

Miniature Telescope (IMT, VisionCare OphthalmicTechnologies,Saratoga,CA), (2) Intraocular Lens for Visually Impaired People (IOL-VIP,IOL-VIP System, Soleko, Pontecorvo, Italy), and (3) Lipschitz Mirror Implant (LMI, Optolight Vision Technology, Herzlia, Israel). The IMT is the only device approved for commercial use in the US. It is implanted in one eye only and it enables patients with end-stage age related macular degeneration to see enlarged views at both distance and near. The internal design allows for a larger field of view than external telescopic devices and the rehabilitation program accompanying the implant supports patients' perceptual adaptation to the 2.7x magnified view. The IMT process requires bi-ocular viewing with the non-implant eye used for wide angle general mobility and the IMT implanted eye used for more detailed activities of daily living such as seeing faces, participating in hobbies, and viewing large print on labels. An increased quality of life score at 6 months post implantation compared to baseline has been demonstrated with the IMT. [38]

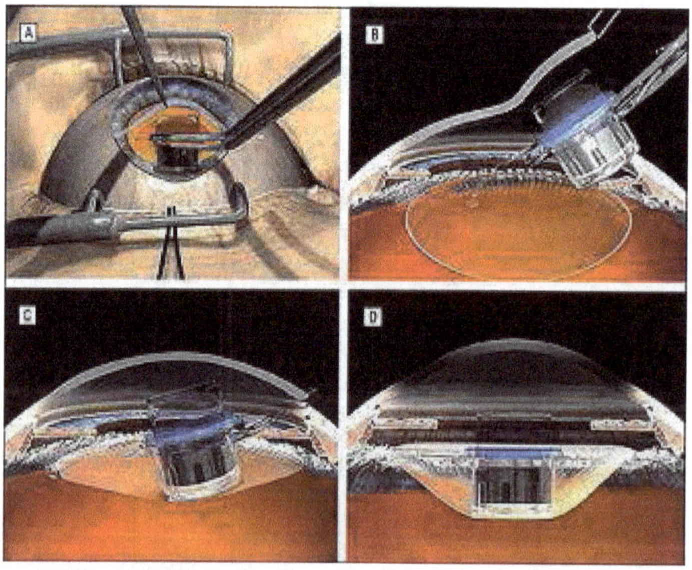

Figure 15. IMT surgical insertion sequence

5.2. *Impact* — Vision enhancement — Non optical

Non-optical vision enhancement has traditionally meant lighting and glare control devices and techniques. These entailed dark glasses, hats with brims, and typoscopes or line guides to cut white page glare while giving peripheral clues to maintain position on the line of letters. The benefits of these devices were subjective and their prescription was done symptomatically with no significant psychometric measure beyond observation of improved performance. This does not diminish their utility, however and a good Occupational Therapist (OT) or low vision trainer can identify useful non-optical devices and teach the techniques of their use in short order with good outcomes.

In recent years, the electronic miniaturization revolution which has given the world cell coverage, smart phones, GPS and mobile connectivity tablets for the fully sighted, has also added a great depth to the armamentarium of the low vision rehabilitation practitioner and opened up a whole world of possibilities to partially sighted and blind patients. Accessibility features are imbedded into every smart phone and tablet that allows many more degrees of freedom in accessing information. Global Positioning System (GPS) and mapping programs inform the patient who cannot see street signs or read storefronts just where they are and what businesses are nearby. Directions for walking routes are a few screen swipes away. A quick picture of an approaching bus and a finger gesture that magnifies the photo enables the person to identify the bus number and route. Similarly, menu items can be read independently and people far away recognized unobtrusively. Specialized apps for the patient with low vision are legion, so many in fact that the Braille Institute [39] has an app just to help organize, categorize and find those apps designed for the visually impaired. Some companies have dedicated their whole enterprise to providing tools and devices for these patients. However, the field of electronic accessibility for the partially sighted changes almost daily so any attempt at detailing it is futile. Suffice it to say that annual meetings for doctors and providers for the visually impaired invariably have sessions on the latest advances and the reader should make the effort to keep abreast of the changes in the field in order to provide the best information and treatment to their patients.

5.3. *Impact* — Vision substitution

When the patient's vision has been reduced to the point that some or all of the functional independence measures are no longer positively impacted by vision enhancement devices, techniques or training, there are still avenues of patient benefit open to the low vision rehabilitation practitioner. That is the field of vision substitution where functional independence can be achieved with devices, techniques and training that do not rely on vision. Some of the more common components of vision substitution are Braille, orientation and mobility (O&M) instruction and audible books. Vision substitution and vision enhancement, however, are not mutually exclusive. In some aspects of functional independence, the patient may perform satisfactorily with vision enhancement while in other functional independence categories they may require vision substitution. An example may be someone who is able to read their mail with high dioptric power devices (vision enhancement) yet is unable to enjoy sustained reading. For them, audible books (vision substitution) are a reasonable accommodation. Additionally, there are devices that provide text to speech or to a file form that allows large viewing on a computer monitor or to a refreshable Braille display. GPS devices without a touch screen empower the functionally blind person with the option of safe, extended and independent travel. Students can quickly receive their assignments electronically rather than having to wait for a Braille transcription. Vision loss no longer has to mean functionality loss when the tools and interprofessional resources of vision substitution are employed by the low vision rehabilitation practitioner. However, this remains an area that has potential not yet fully realized.

6. Conclusion

Low vision rehabilitation is a field which is optimally practiced with a comprehensive, inclusive and interprofessional approach involving optometrists, ophthalmologists, occupational therapists, orientation and mobility specialists, social or rehabilitation workers and teachers of the visually impaired. In our paradigm of *Cause, Effect* and *Impact*, diagnosing and treating in the traditional medical model is shown to be frequently inadequate. We need to also look at incorporating the vocational and rehabilitation model. Determining visual ability in *Cause* by measuring visual acuity, visual fields and contrast sensitivity may not sufficiently take into consideration the functional *Effect* upon the patient's independence in their varied activities of daily life. Therefore, the patient history needs to go beyond the standard queries about chief complaint, review of systems and past, family and social history to a more directed functional survey as seen with quantified functional independence measures (FIM). Early interprofessional referrals thus generated can provide crucial input to the development of a rehabilitation plan that is comprehensive and inclusive addressing the *Effect* through activities of daily life and ultimately *Impact* the patient's qualify of life. Even when the options for vision enhancement are no longer sufficient for the patient, independence can be achieved through interdisciplinary referrals for vision substitution devices, techniques and training. It is incumbent upon the eye doctor to either provide low vision rehabilitation services or refer to those who can.

Acronyms and abbreviations

ADL	Activities of Daily Life
AMD	Age-Related Macular Degeneration
CBS	Charles Bonnet Syndrome
CMS	Center for Medicare & Medicaid Services
DM	Diabetes Mellitus
DR	Diabetic Retinopathy
ETDRS	Early Treatment of Diabetic Retinopathy Study
FIM	Functional Independence Measure
GPS	Global Positioning System
HPI	History of Present Illness
HRQOL	Health Related Quality of Life
IMT	Implantable Miniature Telescope
JND	Just Noticeable Difference
LASER	Light Amplification by the Stimulated Emission of Radiation

LogMAR	Logarithm (base 10) of Minimum Angle of Resolution
LOVIT	Low Vision Intervention Trial
LV	Low Vision
LVR	Low Vision Rehabilitation
MAR	Minimum Angle of Resolution
MN Read	Minnesota Reading Charts
NEI-VFQ	National Eye Institute Vision Function Quality
O&M	Orientation and Mobility
OD	Doctor of Optometry
OT	Occupational Therapist
PFSH	Past, Family and Social History
PRL	Preferred Retinal Locus
QOL	Quality of Life
ROS	Review of Systems
SK Read	Smith-Kettlewell Reading Test
SLO	Scanning LASER Ophthalmoscope
TRL	Trained Retinal Locus
TVI	Teacher of the Visually Impaired
VA	Visual Acuity
VRQOL	Vision Related Quality of Life
WHO	World Health Organization

Acknowledgements

The authors would like to thank Precision Vision of La Salle, Illinois for their generous contribution of images used in this chapter.

Author details

Bennett McAllister[1,2] and Rebecca Kammer[1]

1 Low Vision, American Academy of Optometry, USA

2 Primary Care Service, College of Optometry, Western University of Health Sciences, Pomona, California, USA

References

[1] edited by Robert W. Massof, Lorraine Lidoff Issues in Low Vision Rehabilitation: Service Delivery, Policy, and Funding 2001, AFB Press, NY http://books.google.com/books?hl=en&lr=&id=qm3KCDWxougC&oi=fnd&pg=PR7&dq=Massof,+low+vision+rehabilitation,+book&ots=q82s6fsQUT&sig=lFM6GuU_5R-xXYjKM803ZhaOJN0#v=onepage&q=Massof%2C%20low%20vision%20rehabilitation%2C%20book&f=false

[2] Association of Schools and Colleges of Optometry. http://www.opted.org/files/Entry-LevelCompetencies_LowVision.pdf

[3] Owsley C, McGwin G Jr, Lee PP, Wasserman N, Searcey K Characteristics of low-vision rehabilitation services in the United States. Arch Ophthalmol. 2009 May;127(5): 681-9. doi: 10.1001/archophthalmol.2009.55.

[4] WHO. Main Causes of Vision Impairment. http://www.who.int.blindness/causes/priority/en/indes.html

[5] Tranton JH. Nothing More Can Be Done…A Fable for our Times. Ophthalmology Clinics of North America. June 1994 Volume 7 Number 2

[6] Chous AP. Those who aren't what we call them. doi: 10.1016/j.optm.2008.10.009

[7] CDC. Statement on Vision Loss in America. http://www.cdc.gov/visionhealth/data/national.htm

[8] NIH. NEI. Statement on Age-Related Macular Degeneration. http://www.nei,nih.gov/eyedata/amd.asp

[9] CDC. Statement on Diabetes. http://www.cdc.gov/diabetes/statistics/prev/national/figbyage.htm

[10] Bailey IL, Lovie-Kitchin JE. Visual Acuity Testing. From the Laboratory to the Clinic. Vision Research, Volume 90, September 2013 pages 2-9.

[11] Lovie-Kitchin J Reading with low vision: the impact of research on clinical management. Clin Exp Optom. 2011 Mar;94(2):121-32. doi: 10.1111/j.1444-0938.2010.00565.x. Epub 2011 Jan 26

[12] G T Timberlake, E Peli, E A Essock and R A Augliere. Abstract Reading with a macular scotoma. II. Retinal locus for scanning text.Invest. Ophthalmol. Vis. Sci. August 1987 vol. 28 no. 8 1268-1274

[13] Ronald A. Schuchard, PhD Preferred retinal loci and macular scotoma characteristics in patients with age-related macular degeneration *Canadian Journal of Ophthalmology / Journal Canadien d'Ophtalmologie, Volume 40, Issue 3, June 2005, Pages 303-312*

[14] Déruaz A, Goldschmidt M, Whatham AR, Mermoud C, Lorincz EN, Schnider A, Safran AB. A technique to train new oculomotor behavior in patients with central mac-

ular scotomas during reading related tasks using scanning laser ophthalmoscopy: immediate functional benefits and gains retention. BMC Ophthalmol. 2006 Nov 23;6:35.

[15] Nilsson U, Frennesson C, Nilsson S. Patients with AMD and a large absolute central scotoma can be trained successfully to use eccentric viewing, as demonstrated in a scanning laser ophthalmoscope. *Vision Research* [serial online]. July 2003;43(16): 1777-1787.

[16] Helle K. Falkenberg[a,] Gary S. Rubin[b], Peter J. Bex[c]. Acuity, crowding, reading and fixation stability Vision Research Volume 47, Issue 1, January 2007, Pages 126–135

[17] Mandelcorn MS, Podbielski DW, Mandelcorn ED. Fixation stability as a goal in the treatment of macular disease. Can J Ophthalmol. 2013 Oct;48(5):364-7. doi: 10.1016/j.jcjo.2013.05.006. Epub 2013 Sep 2.

[18] Ronald A. Schuchard, PhD Preferred retinal loci and macular scotoma characteristics in patients with age-related macular degeneration *Canadian Journal of Ophthalmology / Journal Canadien d'Ophtalmologie, Volume 40, Issue 3, June 2005, Pages 303-312*

[19] Markowitz S, Reyes S. Microperimetry and clinical practice: an evidence-based review. *Canadian Journal Of Ophthalmology. Journal Canadien D'ophtalmologie* [serial online]. October 2013;48(5):350-357

[20] Kammer R., Poulter C, Clark J. *The Effect of Altered Stimulus Luminance on the Size of Scotomas Mapped with the Fletcher Central Visual Field Test.* ARVO, Florida, May 2009; poster

[21] Pelli DG, Bex P. Testing Vision: From Laboratory Psychophysical Tests to Clinical Evaluation-Measuring Contrast Sensitivity. Vision Research, Volume 90, September 2013 pages 10-14

[22] Colenbrander A, Fletcher D C. The Mixed Contrast Reading card, a new screening test for contrast sensitivity. In: Jones S, Rubin G, Hamlin D, eds. Vision 2005International Congress Series. London, 2006

[23] Book: Low Vision: Research and New Developments in Rehabilitation edited by A. C. Kooijman, IOS press 1994 Chapter: Optimizing illumination for visually impaired persons; comparing subjective and objective criteria. Ch authors: Cornelissen, Kooijman, Schoot, Bootsma, and Wildt

[24] H Lei and R A Schuchard Using two preferred retinal loci for different lighting conditions in patients with central scotomas. Invest. Ophthalmol. Vis. Sci. August 1997 vol. 38 no. 9 1812-1818

[25] Granger CV, Deutsch A, Linn RT. Rasch analysis of the Functional Independence Measure (FIM) Mastery Test. Arch Phys Med Rehabil. 1998 Jan;79(1):52-7.

[26] Young Y, Fan MY, Hebel JR, Boult C. Concurrent validity of administering the functional independence measure (FIM) instrument by interview. Am J Phys Med Rehabil. 2009 Sep;88(9):766-70. doi: 10.1097/PHM.0b013e3181a9f1d6.

[27] [27]Khadka J, McAlinden C, Pesudovs K. Quality assessment of ophthalmic questionnaires: review and recommendations. Optom Vis Sci. 2013 Aug;90(8):720-44. doi: 10.1097/OPX.0000000000000001.

[28] (no authors listed) The World Health Organization Quality of Life Assessment (WHOQOL): Position paper from the World Health Organization. Soc Sci Med. 1995 Nov;41(10):1403-9

[29] http://www.cdc.gov/hrqol/concept.htm

[30] de Boer MR, Moll AC, de Vet HC, Terwee CB, Volker-Dieben HJ, van Rens GH. Psychometric Properties of Vision-Related Quality of Life Questionnaires: a Systematic Review. Ophthalmic Physician Opt. 2004 Jul;24(4):257-73

[31] Eramudugolla R, Wood J, Anstery KJ. Co-Morbidity of Depression and Anxiety in Common Age-Related Eye Diseases. Frontiers in Aging Neuroscience. October 2013 doi: 10.3389/fnagi.2013.00056

[32] Owsley C. Aging and vision. Vision Res. 2011 Jul 1;51(13):1610-22. doi: 10.1016/j.visres.2010.10.020. Epub 2010 Oct 23.

[33] Renaud J, Bédard E Depression in the elderly with visual impairment and its association with quality of life. Clin Interv Aging. 2013;8:931-43. doi: 10.2147/CIA.S27717. Epub 2013 Jul 19.

[34] Rees G, Mellor D, Heenan M, Fenwick E, Keeffe JE, Marella M, Lamoureux EL. Depression training program for eye health and rehabilitation professionals. Optom Vis Sci. 2010 Jul;87(7):494-500. doi: 10.1097/OPX.0b013e3181df5286.

[35] [35] Khan JC, Shahid H, Thurlby DA, Yates JRW, and Moore AT. Charles Bonnet Syndrome in Age-Related Macular Degeneration: The Nature and Frequency of Images in Subjects with End-Stage Disease. *Ophthalmic Epidemiology,* 15:202–208ISSN: 0928-6586 print / 1744-5086 online Copyright c 2008 Informa Healthcare USA, Inc. DOI: 10.1080/09286580801939320 p.202-208

[36] [36] Ffytche DH, Howard RJ, Brammer MJ, David A, Woodruff P, Williams S. The anatomy of conscious vision: An fMRI study of visual hallucinations. *Nat Neurosci.* 1998;1:738–42.

[37] Liu CJ, Brost MA, Horton VE, Kenyon SB, Mears KE. Occupational therapy interventions to improve performance of daily activities at home for older adults with low vision: a systematic review. Am J Occup Ther. 2013 May-Jun;67(3):279-87. doi: 10.5014/ajot.2013.005512.

[38] Singer A, Amir N., Herro A., Porbandarwalla S., Pollard J. Improving quality of life in patients wit end-stage age-related macular degeneration: focus on miniature ocular implants. Clinical Ophthalmology 2012:6 33–39

[39] Braille Institute. Visually Impaired Apps. https://itunes.apple.com/us/app/via-by-braille-institute/id528499232?mt=8 http://www.who.int/blindness/causes/priority/en/index5.html

6

New Understandings on Pathogenesis of Dry Eye — From Animal Models to Clinical Therapy

Cintia S. de Paiva, Andrew J.W. Huang,
De-Quan Li and Stephen C. Pflugfelder

1. Introduction

As defined by the International Dry Eye Workshop, dry eye is a multifactorial disease of the tears and ocular surface with symptoms of discomfort, visual disturbance, and tear film instability with potential damage to the ocular surface resulting in a dysfunctional lacrimal functional unit [1]. It is one of the most common medical problems that affects 6 to 44 million people in the United States based on reported prevalence figures of 4 to 33% from large epidemiological studies [2-4].

Dry eye affects quality of vision and quality of life. It is also associated with a significant financial burden to the individual and society [5, 6]. It has been shown that dry eye significantly decreases work productivity among office workers, by preventing them from performing at their full potential [7]. The cost of work performance loss associated with dry eye was estimated to be between $10-15 million/year in Japan [7].

The corneal surface irregularity in dry eye degrades visual function by decreasing contrast sensitivity and functional visual acuity [8]. Visual impairment is one of the 10 most common disabilities and vision impacts mobility, independence and quality of life. The presence of dry eye was found to significantly impact the ability to perform daily activities such as reading, using a computer and driving [9]. Visual impairments associated with dry eye disease have been associated with falls and hip fractures in the elderly [10], and complications from these falls is the leading cause of death from injury in men and women over the age of 65 [11]. As vision deteriorates, one's ability to perform activities of daily living becomes exceedingly more difficult. Using time trade off techniques, Schiffman and colleagues calculated that patients with severe dry eye expecting to live 10 years or more, were willing to give up 1.6 years of that time to be disease free [12], an amount similar to patients with moderate to severe angina [13]. Even though dry eye is a chronic disease, dry eye patients often complain about daily exacerbations. One frequent complaint is worsening of irritation symptoms and vision after prolonged use of a computer or grocery shopping.

While its pathogenesis has not been fully elucidated, it has been shown that changes in tear composition including increased proinflammatory cytokines, chemokines, metalloproteinases, increased expression of immune activation and adhesion molecules by the conjunctival epithelium and increased number of T lymphocytes in the conjunctiva play a pathogenic role in both dry eye patients and in animal models [14-21]. Increased knowledge has shown that inflammation is responsible in part for the irritation symptoms, ocular surface epithelial disease including loss of goblet cell, conjunctival metaplasia, and altered corneal epithelial barrier function in dry eye. This book chapter will discuss diverse pathogenic aspects of dry eye.

2. Experimental animal models of dry eye

There are several animal models of dry eye currently used throughout the world. They have been used to evaluate the natural history of the disease, to elucidate pathogenic mechanisms (risk factors and molecular mediators, pathways) and also to evaluate efficacy of therapeutic candidates. Models of dry eye rely on decreasing tear volume and production. To achieve that, surgical excision of the lacrimal gland, injection of pro-inflammatory cytokine IL-1 or isolated lymphocytes into the lacrimal gland, pharmacological blockade of lacrimal gland secretion have been used [22-24]. Autoimmune strains have also been studied. These strains have age-related lymphocytic infiltration of the lacrimal and salivary glands and ocular surface inflammation mimicking Sjögren's syndrome to a certain extent. These include the non-obese diabetic (NOD), MRL/Lpr, NZB/W F1 mouse, and TGF-β1, CD25 and Thrombospondin knock-out (KO) strains [25-32].

We have developed an inducible experimental murine dry eye model where wild-type mice are subjected to an environmental stress for five or ten days and lacrimal gland secretion is pharmacologically inhibited by administration of scopolamine. Mice are kept in an environmentally controlled room where relative humidity is kept below 30% at all times. Mice subjected to this experimental model develop conjunctival goblet cell (GC) loss and increased CD4+T cell infiltration in the conjunctival epithelium (Figure 1A) and increased expression of inflammatory mediators, corneal barrier disruption measured by a fluorescent dye (Figure 1B) similar to human dry eye patients (Figure 1C). Since the initial studies, this experimental model has been used extensively by us and other groups within the US but also worldwide. A significant body of evidence providing insight into the pathogenesis of dry eye has been derived from this animal model and will be discussed in more detailed in the sequential topics.

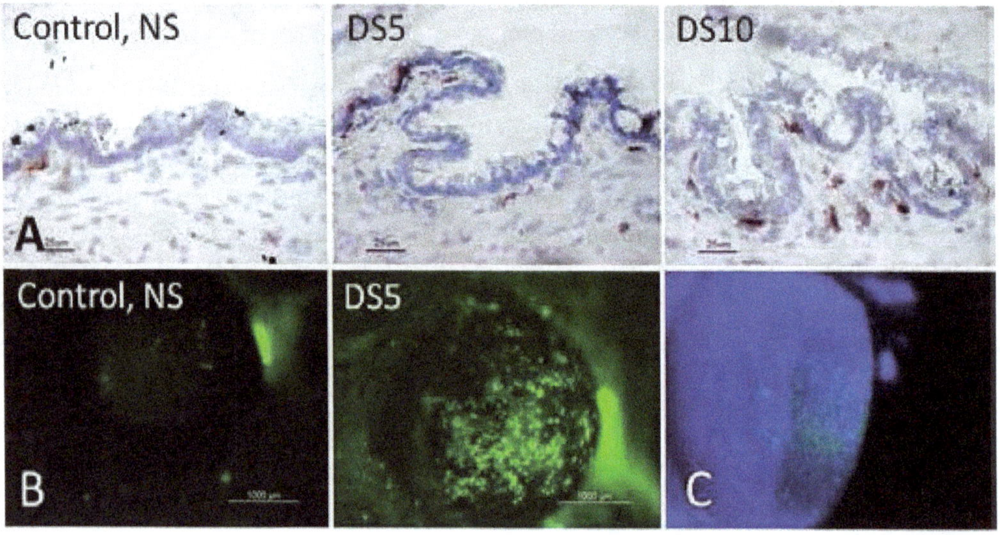

Figure 1. A. Representative images of immunohistochemical CD4+staining (red cells) in the goblet cell rich area of the conjunctiva of C57BL/6 mice without desiccating stress (control, non-stressed, NS) and with desiccating stress for 5 or 10 days (DS5 or DS10, respectively). **B.** Representative images of Oregon-Green-Dextran corneal staining in C57BL/6 mice without desiccating stress (control, non-stressed "NS") and with desiccating stress for 5 days (DS5). **C.** Representative image of human cornea stained with sodium fluorescein and visualized under a blue filter showing punctate dry spots in central cornea.

3. Role of tear hyperosmolarity

Hyperosmolarity has been shown to be a potent pro-inflammatory stimulus involved in the pathogenesis of the ocular surface disease of dry eye, termed keratoconjunctivitis sicca (KCS). Von Bahr was the first to suggest in 1941 that tear film osmolarity is dependent on tear secretion and evaporation, and that decreased secretion would lead to increased osmolarity [33]. Balik appears to have been the first to suggest in 1952 that the corneal and conjunctival changes in KCS could be explained on the basis of an increased "concentration of sodium chloride" in the tear film [34]. It would not be until two decades later that Mishima and colleagues were able to evaluate tear osmolarity and found an elevation of about 25 mOsm/liter in six eyes with KCS [35]. Subsequent studies reported significantly increased tear fluid osmolarity in patients with KCS, with the mean value 343 ± 32 (SD) mOsM, and the ranging up to 441 mOsM [36]. Based on its sensitivity and specificity, tear osmolarity was proposed as a gold standard diagnostic test for dry eye by Farris in 1992 [37], which was further evidenced by the fact that the use of sodium hyaluronate eye drops with pronounced hypotonicity showed greater therapeutic efficacy on the severity of Sjögren's syndrome associated KCS than isotonic solutions [38].

In rabbit dry eye models, the elevated tear film osmolarity caused decreased corneal glycogen and reduced conjunctival goblet cell density, as well as pathological changes in the corneal epithelium, such as increased desquamation, decreased intercellular connections, blunting and loss of microplicae, cell membrane disruptions and cellular swelling [39-41]. In mice following 2 days of DS, tear volume significantly decreased from 0.066ul to 0.026ul in C57BL/6J and 0.093ul to 0.028ul in BALB/c mice while tear osmolarity concomitantly and significantly increased from 177 to 300 mOsM in C57BL/6J mice, and nearly doubled from 285 to 559 mOsM in BALB/C mice. Topical treatment of ocular surface with hypertonic saline (500 mOsM) was found to stimulate expression and production of interleukin (IL)-1β, tumor necrosis factor (TNF) α and MMP-9 by the corneal and conjunctival epithelia, when compared with age matched controls and mice treated with iso-osmolar (305 mOsM) balanced salt solution [42, 43]. In our murine dry eye model [44], the stimulated expression of pro-inflammatory mediator, TNF-α, IL-1β and MMP-9 was observed [45]. The mitogen-activated protein kinases (MAPKs) are well conserved signaling pathways that include extracellular signal regulated kinases (ERK), c-Jun N-terminal kinases (JNK) and p38 MAPK [46-48]. Interestingly, the levels of phosphorylated JNK1/2, ERK1/2, and p38 MAPKs in the corneal and conjunctival epithelia were markedly increased in mice treated with hypertonic saline [45].

In human corneal epithelial cultures, the expression and production of a number of pro-inflammatory mediators, IL-1β, TNF-α, IL-8, and MMPs, including gelatinase MMP-9, collagenases MMP-1 and MMP-13, and stromelysin MMP-3 were progressively increased as the media osmolarity increased from 312 mOsM to 500 mOsM [49, 50]. Activated phospor (p)-JNK-1/p-JNK-2 and p-ERK-1/p-ERK-2 were also detected by Western blot and peaked at 60 minutes in cells exposed to hypertonic media. The levels of p-JNK-1/p-JNK-2 and p-ERK1/p-ERK2 were positively correlated with the medium osmolarity. The inhibitors for JNK or ERK pathways, SB202190, PD98059 and doxycycline markedly suppressed the levels of phosphor-JNKs and/or ERKs, as well as these proinflammatory markers. Other investigators also showed that hyperosmolarity induced the pro-inflammatory cytokine and chemokines IL-6, IL-8 and monocyte chemotactic protein-1 in cultured human corneal epithelial cells [51]. The efficacy of doxycycline in treating ocular surface diseases may be due to its ability to suppress JNK and ERK signaling activation and inflammatory mediator production in the corneal epithelium.

Another hallmark of dry eye is cornea and conjunctiva metaplasia, where the normal epithelium undergoes terminal differentiation and becomes keratinized [52]. The cornea is a highly transparent tissue and this abnormal keratinization process can lead to corneal irregularity and blurred vision [53, 54]. In mice, we observed that desiccating stress induces expression of cornified envelope proteins, including involucrin and small proline-rich proteins 2a and 2b in both cornea and conjunctiva [21, 55]. We also observed that stress-associated pathway, such as JNK, ERK and p38 MAPK are activated in hours after desiccating stress starts [21, 43, 45].

We found increased levels of active phosphorylated JNK1 and JNK2 (JNK2 JNK1) in ocular surface epithelia treated with hypertonic saline in vivo and in cultured human corneal epithelial cells exposed to hyperosmolar media [45, 49, 56]. In vivo, we showed that the JNK2 protein but not JNK1, appears to have an essential role in desiccation-induced corneal epithelial disease by stimulating production of MMP-1, MMP-9, and cornified envelope precursors as JNK2KO mice were resistant to dry eye-induced changes [20].

4. Role of matrix metalloproteinases

The hallmark of dry eye disease is the increased permeability of corneal epithelium to fluorescent dyes, clinically observed as fluorescent punctate spots. Because epithelial corneal disease is responsible for the irritation and blurred vision symptoms reported by most dry eye patients, corneal epithelium health is very important. The epithelium is not bystander, but actively responds to desiccating stress by secreting inflammatory cytokines, chemokimes and matrix metalloproteinases (MMPs).

Matrix degrading enzymes including MMPs have been identified as important factors in the inflammatory and wound healing response of the ocular surface, particularly in dry eye and ocular burns. Their induction during wound healing is thought to play a role in extracellular matrix remodeling, cytokine activation, and regulation of angiogenesis [57]. The MMP family includes more than 25 members that can be divided into collagenases that degrade fibrillar collagen types I, II, and III (MMP-1, -8, -13); gelatinases that degrade collagen types IV, V, and VII and X as well as decorin, fibronectin, and laminin, that are found in basement membranes (MMP-2,-9); stromelysins (MMP-3, and -10); matrilysins that degrade proteoglycans, laminin, and glycoproteins (MMP-7 and -26); and the membrane-type MMPs that are bound to epithelial cell membranes, and can activate MMPs, according to their structure and substrate specificity (MMPs 14-17, and -24) [58-61]. Collectively they are able to degrade the entire extracellular matrix and basement membranes components. Barely detected in an unwounded cornea, MMPs are strongly induced during wound healing. Among these, MMP–9 plays a prominent role being produced by stressed cornea and conjunctival epithelial cells and has both matrix degrading and pro-inflammatory activities [62-64].

Several members of MMPs have been found to increase in the corneal epithelium after experimental dry eye and MMP-9 (Figure 2) [57]. MMP-9 has been found in tear fluid of dry eye patients [65]. Of special interest, we have shown that epithelium-secreted MMP-9 after experimental dry eye activates TGF-β [66], breaks-down the apical corneal epithelial tight junctions (Figure 3), facilitating corneal barrier dysfunction [21, 57, 67] and accelerating corneal desquamation [68].

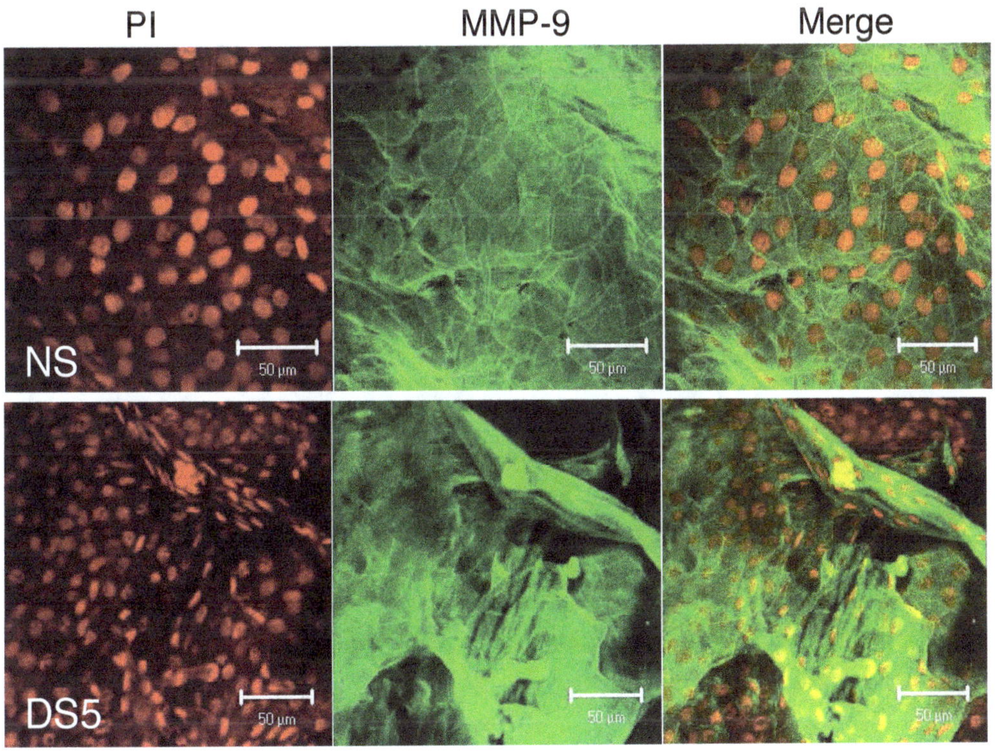

Figure 2. Laser scanning confocal microscopy of wholemount murine corneas stained for MMP-9 (in green) with propidium iodide nuclear counterstaining (PI, in red), organized into non-stressed (NS) and desiccating stress for 5 days (DS5).

MMP-9 knock-out mice are resistant to these changes, but exogenous topical administration of MMP-9 to MMP-9KO mice induced increased corneal permeability in similar range to wild-type control mice. Moreover, cultured human corneal epithelial cells treated with MMP-9 showed breakdown of tight junction proteins, notably occludin [67]. In human dry eye patients, increased MMP-9 mRNA transcripts in conjunctiva and increased MMP-9 activity in tears was noted compared to normal subjects; increased MMP-9 activity in tears positively correlated with symptom score, cornea and conjunctiva staining, low contrast visual acuity and inversely correlated with tear-break-up [54]. In a group of dry eye patients, we observed that tear MMP-9 activity levels increased as the severity of corneal disease progressed (Table 1) [54].

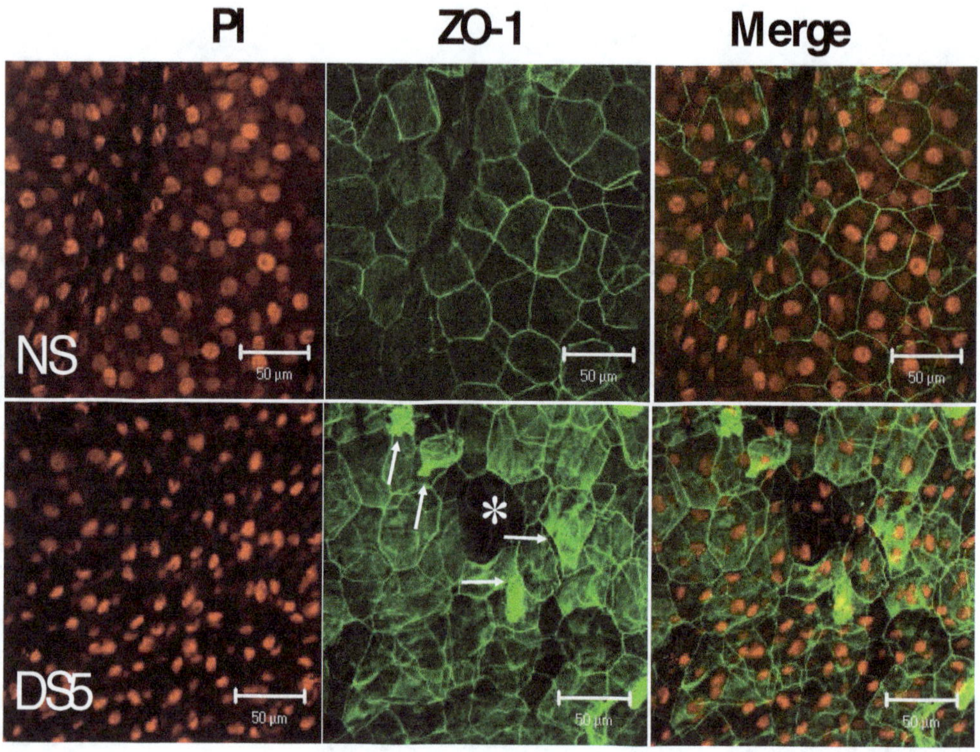

Figure 3. Laser scanning confocal microscopy of wholemount murine corneas stained for zona occludens 1 (ZO-1, in green) with propidium iodide nuclear counterstaining (PI, in red), organized into non-stressed (NS) and desiccating stress for 5 days (DS5). The NS controls show uniform cell with membrane staining while the DS5 corneas have increased apical cell loss (asterisk) and increase desquamation (arrows show either broken ZO-1 or cells that are rolling up).

Group	MMP-9 Activity (ng/mL)
Normal (n=18)	8.39 ± 4.70
Dysfunctional tear syndrome 1 (n=10)	62.40 ± 49.33**
Dysfunctional tear syndrome 2 (n=20)	58.84 ± 49.46**
Dysfunctional tear syndrome 3 (n=07)	116.99 ± 138.18**
Dysfunctional tear syndrome 4 (n=11)	360.25 ± 168.83**◆◆

Note: DTS=dysfunctional tear syndrome ** *P*<0.004 versus normal;◆◆*P* <0.007 versus normal and the other severity based DTS groups

Table 1. Tear MMP-9 activity levels among normal subjects and dry eye patients stratified by 4 levels of severity according to the Delphi Panel [69] [range from DTS1 (very mild) to DTS4 (severe dry eye)]

5. The conjunctiva acts as an exogenous lymphoid tissue

Similar to other mucosal tissues, the conjunctiva is covered with epithelium containing dendritic antigen presenting cells and a variety of intraepithelial lymphocyte (IEL) populations, lymphocytes that reside outside the lymphoid organs and in contact with epithelial cells in the gut, skin and lungs [70]. To date, several subsets of IELs have been identified in the mouse and human conjunctiva, including CD4$^+$, CD8$^+$, gammadelta $(\gamma\delta)^+$and NK$^+$ cells[71-74]. The CD103 integrin has been used as a marker for IEL in different mucosal sites because it mediates homing and retention of lymphocytes to the epithelium. Its ligand, E-cadherin is highly expressed on mucosal epithelial cells [75, 76].

An important breakthrough in recent studies is the discovery of a link between the ocular surface epithelium and immune cells. Soluble factors from immune cells have been found to be either pathogenic or homeostatic to cornea and conjunctiva epithelium. Early biopsies from Sjögren's Syndrome (SS) patients have shown lymphocytic infiltration in the lacrimal gland and activated T cells have been detected in the conjunctiva dry eye patients [77-82]. Animal studies using the adoptive transfer experiment showed that dry eye can be induced in T cell deficient nude mice that had never been exposed to desiccated stress by adoptively transferring CD4$^+$T cells from dry eye mouse model [83]. This landmark study showed that immunocompetent recipients will only develop disease when regulatory cells are depleted with antibody to CD25 [83]. Taken together, these experiments showed that: 1) dry eye is indeed an autoimmune disease, since goblet cell loss and CD4$^+$T infiltration was seen in naïve mice receiving cells but never subjected to DS; 2) confirmed the pathogenic role of CD4$^+$T cells as adoptive transfer of unfractionated or non-CD4+T cells had minimal effect; 3) showed that CD4$^+$T cells primed in vivo during DS will migrate back to ocular surface tissues and LG; 4) dry eye induces a systemic immune response, as adoptive transfer of splenic CD4$^+$T cells was sufficient to induce disease and 5) provided a mechanism to evaluate different components of the immune system.

T helper (Th) CD4$^+$T cells have been classically divided into Th-1, Th-2 and Th-17. Th-1 responses are important for controlling viral, fungal and intracellular bacterial infections. Th-1 cells are classically identified by the production of interferon-gamma (IFN-γ). Once committed, the Th-1 cells activate macrophages and induce IgG2a production by B cells. Th-2 responses are frequently found in allergic diseases, such as asthma, and are particularly important in the host response to parasites and helminthes in the gut. Th-2 cell differentiation is promoted by interleukin (IL)-4 and it is characterized by production of IL-4, IL-13 and IL-5. The Th-2 committed cells promote IgG1 and IgE class switching and eosinophil recruitment. Th-17 cells are important in responding to extracellular bacterial and fungal pathogens, by recruiting neutrophils and macrophages to infected tissues and have been implicated in autoimmunity [84-86].

Migration of CD4+T cells into the conjunctival and cornea in dry eye disease may be modulated by chemokine ligands produced by the surface epithelium that increase in dryness. Pathogenic CD4 cells that infiltrate the ocular surface tissues express receptors to these ligands [18, 87, 88].

5.1. Th-1 CD4+T cells in dry eye

Th-1 committed CD4+T cells secrete IFN-γ. CXCL9, CXCL10, CXCL11, IFN-γ inducible chemokines, are highly expressed after experimental desiccating stress in both cornea and conjunctiva [87-89] which will in turn attract more Th-1 cells, serving as an amplifying mechanism.

IFN-γ has been proposed as a biomarker for dry eye disease and SS because elevated IFN-γ, either protein or RNA levels, has been detected in tears [90-97], conjunctiva [96-100], saliva [101, 102], lacrimal [26, 103-108], submandibular glands [94, 103, 109-111], and blood [112, 113].

Increased IFN-γ concentration in tears of dry eye patients detected by ELISA was reported more than a decade ago. More sensitive immunoassays, such as Luminex and antibody microarrays used in subsequent studies have confirmed these early results [90, 92-96]. In addition to dry eye, increased tear IFN-γ concentration has also been found in patients with sicca symptoms after bone marrow transplantation [90] and in tears of SS patients [91, 93]. Among the various subsets of dysfunctional tear syndrome, those with meibomian gland disease (MGD) had significantly lower IFN-γ concentration than those without MGD [91, 92] and tear IFN-γ concentration was found to correlate with corneal fluorescein staining score [91]. It is possible that inflamed lacrimal glands in patients with SS are one source for their increased tear IFN-γ.

Similarly to tears [90], increased IFN-γ has been found in saliva of SS patients and its presence correlated with sicca symptoms [101]. Interestingly, increased Th1/Th2 ratios was observed in more severe SS cases [114-116], where increased Th-2 response correlated with milder SS [101, 102, 117, 118]. Virtually every mouse autoimmune model that mimics SS or even environmentally-induced mouse dry eye models have shown increased expression of IFN-γ in LG and submandibular gland [26, 103-109, 118]. Increased expression of IFN-γ mRNA has also been observed in the conjunctiva, both in dry eye patients and mice subjected to dry eye [18, 96-100]. We have shown that IFN-γ induces conjunctiva metaplasia and apoptosis and loss of conjunctival goblet cells [97, 119, 120]. IFN-γKO mice are resistant to dry eye induced changes but reconstitution of KO mice with exogenous IFN-γ induces goblet cell loss in similar magnitude as wild-type mice and this was accompanied by cornification and apoptosis of conjunctival epithelium [97, 120]. It has also been shown that IFN-γ significantly decreases epithelial mucin expression [121]. Adoptive transfer of CD4+T cells from donor mice exposed to desiccating stress that received anti-IFN-γ were less pathogenic to immunodeficient mice recipients, yielding less corneal apoptosis and greater number of PAS+filled goblet cells [119]. Mice that received subconjunctival injections of anti-IFN-γ antibody showed decreased corneal and conjunctival apoptosis [98, 119].

5.2. Th-17 and NK cells in dry eye

IL-17A is the signature cytokine of the new discovered Th subtype, Th-17. The differentiation of Th17 cells from naïve $CD4^{+}T$ cells is regulated by cytokines [122]. Transforming growth factor-β (TGF-β) and IL-6, broadly expressed by many cell types in the body, including dendritic and epithelial cells, are dominant in the initiation of Th17 cell differentiation [122-124]. IL-23, IL-1β and IL-21, which are products of activated dendritic cells, macrophages, activated T cell or inflamed epithelial cells, possibly expand and maintain the differentiated Th17 cells in the presence of IL-6 and TGF-β1 [122, 125, 126]. Furthermore, signal transducer and activator of transcription 3 (STAT3) has been found to mediate the initiation of Th17 cell differentiation by these inducing cytokines [127].

TGF-β is a critical factor in Th-17 differentiation. TGF-β is a pleiotropic cytokine that can have pro- or anti-inflammatory effects depending on the context. It regulates various biologic processes such as embryonic development, cell proliferation and differentiation, extracellular matrix synthesis, immune response, inflammation, and apoptosis [128]. TGF-β1 is produced by the human lacrimal gland (LG) and corneal and conjunctiva epithelia and has been detected in tears [129, 130]. Elevated levels of bioactive TGF-β1 in tears and elevated TGF-β1 mRNA transcripts in conjunctiva and minor salivary glands of human Sjögren's Syndrome (SS) patients has also been reported [18, 78, 131, 132].

We addressed the role of TGF-β in the Th-17 response in the conjunctiva by evaluating TGF-β dominant-negative TGF-β type II receptor (CD4-DNTGFβRII) mice. These mice have a truncated TGF-β receptor in $CD4^+T$ cells, rendering them unresponsive to TGF-β. These mice exhibit an age-related dry eye phenotype at 14 weeks of age; however, when subjected to desiccating stress, we observed that DS improved their corneal barrier function and corneal surface irregularity, increased their number of PAS+GC, and lowered $CD4^+T$ cell infiltration in conjunctiva. In contrast to WT, CD4-DNTGFβRII mice did not generate a Th-17 and Th-1 response, and they failed to upregulate MMP-9, IL-23, IL-17A, RORγT, IFN-γ and T-bet mRNA transcripts in conjunctiva. RAG1KO recipients of adoptively transferred CD4+T cells isolated from DS5 CD4-DNTGFβRII showed milder dry eye phenotype and less conjunctival inflammation than recipients of WT control [19].

Thrombospondin-1 (TSP-1) is an extracellular matrix protein that activates TGF-β1. When covalently bound to TGF-β1, the latency associated peptide (LAP) blocks its active site and renders the molecule inactive. This immature form of TGF-β1 naturally equilibrates with its active state via detachment from LAP. Thrombospondin-1 stabilizes the covalent binding sites on the disassociated LAP, thereby preventing its interaction and subsequent inhibition of TGF-β1 [133]. As a result, increased levels of TSP-1 in the presence of TGF-β1 are linked to greater levels of active TGF-β1 [133, 134]. Interestingly, similar to our findings in the CD4-DNTGFβRII mice, TSP-1KO mice had decreased corneal surface dye staining, increased number of conjunctival goblet cells and low levels of inflammatory cytokine mRNA transcripts in cornea tissue compared to WT mice. We also showed that adoptive transfer of WT bone-marrow DC into TSP-1KO reverted the TSP-1KO resistance to desiccating stress, showing that DC-derived TSP is critical for the immune dry eye phenotype [135].

The corneal epithelium responds quickly to different stressors. Cultured human corneal epithelial cells challenged by hyperosmotic media (450 mOsM), microbial components (polyI:C, flagellin, R837, and other TLR ligands) and TNF-alpha responded by significantly increasing expression of IL-6, TGF-β and IL-1β and IL-23 mRNA transcripts. Interestingly, when incubated with conditioned media of HCECs irritated by polyI:C or TNF-α, $CD4^+$ T cells displayed increased mRNA levels of IL-17A, IL-17F, IL-22, CCL-20, and STAT3, increased IL-17 protein in the supernatant, and increased numbers of IL-17-producing T cells (Th17 cells). These findings demonstrate for the first time that Th17 differentiation can be promoted by cytokines produced by corneal epithelium that are exposed to hyperosmotic, microbial, and inflammatory stimuli [136].

Th17 cells can be identified by expression of CCR6 surface receptors [137-139]. CCR6 only ligand known, CCL20, is highly expressed after injuries to epithelium, including experimental desiccating stress [18]. Dry eye has been demonstrated to cause inflammation on the ocular surface, evidenced by increased levels of inflammatory cytokines (IL-1, IL-6, IL-17 and TNF-α) in the tear fluid and corneal and conjunctival epithelium, and an increased infiltration of DCs and T lymphocytes in the conjunctiva [18, 79, 83, 96, 136, 140-144]. Increased levels of IL-17, IL-23 and IL-6 were also found in saliva and salivary glands biopsies obtained from patients with the severe autoimmune dry eye condition, Sjögren's syndrome [145-147].

Evidence in mouse models of dry eye indicates that IL-17 stimulates production of MMP-3 and MMP-9 that contribute to disruption of corneal epithelial barrier function. Recent studies have shown that antibody neutralization of IL-17 ameliorated corneal barrier disruption in mice subjected to desiccating stress [18, 148] and decreased expression of MMP-3 and-9 mRNA transcripts in the corneal epithelium [18], providing a definitive link between epithelial and immune cells in this process.

5.3. Goblet Cells in dry eye

The conjunctival epithelium is part of the few tissues in the body where goblet cells are present, including the gut and the airway epithelia. Goblet cell loss is another clinical characteristic of ocular surface diseases, including dry eye, Stevens-Johnson and ocular graft-versus-host-diseases [149, 150]. Both NK and NKT cells are resident cells in conjunctiva [142]. NK cells are a subtype of lymphocytes that lack expression of the antigen receptors expressed by B and T cells; their name is derived from their ability to recognize and kill malignant cells. NKT cells are defined as NK cells that express conventional T cell receptor (TCR). Both cell types are important source of inflammatory cytokines, notably after encountering pathogens (viruses, bacteria and protozoans). NKT cells have been involved in mucosal immunity and in a variety of inflammatory/autoimmune diseases, such as experimental murine and human ulcerative colitis, asthma, multiple sclerosis and skin diseases (atopic dermatitis, psoriasis) [151-153].

Using isolation techniques, we identified that NKT-derived IL-13 is trophic factor for conjunctival goblet cells, as IL-13KO and STAT6KO strains had lower goblet cell density than their wild-type control mice [154]. In experimental murine dry eye, IL-13 significantly decreased in tears after 5 and 10 days in Th-1 prone C57BL/6 mice, while it increased in BALB/C mice that have been found to develop less severe corneal and conjunctival disease in response to desiccating stress [96].

NK cells participate in the initiation of the immune response by releasing IFN-γ [99] and IL-17A and by decreasing dendritic cell activation [142]. NK cells have been implicated in both the regulation and immunopathogenesis of dry eye disease since they are an early source of IFN-γ during the induction phase of experimental dry eye disease [99]. Systemic depletion of NK cells prior and during DS led to a decrease in the frequency of total and activated DCs, a decrease in T helper-17(+) cells in the cervical lymph nodes and generation of less pathogenic $CD4^+T$ cells. B6.nude recipient mice of adoptively transferred $CD4^+T$ cells isolated from NK-depleted DS5 donor mice showed significantly less corneal barrier disruption, lower levels of IL-17A, CCL20 and MMP-3 in the cornea epithelia compared to recipients of control $CD4^+T$ cells [142].

5.4. Regulatory T Cells in dry eye

Resident $CD8^+T$ cells have been found in the epithelium and stroma of normal human and mouse conjunctiva [97, 155], but their function remains unknown. In non-ocular tissues, $CD8^+T$ cells have been found to have an immunoregulatory function. In the Lewis rat, peripheral tolerance to orally administered antigens was mediated by TGF-β secreting $CD8^+T$ cells [156, 157]. In the iris, $CD8^+T$ cells once activated in the presence of parenchymal cells, expressed and secreted enhanced amounts of TGF-β2 [158]. In certain conjunctival inflammatory conditions, including graft-versus-host disease, Sjögren's syndrome and human and experimental murine keratoconjunctivitis, a significant decrease in $CD8^+T$ cells with concomitant increase in CD4/CD8 ratio in the conjunctiva has been observed [74, 97, 159].

We have identified that $CD8^+$ T cells can also function as regulatory cells. $CD8^+$ T cell depletion promoted generation of IL-17A producing $CD4^+T$ cells via activation of dendritic cells in both the ocular surface and draining cervical lymph nodes in C57BL/6 mice subjected to DS. T cell-deficient nude recipient mice receiving adoptively transferred $CD4^+T$ cells from $CD8^+$cell-depleted donors exposed to DS displayed increased $CD4^+T$ cell infiltration and elevated IL-17A and CCL20 levels in the ocular surface, which was associated with greater corneal barrier disruption. Enhanced DS-specific corneal barrier disruption in CD8-depleted donor mice correlated with a Th17-mediated expression of MMP-3 and 9 in the recipient corneal epithelium. Co-transfer of $CD8^+CD103^+$Tregs did not affect the ability of DS-specific pathogenic $CD4^+T$ cells to infiltrate and cause ocular surface disease in the nude recipients, showing that $CD8^+$cells regulate the afferent arm of DS-induced immune response. In summary, $CD8^+$regulatory cells suppress generation of a pathogenic Th17 response that plays a pivotal role in DS-induced disruption of corneal barrier function [160].

6. Therapeutic strategies: from bench side to clinic

Traditionally, dry eye was treated with palliative solutions and frequent instillation of artificial tears. With the change of paradigm and recognition of the role of inflammation in the disease, several other modalities of treatment entered the pipeline. Animal models have suggested potential agents/pathways.

Anti-protease therapy is very effective in treating dry eye associated corneal epithelial disease. Previously reported studies using our experimental dry eye model demonstrated that the

MMP inhibitor doxycycline and the steroid methylprednisolone was efficacious in decreasing gelatinolytic activity and levels of MMP-9 transcripts in corneal epithelium, as well as preventing the dry eye-induced increase in inflammatory cytokines IL-1 and TNF-α [161]. Doxycycline also improved corneal surface regularity and improved corneal barrier function [21]. At the cellular level, doxycycline preserved apical epithelial cell area and the tight-junction protein occludin, resulting in a decreased number of desquamating epithelial cells from the surface of the cornea [21, 68]. The inhibitory effect of doxycycline on MMP-9 was also confirmed on osmotically stressed cultured human corneal epithelial cells [67]. While there is no FDA approved anti-inflammatory agents, both steroid and doxycycline eyedrops have also been used with success in human dry eye patients [162, 163].

It has also been shown that manipulation of afferent (migration of DC into the regional lymph nodes) or efferent (migration of differentiated cells from the nodes and into the cornea and conjunctiva) can ameliorate development of dry eye disease [137, 164-167] indicating that therapeutic strategies that interfere with various points in this immune circle may have clinical significance.

Cyclosporine A 0.01 % emulsion (CsA), the only FDA-approved drug to treat dry-eye disease has been shown to modulate several arms of the immune response by decreasing HLA-DR expression in conjunctiva of dry eye patients [16, 168, 169] and decreasing expression of IL-17A and IFN-γ in conjunctiva of animals after desiccating stress [18]. One beneficial side effect from Cyclosporine emulsion is its significant effect increasing the amount of goblet cells in human patients. We observed similar findings in our animal model as well: CsA topical treatment prevented goblet cell loss, maintained the number of NK+cells in the conjunctiva increased IL-13 mRNA in NK+cells, and decreased IFN-γ and IL-17A mRNA transcripts in NK+and NK- populations, showing that CsA can act in both epithelial and immune compartments [154].

Novel therapeutic strategies based on the interruption of migration of Th17$^+$CCR6$^+$cells to the ocular surface or production of IL-17 have been shown to ameliorated dry eye disease in animal models of dry eye [18, 137, 142, 148, 165]. Exogenous administration of IL-13 to wild-type mice subjected to desiccating stress for 5 days prevented DS-induced goblet cell loss [154]. Recently, it has been made clear that strategies to neutralize IFN-γ may inhibit development of corneal and conjunctival disease in experimental dry eye. Neutralization of NK cells, early producers of IFN-γ (NK cells) following desiccating stress was found to decrease corneal fluorescein staining and inflammatory cytokine expression in the cornea and conjunctiva [99, 142] and also to decrease the Th-17 response.

7. Conclusions

This book chapter described the most recent advances in understanding the pathogenesis of dry eye disease. A significant amount of work has been performed using an environmentally-induced murine dry eye model. Inflammation is now recognized as important player in dry eye. While there is just one FDA-approved drug to treat dry eye, several other drugs are in the pipeline addressing different aspects of the disease and are potential new therapeutics.

Author details

Cintia S. de Paiva[1], Andrew J.W. Huang[2], De-Quan Li[1] and Stephen C. Pflugfelder[1*]

*Address all correspondence to: stevenp@bcm.edu

1 The Ocular Surface Center, Cullen Eye Institute, Department of Ophthalmology, Baylor College of Medicine, USA

2 Department of Ophthalmology and Visual Sciences, School of Medicine, Washington University, St. Louis, MO, USA

References

[1] Epidemiology Subcommittee: The definition and classification of dry eye disease: report of the Definition and Classification Subcommittee of the International Dry Eye WorkShop (2007). *Ocul Surf* 2007,5(2): 75-92.

[2] Moss SE, Klein R, Klein BE: Incidence of dry eye in an older population. *Arch Ophthalmol* 2004,122: 369-373.

[3] Schein OD, Munoz B, Tielsch JM, Bandeen-Roche K, West S: Prevalence of dry eye among the elderly. *Am J Ophthalmol* 1997,124: 723-728.

[4] Schaumberg DA, Sullivan DA, Buring JE, Dana MR: Prevalence of dry eye syndrome among US women. *Am J Ophthalmol* 2003,136: 318-326.

[5] Pflugfelder SC: Prevalence, burden, and pharmacoeconomics of dry eye disease. *Am J Manag Care* 2008,14: S102-S106.

[6] Yu J, Asche CV, Fairchild CJ: The economic burden of dry eye disease in the United States: a decision tree analysis. *Cornea* 2011,30: 379-387.

[7] Yamada M, Mizuno Y, Shigeyasu C: Impact of dry eye on work productivity. *Clinicoecon Outcomes Res* 2012,4: 307-312.

[8] Maeda N, Sato S, Watanabe H, Inoue Y, Fujikado T, Shimomura Y, Tano Y: Prediction of letter contrast sensitivity using videokeratographic indices. *Am J Ophthalmol* 2000,129: 759-763.

[9] Miljanovic B, Dana R, Sullivan DA, Schaumberg DA: Impact of dry eye syndrome on vision-related quality of life. *Am J Ophthalmol* 2007,143: 409-415.

[10] Ivers RQ, Cumming RG, Mitchell P, Attebo K: Visual impairment and falls in older adults: the Blue Mountains Eye Study. *J Am Geriatr Soc* 1998,46: 58-64.

[11] Sattin RW: Falls among older persons: a public health perspective. *Annu Rev Public Health* 1992,13: 489-508.

[12] Schiffman RM, Walt JG, Jacobsen G, Doyle JJ, Lebovics G, Sumner W: Utility assessment among patients with dry eye disease. *Ophthalmology* 2003,110: 1412-1419.

[13] Harris RA, Nease RF, Jr.: The importance of patient preferences for comorbidities in cost-effectiveness analyses. *J Health Econ* 1997,16: 113-119.

[14] Pflugfelder SC: Differential diagnosis of dry eye conditions. *Adv Dent Res* 1996,10: 9-12.

[15] Lemp MA: Evaluation and differential diagnosis of keratoconjunctivitis sicca. *J Rheumatol Suppl* 2000,61: 11-14.

[16] Brignole F, Pisella PJ, Goldschild M, De Saint JM, Goguel A, Baudouin C: Flow cytometric analysis of inflammatory markers in conjunctival epithelial cells of patients with dry eyes. *Invest Ophthalmol Vis Sci* 2000,41: 1356-1363.

[17] Kunert KS, Tisdale AS, Gipson IK: Goblet cell numbers and epithelial proliferation in the conjunctiva of patients with dry eye syndrome treated with cyclosporine. *Arch Ophthalmol* 2002,120: 330-337.

[18] de Paiva CS, Chotikavanich S, Pangelinan SB, Pitcher JI, Fang B, Zheng X, Ma P, Farley WJ, Siemasko KS, Niederkorn JY, Stern ME, Li D-Q, Pflugfelder SC: IL-17 disrupts corneal barrier following desiccating stress. *Mucosal Immunology* 2009, May; 2(3): 243-53

[19] de Paiva CS, Volpe EA, Gandhi NB, Zhang X, Zheng X, Pitcher JD, III, Farley WJ, Stern ME, Niederkorn JY, Li DQ, Flavell RA, Pflugfelder SC: Disruption of TGF-beta Signaling Improves Ocular Surface Epithelial Disease in Experimental Autoimmune Keratoconjunctivitis Sicca. *PLoS One* 2011,6: e29017. Epub 2011 Dec 14.

[20] de Paiva CS, Pangelinan SB, Chang E, Yoon KC, Farley WJ, Li DQ, Pflugfelder SC: Essential role for c-Jun N-terminal kinase 2 in corneal epithelial response to desiccating stress. *Arch Ophthalmol* 2009,127: 1625-1631.

[21] de Paiva CS, Corrales RM, Villarreal AL, Farley W, Li DQ, Stern ME, Pflugfelder SC: Apical corneal barrier disruption in experimental murine dry eye is abrogated by methylprednisolone and doxycycline. *Invest Ophthalmol Vis Sci* 2006,47: 2847-2856.

[22] Pitcher JI, de Paiva CS, Pelegrino FSA, McClellan AJ, Raince JK, Pangelinan SB, Rahimy E, Farley JW, Stern ME, Li D-Q, Pflugfelder SC: Pharmacological cholinergic blockade stimulates inflammatory cytokine production in the mouse lacrimal gland. *Invest Ophthalmol Vis Sci* 2011,16: 3221-7.

[23] Zoukhri D, Macari E, Kublin CL: A single injection of interleukin-1 induces reversible aqueous-tear deficiency, lacrimal gland inflammation, and acinar and ductal cell proliferation. *Exp Eye Res* 2007,84: 894-904.

[24] Mircheff AK, Wang Y, Thomas PB, Nakamura T, Samant D, Trousdale MD, Warren DW, Ding C, Schechter JE: Systematic variations in immune response-related gene transcript abundance suggest new questions about environmental influences on lacrimal gland immunoregulation. *Curr Eye Res* 2011,36: 285-294.

[25] Van Blokland SC, Versnel MA: Pathogenesis of Sjogren's syndrome: characteristics of different mouse models for autoimmune exocrinopathy. *Clin Immunol* 2002,103: 111-124.

[26] de Paiva CS, Hwang CS, Pitcher JD, III, Pangelinan SB, Rahimy E, Chen W, Yoon KC, Farley WJ, Niederkorn JY, Stern ME, Li DQ, Pflugfelder SC: Age-related T-cell cytokine profile parallels corneal disease severity in Sjogren's syndrome-like keratoconjunctivitis sicca in CD25KO mice. *Rheumatology (Oxford)* 2010,49: 246-258.

[27] Yang Z, Mu Z, Dabovic B, Jurukovski V, Yu D, Sung J, Xiong X, Munger JS: Absence of integrin-mediated TGFbeta1 activation in vivo recapitulates the phenotype of TGFbeta1-null mice. *J Cell Biol* 2007,176: 787-793.

[28] Cha S, Peck AB, Humphreys-Beher MG: Progress in understanding autoimmune exocrinopathy using the non-obese diabetic mouse: an update. *Crit Rev Oral Biol Med* 2002,13: 5-16.

[29] Sharma R, Bagavant H, Jarjour WN, Sung SS, Ju ST: The role of Fas in the immune system biology of IL-2R alpha knockout mice: interplay among regulatory T cells, inflammation, hemopoiesis, and apoptosis. *J Immunol* 2005,175: 1965-1973.

[30] McCartney-Francis NL, Mizel DE, Redman RS, Frazier-Jessen M, Panek RB, Kulkarni AB, Ward JM, McCarthy JB, Wahl SM: Autoimmune Sjogren's-like lesions in salivary glands of TGF-beta1-deficient mice are inhibited by adhesion-blocking peptides. *J Immunol* 1996,157: 1306-1312.

[31] McCartney-Francis NL, Mizel DE, Frazier-Jessen M, Kulkarni AB, McCarthy JB, Wahl SM: Lacrimal gland inflammation is responsible for ocular pathology in TGF-beta 1 null mice. *Am J Pathol* 1997,151: 1281-1288.

[32] Shull MM, Ormsby I, Kier AB, Pawlowski S, Diebold RJ, Yin M, Allen R, Sidman C, Proetzel G, Calvin D,.: Targeted disruption of the mouse transforming growth factor-beta 1 gene results in multifocal inflammatory disease. *Nature* 1992,359: 693-699.

[33] Von Bahr G: Konnte der flussigkeitsabgang durch die cornea von physiologischer bedeutung sein? *Acta Ophthalmol* 1941,19: 125-134.

[34] BALIK J: The lacrimal fluid in keratoconjunctivitis sicca; a quantitative and qualitative investigation. *Am J Ophthalmol* 1952,35: 1773-1782.

[35] Mishima S, Kubota Z, Farris RL. The tear flow dynamics in normal and in keratoconjunctivitis sicca cases. 1971:1801-1805.

[36] Gilbard JP, Farris RL, Santamaria J: Osmolarity of tear microvolumes in keratoconjunctivitis sicca. *Arch Ophthalmol* 1978,96: 677-681.

[37] Farris RL: Tear osmolarity-a new gold standard? *Adv Exp Med Biol* 1994,350: 495-503.

[38] Aragona P, Di Stefano G, Ferreri F, Spinella R, Stilo A: Sodium hyaluronate eye drops of different osmolarity for the treatment of dry eye in Sjogren's syndrome patients. *Br J Ophthalmol* 2002,86: 879-884.

[39] Gilbard JP, Rossi SR, Gray KL, Hanninen LA, Kenyon KR: Tear film osmolarity and ocular surface disease in two rabbit models for keratoconjunctivitis sicca. *Invest Ophthalmol Vis Sci* 1988,29: 374-378.

[40] Gilbard JP, Rossi SR, Gray KL, Hanninen LA: Natural history of disease in a rabbit model for keratoconjunctivitis sicca. *Acta Ophthalmol Suppl* 1989,192: 95-101.

[41] Gilbard JP, Carter JB, Sang DN, Refojo MF, Hanninen LA, Kenyon KR: Morphologic effect of hyperosmolarity on rabbit corneal epithelium. *Ophthalmology* 1984,91: 1205-1212.

[42] de Paiva CS, Corrales RM, Villarreal AL, Farley W, D.-Q L, Stern ME, Pflugfelder SC: Corticosteroid and doxycycline suppress MMP-9 and inflammatory cytokine expression, MAPK activation in the corneal epithelium in experimental dry eye. *Exp Eye Res* 2006,83: 526-535.

[43] Luo L, Li DQ, Corrales RM, Pflugfelder SC: Hyperosmolar saline is a proinflammatory stress on the mouse ocular surface. *Eye & Contact Lens* 2005,31(5): 186-93.

[44] Dursun D, Wang M, Monroy D, Li DQ, Lokeshwar BL, Stern M, Pflugfelder SC: Experimentally induced dry eye produces ocular surface inflammation and epithelial disease. *Adv Exp Med Biol* 2002,506: 647-655.

[45] Luo L, Li DQ, Doshi A, Farley W, Corrales RM, Pflugfelder SC: Experimental dry eye stimulates production of inflammatory cytokines and MMP-9 and activates MAPK signaling pathways on the ocular surface. *Invest Ophthalmol Vis Sci* 2004,45: 4293-4301.

[46] Kyriakis JM, Banerjee P, Nikolakaki E, Dai T, Rubie EA, Ahmad MF, Avruch J, Woodgett JR: The stress-activated protein kinase subfamily of c-Jun kinases. *Nature* 1994,369: 156-160.

[47] Galcheva-Gargova Z, Derijard B, Wu IH, Davis RJ: An osmosensing signal transduction pathway in mammalian cells. *Science* 1994,265: 806-808.

[48] Rosette C, Karin M: Ultraviolet light and osmotic stress: activation of the JNK cascade through multiple growth factor and cytokine receptors. *Science* 1996,274: 1194-1197.

[49] Li DQ, Chen Z, Song XJ, Luo L, Pflugfelder SC: Stimulation of matrix metalloproteinases by hyperosmolarity via a JNK pathway in human corneal epithelial cells. *Invest Ophthalmol Vis Sci* 2004,45: 4302-4311.

[50] Li DQ, Luo L, Chen Z, Kim HS, Song XJ, Pflugfelder SC: JNK and ERK MAP kinases mediate induction of IL-1beta, TNF-alpha and IL-8 following hyperosmolar stress in human limbal epithelial cells. *Exp Eye Res* 2006,82: 588-596.

[51] Cavet ME, Harrington KL, Ward KW, Zhang JZ: Mapracorat, a novel selective glucocorticoid receptor agonist, inhibits hyperosmolar-induced cytokine release and MAPK pathways in human corneal epithelial cells. *Mol Vis* 2010,16: 1791-1800.

[52] Pflugfelder SC, Huang AJW, Schuchovski PT, Pereira IC, Tseng SCG: Conjunctival cytological features of primary Sjogren syndrome. *Ophthalmology* 1990,97: 985-991.

[53] de Paiva CS, Lindsey JL, Pflugfelder SC: Assessing the severity of keratitis sicca with videokeratoscopic indices. *Ophthalmology* 2003,110: 1102-1109.

[54] Chotikavanich S, de Paiva CS, D.-Q L, Chen JJ, Bian F, Farley WJ, Pflugfelder SC: Production and Activity of Matrix Metalloproteinase-9 on the Ocular Surface Increase in Dysfunctional Tear Syndrome. *Invest Ophthalmol Vis Sci* 2009, 50(7):-3203.

[55] Corrales RM, de Paiva CS, Li DQ, Farley WJ, Henriksson JT, Bergmanson JP, Pflugfelder SC: Entrapment of conjunctival goblet cells by desiccation-induced cornification. *Invest Ophthalmol Vis Sci* 2011,52: 3492-3499.

[56] Luo L, Li DQ, Pflugfelder SC. Hyperosmolarity-induced apoptosis in human corneal epithelial cells is mediated by cytochrome c and MAPK pathways. *Cornea* 2007, 26:452-460.

[57] Corrales RM, Stern ME, de Paiva CS, Welch J, Li DQ, Pflugfelder SC: Desiccating stress stimulates expression of matrix metalloproteinases by the corneal epithelium. *Invest Ophthalmol Vis Sci* 2006,47: 3293-3302.

[58] Nagase H, Woessner JF, Jr.: Matrix metalloproteinases. *J Biol Chem* 1999,274: 21491-21494.

[59] Johnson LL, Dyer R, Hupe DJ: Matrix metalloproteinases. *Curr Opin Chem Biol* 1998,2: 466-471.

[60] Visse R, Nagase H: Matrix metalloproteinases and tissue inhibitors of metalloproteinases: structure, function, and biochemistry. *Circ Res* 2003,92: 827-839.

[61] Brejchova K, Liskova P, Hrdlickova E, Filipec M, Jirsova K: Matrix metalloproteinases in recurrent corneal melting associated with primary Sjorgen's syndrome. *Mol Vis* 2009,15: 2364-2372.

[62] Fini ME, Girard MT, Matsubara M: Collagenolytic/gelatinolytic enzymes in corneal wound healing. *Acta Ophthalmol Suppl* 1992: 26-33.

[63] Matsubara M, Girard MT, Kublin CL, Cintron C, Fini ME: Differential roles for two gelatinolytic enzymes of the matrix metalloproteinase family in the remodelling cornea. *Dev Biol* 1991,147: 425-439.

[64] Matsubara M, Zieske JD, Fini ME: Mechanism of basement membrane dissolution preceding corneal ulceration. *Invest Ophthalmol Vis Sci* 1991,32: 3221-3237.

[65] Afonso AA, Sobrin L, Monroy DC, Selzer M, Lokeshwar B, Pflugfelder SC: Tear fluid gelatinase B activity correlates with IL-1alpha concentration and fluorescein clearance in ocular rosacea. *Invest Ophthalmol Vis Sci* 1999,40: 2506-2512.

[66] Kim HS, Luo L, Pflugfelder SC, Li DQ: Doxycycline Inhibits TGF-{beta}1-Induced MMP-9 via Smad and MAPK Pathways in Human Corneal Epithelial Cells. *Invest Ophthalmol Vis Sci* 2005,46: 840-848.

[67] Pflugfelder SC, Farley W, Luo L, Chen LZ, de Paiva CS, Olmos LC, Li DQ, Fini ME: Matrix metalloproteinase-9 knockout confers resistance to corneal epithelial barrier disruption in experimental dry eye. *Am J Pathol* 2005,166: 61-71.

[68] Beardsely RM, de Paiva CS, Power DF, Pflugfelder SC: Desiccating stress decreases apical corneal epithelial cell size--modulation by the metalloproteinase inhibitor doxycycline. *Cornea* 2008,27: 935-940.

[69] Behrens A, Doyle JJ, Stern L, Chuck RS, McDonnell PJ, Azar DT, Dua HS, Hom M, Karpecki PM, Laibson PR, Lemp MA, Meisler DM, Del Castillo JM, O'Brien TP, Pflugfelder SC, Rolando M, Schein OD, Seitz B, Tseng SC, van SG, Wilson SE, Yiu SC: Dysfunctional tear syndrome: a Delphi approach to treatment recommendations. *Cornea* 2006,25: 900-907.

[70] Jameson JM, Sharp LL, Witherden DA, Havran WL: Regulation of skin cell homeostasis by gamma delta T cells. *Front Biosci* 2004,9: 2640-2651.

[71] Dua HS, Gomes JA, Jindal VK, Appa SN, Schwarting R, Eagle RC, Jr., Donoso LA, Laibson PR: Mucosa specific lymphocytes in the human conjunctiva, corneoscleral limbus and lacrimal gland. *Curr Eye Res* 1994,13: 87-93.

[72] Dua HS, Gomes JA, Donoso LA, Laibson PR: The ocular surface as part of the mucosal immune system: conjunctival mucosa-specific lymphocytes in ocular surface pathology. *Eye (Lond)* 1995,9 (Pt 3): 261-267.

[73] Hingorani M, Metz D, Lightman SL: Characterisation of the normal conjunctival leukocyte population. *Exp Eye Res* 1997,64: 905-912.

[74] Rojas B, Cuhna R, Zafirakis P, Ramirez JM, Lizan-garciia M, Zhao T, Foster CS: Cell populations and adhesion molecules expression in conjunctiva before and after bone marrow transplantation. *Exp Eye Res* 2005,81: 313-325.

[75] Cepek KL, Parker CM, Madara JL, Brenner MB: Integrin alpha E beta 7 mediates adhesion of T lymphocytes to epithelial cells. *J Immunol* 1993,150: 3459-3470.

[76] Cepek KL, Shaw SK, Parker CM, Russell GJ, Morrow JS, Rimm DL, Brenner MB: Adhesion between epithelial cells and T lymphocytes mediated by E-cadherin and the alpha E beta 7 integrin. *Nature* 1994,372: 190-193.

[77] Jones DT, Monroy D, Ji Z, Atherton SS, Pflugfelder SC: Sjogren's syndrome: cytokine and Epstein-Barr viral gene expression within the conjunctival epithelium. *Invest Ophthalmol Vis Sci* 1994,35: 3493-3504.

[78] Pflugfelder SC, Jones D, Ji Z, Afonso A, Monroy D: Altered cytokine balance in the tear fluid and conjunctiva of patients with Sjogren's syndrome keratoconjunctivitis sicca. *Curr Eye Res* 1999,19: 201-211.

[79] Solomon A, Dursun D, Liu Z, Xie Y, Macri A, Pflugfelder SC: Pro-and anti-inflammatory forms of interleukin-1 in the tear fluid and conjunctiva of patients with dry-eye disease. *Invest Ophthalmol Vis Sci* 2001,42: 2283-2292.

[80] Calonge M: The treatment of dry eye. *Surv Ophthalmol* 2001,45 Suppl 2: S227-S239.

[81] Stern ME, Gao J, Schwalb TA, Ngo M, Tieu DD, Chan CC, Reis BL, Whitcup SM, Thompson D, Smith JA: Conjunctival T-cell subpopulations in Sjogren's and non-Sjogren's patients with dry eye. *Invest Ophthalmol Vis Sci* 2002,43: 2609-2614.

[82] Kunert KS, Tisdale AS, Stern ME, Smith JA, Gipson IK: Analysis of topical cyclosporine treatment of patients with dry eye syndrome: effect on conjunctival lymphocytes. *Arch Ophthalmol* 2000,118: 1489-1496.

[83] Niederkorn JY, Stern ME, Pflugfelder SC, de Paiva CS, Corrales RM, Gao J, Siemasko K: Desiccating Stress Induces T Cell-Mediated Sjogren's Syndrome-Like Lacrimal Keratoconjunctivitis. *J Immunol* 2006,176: 3950-3957.

[84] Happel KI, Dubin PJ, Zheng M, Ghilardi N, Lockhart C, Quinton LJ, Odden AR, Shellito JE, Bagby GJ, Nelson S, Kolls JK: Divergent roles of IL-23 and IL-12 in host defense against Klebsiella pneumoniae. *J Exp Med* 2005,202: 761-769.

[85] Chung DR, Kasper DL, Panzo RJ, Chitnis T, Grusby MJ, Sayegh MH, Tzianabos AO: CD4+T cells mediate abscess formation in intra-abdominal sepsis by an IL-17-dependent mechanism. *J Immunol* 2003,170: 1958-1963.

[86] Huang W, Na L, Fidel PL, Schwarzenberger P: Requirement of interleukin-17A for systemic anti-Candida albicans host defense in mice. *J Infect Dis* 2004,190: 624-631.

[87] Yoon KC, Park CS, You IC, Choi HJ, Lee KH, Im SK, Park HY, Pflugfelder SC: Expression of CXCL9,-10,-11, and CXCR3 in the tear film and ocular surface of patients with dry eye syndrome. *Invest Ophthalmol Vis Sci* 2010,51: 643-650.

[88] Yoon KC, de Paiva CS, Qi H, Chen Z, Farley WJ, Li DQ, Pflugfelder SC: Expression of th-1 chemokines and chemokine receptors on the ocular surface of C57BL/6 mice: effects of desiccating stress. *Invest Ophthalmol Vis Sci* 2007,48: 2561-2569.

[89] Choi W, Li Z, Oh HJ, Im SK, Lee SH, Park SH, You IC, Yoon KC: Expression of CCR5 and its ligands CCL3,-4, and-5 in the tear film and ocular surface of patients with dry eye disease. *Curr Eye Res* 2012,37: 12-17.

[90] Riemens A, Stoyanova E, Rothova A, Kuiper J: Cytokines in tear fluid of patients with ocular graft-versus-host disease after allogeneic stem cell transplantation. *Mol Vis* 2012,18: 797-802.

[91] Lam H, Blieden L, de Paiva CS, Farley WJ, Stern ME, Pflugfelder SC: Tear Cytokine Profiles in Dysfunctional Tear Syndrome. *Am J Ophthalmol* 2009, 147: 198-205. Nov. 5 [Epub ahead of print].

[92] Enriquez-de-Salamanca A, Castellanos E, Stern ME, Fernandez I, Carreno E, Garcia-Vazquez C, Herreras JM, Calonge M: Tear cytokine and chemokine analysis and clinical correlations in evaporative-type dry eye disease. *Mol Vis* 2010,16: 862-873.

[93] Massingale ML, Li X, Vallabhajosyula M, Chen D, Wei Y, Asbell PA: Analysis of inflammatory cytokines in the tears of dry eye patients. *Cornea* 2009,28: 1023-1027.

[94] Mrugacz M, Kaczmarski M, Bakunowicz-Lazarczyk A, Zelazowska B, Wysocka J, Minarowska A: IL-8 and IFN-gamma in tear fluid of patients with cystic fibrosis. *J Interferon Cytokine Res* 2006,26: 71-75.

[95] Boehm N, Riechardt AI, Wiegand M, Pfeiffer N, Grus FH: Proinflammatory cytokine profiling of tears from dry eye patients by means of antibody microarrays. *Invest Ophthalmol Vis Sci* 2011,52: 7725-7730.

[96] Corrales RM, Villarreal A, Farley W, Stern ME, Li DQ, Pflugfelder SC: Strain-related cytokine profiles on the murine ocular surface in response to desiccating stress. *Cornea* 2007,26: 579-584.

[97] de Paiva CS, Villarreal AL, Corrales RM, Rahman HT, Chang VY, Farley WJ, Stern ME, Niederkorn JY, Li DQ, Pflugfelder SC: Dry Eye-Induced Conjunctival Epithelial Squamous Metaplasia Is Modulated by Interferon-{gamma}. *Invest Ophthalmol Vis Sci* 2007,48: 2553-2560.

[98] Zhang X, Chen W, de Paiva CS, Corrales RM, Volpe EA, McClellan AJ, Farley WJ, Li DQ, Pflugfelder SC: Interferon-{gamma} Exacerbates Dry Eye Induced Apoptosis in Conjunctiva via Dual Apoptotic Pathways. *Invest Ophthalmol Vis Sci* 2011.

[99] Chen Y, Chauhan SK, Saban DR, Sadrai Z, Okanobo A, Dana R: Interferon-{gamma}-secreting NK cells promote induction of dry eye disease. *J Leukoc Biol* 2011,89: 965-972.

[100] Chen Z, Mok H, Pflugfelder SC, Li DQ, Barry MA: Improved transduction of human corneal epithelial progenitor cells with cell-targeting adenoviral vectors. *Exp Eye Res* 2006,83: 798-806.

[101] Kang EH, Lee YJ, Hyon JY, Yun PY, Song YW: Salivary cytokine profiles in primary Sjogren's syndrome differ from those in non-Sjogren sicca in terms of TNF-alpha levels and Th-1/Th-2 ratios. *Clin Exp Rheumatol* 2011,29: 970-976.

[102] Pertovaara M, Antonen J, Hurme M: Th2 cytokine genotypes are associated with a milder form of primary Sjogren's syndrome. *Ann Rheum Dis* 2006,65: 666-670.

[103] Hayashi T, Shimoyama N, Mizuno T: Destruction of salivary and lacrimal glands by Th1-polarized reaction in a model of secondary Sjogren's syndrome in lupus-prone female NZB x NZWF(1) mice. *Inflammation* 2012,35: 638-646.

[104] Ogawa N, Ping L, Zhenjun L, Takada Y, Sugai S: Involvement of the interferon-gamma-induced T cell-attracting chemokines, interferon-gamma-inducible 10-kd protein (CXCL10) and monokine induced by interferon-gamma (CXCL9), in the salivary gland lesions of patients with Sjogren's syndrome. *Arthritis Rheum* 2002,46: 2730-2741.

[105] Viau S, Pasquis B, Maire MA, Fourgeux C, Gregoire S, Acar N, Bretillon L, Creuzot-Garcher CP, Joffre C: No consequences of dietary n-3 polyunsaturated fatty acid deficiency on the severity of scopolamine-induced dry eye. *Graefes Arch Clin Exp Ophthalmol* 2011,249: 547-557.

[106] Jie G, Jiang Q, Rui Z, Yifei Y: Expression of interleukin-17 in autoimmune dacryoadenitis in MRL/lpr mice. *Curr Eye Res* 2010,35: 865-871.

[107] Rahimy E, Pitcher JD, III, Pangelinan SB, Chen W, Farley WJ, Niederkorn JY, Stern ME, Li DQ, Pflugfelder SC, de Paiva CS: Spontaneous autoimmune dacryoadenitis in aged CD25KO mice. *Am J Pathol* 2010,177: 744-753.

[108] Pelegrino FS, Volpe EA, Gandhi NB, Li DQ, Pflugfelder SC, de Paiva CS: Deletion of interferon-gamma delays onset and severity of dacryoadenitis in CD25KO mice. *Arthritis Res Ther* 2012,14: R234.

[109] Kohashi M, Ishimaru N, Arakaki R, Hayashi Y: Effective treatment with oral administration of rebamipide in a mouse model of Sjogren's syndrome. *Arthritis Rheum* 2008,58: 389-400.

[110] Koarada S, Haruta Y, Mitamura M, Morito F, Tada Y, Ohta A, Nagasawa K: Ex vivo CD(+) T-cell cytokine expression from patients with Sjogren's syndrome following in vitro stimulation to induce proliferation. *Rheumatology (Oxford)* 2006,45: 392-399.

[111] Brookes SM, Price EJ, Venables PJ, Maini RN: Interferon-gamma and epithelial cell activation in Sjogren's syndrome. *Br J Rheumatol* 1995,34: 226-231.

[112] Szodoray P, Gal I, Barath S, Aleksza M, Horvath IF, Gergely P, Jr., Szegedi G, Nakken B, Zeher M: Immunological alterations in newly diagnosed primary Sjogren's syndrome characterized by skewed peripheral T-cell subsets and inflammatory cytokines. *Scand J Rheumatol* 2008,37: 205-212.

[113] Hagiwara E, Pando J, Ishigatsubo Y, Klinman DM: Altered frequency of type 1 cytokine secreting cells in the peripheral blood of patients with primary Sjogren's syndrome. *J Rheumatol* 1998,25: 89-93.

[114] Konttinen YT, Kemppinen P, Koski H, Li TF, Jumppanen M, Hietanen J, Santavirta S, Salo T, Larsson A, Hakala M, Sorsa T: T(H)1 cytokines are produced in labial salivary glands in Sjogren's syndrome, but also in healthy individuals. *Scand J Rheumatol* 1999,28: 106-112.

[115] Ajjan RA, McIntosh RS, Waterman EA, Watson PF, Franklin CD, Yeoman CM, Weetman AP: Analysis of the T-cell receptor Valpha repertoire and cytokine gene expression in Sjogren's syndrome. *Br J Rheumatol* 1998,37: 179-185.

[116] Giron-Gonzalez JA, Baturone R, Soto MJ, Marquez M, Macias I, Montes de OM, Medina F, Chozas N, Garcia-Perez S: Implications of immunomodulatory interleukins for the hyperimmunoglobulinemia of Sjogren's syndrome. *Cell Immunol* 2009,259: 56-60.

[117] van Woerkom JM, Kruize AA, Wenting-van Wijk MJ, Knol E, Bihari IC, Jacobs JW, Bijlsma JW, Lafeber FP, van Roon JA: Salivary gland and peripheral blood T helper 1 and 2 cell activity in Sjogren's syndrome compared with non-Sjogren's sicca syndrome. *Ann Rheum Dis* 2005,64: 1474-1479.

[118] Mitsias DI, Tzioufas AG, Veiopoulou C, Zintzaras E, Tassios IK, Kogopoulou O, Moutsopoulos HM, Thyphronitis G: The Th1/Th2 cytokine balance changes with the progress of the immunopathological lesion of Sjogren's syndrome. *Clin Exp Immunol* 2002,128: 562-568.

[119] Zhang X, Chen W, de Paiva CS, Volpe EA, Gandhi NB, Farley WJ, Li DQ, Niederkorn JY, Stern ME, Pflugfelder SC: Desiccating Stress Induces CD4(+) T-Cell-Mediated Sjogren's Syndrome-Like Corneal Epithelial Apoptosis via Activation of the Extrinsic Apoptotic Pathway by Interferon-gamma. *Am J Pathol* 2011,179: 1807-1814.

[120] Zhang X, Chen W, de Paiva CS, Corrales RM, Volpe EA, McClellan AJ, Farley WJ, Li DQ, Pflugfelder SC: Interferon-gamma exacerbates dry eye-induced apoptosis in conjunctiva through dual apoptotic pathways. *Invest Ophthalmol Vis Sci* 2011,52: 6279-6285.

[121] Albertsmeyer AC, Kakkassery V, Spurr-Michaud S, Beeks O, Gipson IK: Effect of pro-inflammatory mediators on membrane-associated mucins expressed by human ocular surface epithelial cells. *Exp Eye Res* 2010,90: 444-451.

[122] Veldhoen M, Hocking RJ, Atkins CJ, Locksley RM, Stockinger B: TGFbeta in the context of an inflammatory cytokine milieu supports de novo differentiation of IL-17-producing T cells. *Immunity* 2006,24: 179-189.

[123] Bettelli E, Carrier Y, Gao W, Korn T, Strom TB, Oukka M, Weiner HL, Kuchroo VK: Reciprocal developmental pathways for the generation of pathogenic effector TH17 and regulatory T cells. *Nature* 2006,441: 235-238.

[124] Mangan PR, Harrington LE, O'Quinn DB, Helms WS, Bullard DC, Elson CO, Hatton RD, Wahl SM, Schoeb TR, Weaver CT: Transforming growth factor-beta induces development of the T(H)17 lineage. *Nature* 2006,441: 231-234.

[125] Korn T, Mitsdoerffer M, Croxford AL, Awasthi A, Dardalhon VA, Galileos G, Vollmar P, Stritesky GL, Kaplan MH, Waisman A, Kuchroo VK, Oukka M: IL-6 controls Th17 immunity in vivo by inhibiting the conversion of conventional T cells into Foxp3+regulatory T cells. *Proc Natl Acad Sci U S A* 2008,105: 18460-18465.

[126] Nurieva RI, Chung Y, Hwang D, Yang XO, Kang HS, Ma L, Wang YH, Watowich SS, Jetten AM, Tian Q, Dong C: Generation of T follicular helper cells is mediated by interleukin-21 but independent of T helper 1, 2, or 17 cell lineages. *Immunity* 2008,29: 138-149.

[127] Yang XO, Panopoulos AD, Nurieva R, Chang SH, Wang D, Watowich SS, Dong C: STAT3 regulates cytokine-mediated generation of inflammatory helper T cells. *J Biol Chem* 2007,282: 9358-9363.

[128] Li MO, Wan YY, Sanjabi S, Robertson AK, Flavell RA: Transforming growth factor-beta regulation of immune responses. *Annu Rev Immunol* 2006,24: 99-146.

[129] Gupta A, Monroy D, Ji Z, Yoshino K, Huang AJW, Pflugfelder SC: Transforming growth factor beta-1 and beta-2 in human tear fluid. *Curr Eye Res* 1996,15: 605-614.

[130] Yoshino K, Garg R, Monroy D, Ji Z, Pflugfelder SC: Production and secretion of transforming growth factor beta (TGF-β) by the human lacrimal gland. *Curr Eye Res* 1996,15: 615-624.

[131] Zheng X, de Paiva CS, Rao K, Li DQ, Farley WJ, Stern M, Pflugfelder SC: Evaluation of the transforming growth factor-beta activity in normal and dry eye human tears by CCL-185 cell bioassay. *Cornea* 2010,29: 1048-1054.

[132] Sun D, Emmert-Buck MR, Fox PC: Differential cytokine mRNA expression in human labial minor salivary glands in primary Sjogren's syndrome. *Autoimmunity* 1998,28: 125-137.

[133] Murphy-Ullrich JE, Poczatek M: Activation of latent TGF-beta by thrombospondin-1: mechanisms and physiology. *Cytokine Growth Factor Rev* 2000,11: 59-69.

[134] Turpie B, Yoshimura T, Gulati A, Rios JD, Dartt DA, Masli S: Sjogren's syndrome-like ocular surface disease in thrombospondin-1 deficient mice. *Am J Pathol* 2009,175: 1136-1147.

[135] Gandhi NB, Su Z, Zhang X, Volpe EA, Pelegrino FS, Rahman SA, Li DQ, Pflugfelder SC, de Paiva CS: Dendritic cell-derived thrombospondin-1 is critical for the generation of the ocular surface Th17 response to desiccating stress. *J Leukoc Biol* 2013, 94:1293-301.

[136] Zheng X, Bian F, Ma P, de Paiva CS, Stern M, Pflugfelder SC, Li DQ: Induction of Th17 differentiation by corneal epithelial-derived cytokines. *J Cell Physiol* 2009,2009 Sep 10;222(1): 95-102.

[137] Coursey TG, Gandhi NB, Volpe EA, Pflugfelder SC, de Paiva CS. CCR6 KO Mice Are Resistant To Dry Eye Disease. *PLoS One* 2013, 8: e78508.

[138] Wang C, Kang SG, Lee J, Sun Z, Kim CH: The roles of CCR6 in migration of Th17 cells and regulation of effector T-cell balance in the gut. *Mucosal Immunol* 2009,2: 173-183.

[139] Hirota K, Yoshitomi H, Hashimoto M, Maeda S, Teradaira S, Sugimoto N, Yamaguchi T, Nomura T, Ito H, Nakamura T, Sakaguchi N, Sakaguchi S: Preferential recruitment of CCR6-expressing Th17 cells to inflamed joints via CCL20 in rheumatoid arthritis and its animal model. *J Exp Med* 2007,204: 2803-2812.

[140] Pflugfelder SC: Anti-inflammatory therapy of dry eye. *Am J Ophthalmol* 2004,137: 337-342.

[141] Turner K, Pflugfelder SC, Ji Z, Feuer WJ, Stern M, Reis BL: Interleukin-6 levels in the conjunctival epithelium of patients with dry eye disease treated with cyclosporine ophthalmic emulsion. *Cornea* 2000,19: 492-496.

[142] Zhang X, Volpe EA, Gandhi NB, Schaumburg CS, Siemasko KF, Pangelinan SB, Kelly SD, Hayday AC, Li DQ, Stern ME, Niederkorn JY, Pflugfelder SC, de Paiva CS: NK cells promote Th-17 mediated corneal barrier disruption in dry eye. *PLoS One* 2012,7: e36822.

[143] Zheng X, de Paiva CS, Li DQ, Farley WJ, Pflugfelder SC: Desiccating stress promotion of Th17 differentiation by ocular surface tissues through a dendritic cell-mediated pathway. *Invest Ophthalmol Vis Sci* 2010,51: 3083-3091.

[144] Solomon A, Rosenblatt M, Monroy D, Ji Z, Pflugfelder SC, Tseng SC: Suppression of interleukin 1alpha and interleukin 1beta in human limbal epithelial cells cultured on the amniotic membrane stromal matrix. *Br J Ophthalmol* 2001,85: 444-449.

[145] Katsifis GE, Rekka S, Moutsopoulos NM, Pillemer S, Wahl SM: Systemic and local interleukin-17 and linked cytokines associated with Sjogren's syndrome immunopathogenesis. *Am J Pathol* 2009,175: 1167-1177.

[146] Sakai A, Sugawara Y, Kuroishi T, Sasano T, Sugawara S: Identification of IL-18 and Th17 cells in salivary glands of patients with Sjogren's syndrome, and amplification of IL-17-mediated secretion of inflammatory cytokines from salivary gland cells by IL-18. *J Immunol* 2008,181: 2898-2906.

[147] Nguyen CQ, Hu MH, Li Y, Stewart C, Peck AB: Salivary gland tissue expression of interleukin-23 and interleukin-17 in Sjogren's syndrome: findings in humans and mice. *Arthritis Rheum* 2008,58: 734-743.

[148] Chauhan SK, El AJ, Ecoiffier T, Goyal S, Zhang Q, Saban DR, Dana R: Autoimmunity in dry eye is due to resistance of Th17 to Treg suppression. *J Immunol* 2009,182: 1247-1252.

[149] Nakamura T, Nishida K, Dota A, Matsuki M, Yamanishi K, Kinoshita S: Elevated expression of transglutaminase 1 and keratinization-related proteins in conjunctiva in severe ocular surface disease. *Invest Ophthalmol Vis Sci* 2001,42: 549-556.

[150] Pflugfelder SC, Tseng SCG, Yoshino K, Monroy D, Felix C, Reis BL: Correlation of goblet cell density and mucosal epithelial membrane mucin expression with rose bengal staining in patients with ocular irritation. *Ophthalmology* 1997,104: 223-235.

[151] Fuss IJ, Strober W: The role of IL-13 and NK T cells in experimental and human ulcerative colitis. *Mucosal Immunol* 2008,1 Suppl 1: S31-S33.

[152] Middendorp S, Nieuwenhuis EE: NKT cells in mucosal immunity. *Mucosal Immunol* 2009,2: 393-402.

[153] Matangkasombut P, Pichavant M, Dekruyff RH, Umetsu DT: Natural killer T cells and the regulation of asthma. *Mucosal Immunol* 2009,2: 383-392.

[154] de Paiva CS, Raince JK, McClellan AJ, Shanmugam KP, Pangelinan SB, Volpe EA, Corrales RM, Farley WJ, Corry DB, Li DQ, Pflugfelder SC: Homeostatic control of conjunctival mucosal goblet cells by NKT-derived IL-13. *Mucosal Immunol* 2011,4(4): 397-408. doi: 10.1038/mi.2010.82. Epub 2010 Dec 22.

[155] Sacks EH, Wieczorek R, Jakobiec FA, Knowles DM: Lymphocytic subpopulations in the normal human conjunctiva. A monoclonal antibody study. *Ophthalmology* 1986,93: 1276-1283.

[156] Lider O, Santos LM, Lee CS, Higgins PJ, Weiner HL: Suppression of experimental autoimmune encephalomyelitis by oral administration of myelin basic protein. II. Suppression of disease and in vitro immune responses is mediated by antigen-specific CD8+T lymphocytes. *J Immunol* 1989,142: 748-752.

[157] Miller A, Lider O, Weiner HL: Antigen-driven bystander suppression after oral administration of antigens. *J Exp Med* 1991,174: 791-798.

[158] Sugita S, Ng TF, Schwartzkopff J, Streilein JW: CTLA-4+CD8+T cells that encounter B7-2+iris pigment epithelial cells express their own B7-2 to achieve global suppression of T cell activation. *J Immunol* 2004,172: 4184-4194.

[159] Raphael M, Bellefqih S, Piette JC, Le HP, Debre P, Chomette G: Conjunctival biopsy in Sjogren's syndrome: correlations between histological and immunohistochemical features. *Histopathology* 1988,13: 191-202.

[160] Zhang X, Schaumburg CS, Coursey TG, Siemasko KF, Volpe EA, Gandhi NB, D.-Q L, Niederkorn JY, Stern ME, Pflugfelder SC, de Paiva CS. $CD8^{+}$Cells Regulate the T

helper-17 Response in an Experimental Murine Model of Sjögren Syndrome. Mucosal Immunol. 2014, 7:417-27.

[161] de Paiva CS, Corrales RM, Villarreal AL, Farley WJ, Li DQ, Stern ME, Pflugfelder SC: Corticosteroid and doxycycline suppress MMP-9 and inflammatory cytokine expression, MAPK activation in the corneal epithelium in experimental dry eye. *Exp Eye Res* 2006,83: 526-535.

[162] Pflugfelder SC, Maskin SL, Anderson B, Chodosh J, Holland EJ, de Paiva CS, Bartels SP, Micuda T, Proskin HM, Vogel R: A randomized, double-masked, placebo-controlled, multicenter comparison of loteprednol etabonate ophthalmic suspension, 0.5%, and placebo for treatment of keratoconjunctivitis sicca in patients with delayed tear clearance. *Am J Ophthalmol* 2004,138: 444-457.

[163] Dursun D, Kim MC, Solomon A, Pflugfelder SC: Treatment of recalcitrant recurrent corneal erosions with inhibitors of matrix metalloproteinase-9, doxycycline and corticosteroids. *Am J Ophthalmol* 2001,132: 8-13.

[164] Schaumburg CS, Siemasko KF, de Paiva CS, Pflugfelder ME, Stern ME: Ocular Surface Antigen Presenting Cells are Necessary for Activation of Autoreactive T cells and Development of Autoimmune Lacrimal Keratoconjunctivtis. *J Immunol* 2011,187(7): 3653-3662.

[165] Sadrai Z, Stevenson W, Okanobo A, Chen Y, Dohlman TH, Hua J, Amparo F, Chauhan SK, Dana R: PDE4 inhibition suppresses IL-17-associated immunity in dry eye disease. *Invest Ophthalmol Vis Sci* 2012,53: 3584-3591.

[166] Lee HS, Chauhan SK, Okanobo A, Nallasamy N, Dana R: Therapeutic Efficacy of Topical Epigallocatechin Gallate in Murine Dry Eye. *Cornea* 2011,30(12): 1465-1472.

[167] Goyal S, Chauhan SK, Zhang Q, Dana R: Amelioration of murine dry eye disease by topical antagonist to chemokine receptor 2. *Arch Ophthalmol* 2009,127: 882-887.

[168] Baudouin C, Brignole F, Pisella PJ, De Jean MS, Goguel A: Flow cytometric analysis of the inflammatory marker HLA DR in dry eye syndrome: results from 12 months of randomized treatment with topical cyclosporin A. Adv Exp Med Biol 2002,506: 761-769.

[169] Brignole F, Pisella PJ, De Saint JM, Goldschild M, Goguel A, Baudouin C: Flow cytometric analysis of inflammatory markers in KCS: 6-month treatment with topical cyclosporin A. Invest Ophthalmol Vis Sci 2001,42: 90-95.

7

Advances in Pathogenesis of Behcet's Disease and Vogt-Koyanagi-Harada Syndrome

Peizeng Yang, Chaokui Wang, Shengping Hou,
Bo Lei, Aize Kijlstra and De-Quan Li

1. Introduction

Uveitis is one of the leading causes of blindness in the world. It is estimated that uveitis accounts for 10%-15% of the blindness in the western world [1]. More importantly, the blindness caused by uveitis is mostly permanent and irreversible since the retina and optic nerve are damaged by inflammation.

Uveitis was previously defined as inflammation of the uveal tract, which is classically composed of the iris, ciliary body and choroid. Yet in common practice, uveitis refers to inflammation involving any intraocular structure and therefore carries the following names: iritis, iridocyclitis, parsplanitis, posterior uveitis, choroiditis, retinitis and retinal vasculitis. It is usually classified into infectious and noninfectious origins on the basis of predominant etiological characteristics. Behcet's disease (BD) is thought to be an autoinflammatory disease, while Vogt-Koyanagi-Harada (VKH) syndrome is an autoimmune disease. Therefore, we chose BD and VKH, which are two important representative entities among the noninfectious uveitis class, to discuss the recent advances in our knowledge on the pathogenesis of uveitis.

BD is a chronic systemic autoinflammatory disease, characterized by recurrent uveitis, skin lesions, oral and genital mucous ulcers, as well as some complications in central nervous system, gastrointestinal tract and thrombotic events [2]. A high prevalence of BD has been reported along the ancient Silk Road [3], from Asia to the Mediterranean basin countries, such as Turkey, Iraq, Iran, Korea and Japan. The clinical features of BD have been well documented in publications originating from the high incidence countries. Our research group has evaluated the clinical characteristics and associated ocular complications in a large group of consecutive Chinese BD patients and found that most patients presented a bilateral nongranulomatous anterior, posterior, or panuveitis with a chronic and relapsing course. Uveitis occurred mostly in male patients and in the age group from the second to fifth decade of life. Oral aphthae (100%), skin lesions (78%), and genital ulcers (57.9%) were the typical extraocular findings in patients with BD [4].

VKH syndrome is a well-established immune-mediated multi-organ disorder characterized by a bilateral granulomatous panuveitis frequently associated with extraocular findings including poliosis, vitiligo, alopecia, and central nervous system and auditory signs [5]. It is an autoimmune disease against melanocyte-associated antigens in genetically susceptible individuals. VKH mainly affects certain pigmented races, such as Asians and Native Americans [5-6]. Four clinical stages of uveitis could be developed in patients with VKH syndrome: prodromal, acute, convalescent, and chronic recurrent stages. A clinical analysis based on a large group (n=410) of uveitis patients with VKH syndrome performed by our group showed that the disease was diagnosed most often in young people without a gender predisposition. The intraocular manifestations typically began with choroiditis or chorioretinitis, serous retinal detachment, and optic disc edema, and then proceeded to anterior uveitis if appropriate treatment was not given during the first 2 weeks. Eventually, the eyes developed a recurrent generalized granulomatous uveitis. With regard to the extraocular manifestations, meningismus signs, tinnitus, and abnormal touch sensitivity of the hair frequently occurred before or concurrently with ocular involvement, whereas vitiligo and poliosis usually appear after the uveitis attack [7]. This is possibly due to the autoimmune attack against melanocytes at different sites of the body.

Although the etiology and pathogenesis of BD and VKH syndrome is not completely known, it is hypothesized that abnormalities in the regulation of the immune system and an immunogenetic predisposition are involved in the development of these diseases. Deregulation of Th1, Th17 and regulatory T cells and abnormalities in the associated molecules were found to be involved in the development of these diseases. Recently, two large genome-wide association studies (GWAS) from Japan and Turkey reported an association between single nucleotide polymorphism (SNP) of IL-10, IL-23R/IL-12RB2 gene and BD [8-9]. HLA-DR4 and HLA-DRw53 were reported to be highly associated with VKH syndrome [10], implicating that genetic factors contributed to the pathogenesis of BD and VKH syndrome. The aim of this chapter is to expound the pathogenesis of BD and VKH syndrome with emphasis on new insights in the area of immunoregulation and immunogenetics.

2. Th1 cells and cytokines in Behcet's disease and VKH syndrome

Th1 cells were the first subtype of T help cells that was reported to be involved in the pathogenesis of autoimmune diseases. IFN-γ is the hallmark cytokine of Th1 cells. A number of studies have determined the role of the Th1 cell and its specific cytokine repertoire in the pathogenesis of BD and VKH syndrome. The increased levels of IFN-γ and T-bet, which is considered as the critical transcriptional factor for Th1 cells, have been observed in the peripheral blood of the patients with active uveitis of BD and VKH syndrome [11-14]. Our study found that S-Ag specific T cells may be involved in the pathogenesis of BD via the production of Th1-dominant cytokines, but not Th17 cytokines [15]. The increased levels of Th1 cell specific cytokines and chemokines in the cerebrospinal fluid (CSF) of VKH patients and in the lesions of active BD patients were also reported [16-17]. El-Asrar et al found an increased levels of IFN-γ in the aqueous humor samples of uveitis from BD, VKH syndrome and HLA-B27-associated uveitis as compared with normal controls; and importantly, the levels of IFN-γ were higher in BD patients than in VKH and HLA-B27-associated uveitis [18], which suggests that IFN-γ may play more important role in the pathogenesis of BD.

In the murine uveitis models, previous reports suggested that Th1 played a pathogenic role during experimental autoimmune uveitis (EAU) development. It was shown that mice neutralized with monoclonal antibodies to IL-12, which drives Th1 differentiation, did not develop EAU [19]. In order to detect whether constitutive ocular expression of IFN-γ influences the course of EAU, Egwuagu et al generated transgenic rats with targeted expression of IFN-γ in the eye and found that IFN-γ markedly accelerated the onset and exacerbated the severity of rat EAU [20]. However, it has been reported that IFN-γ can also provide a protective role in this model. Genetic deletion or neutralization with antibodies against endogenous IFN-γ did not lead to a resistance of EAU induction and development, but rather aggravated the severity of uveitis [21-22]. Mice treated with IL-12 during the first week after immunization appeared to protect the animals from EAU through an IFN-γ-dependent mechanism. It has now been demonstrated that the role of IFN-γ in the development of uveitis is dependent on the stage of disease and the model of EAU that is being studied. IFN-γ confers protection when it is produced during the early stage of the disease. Th1 cells play an essential pathogenic role in the induction of the so called dendritic cell (DC) EAU model, which is induced by the infusion of uveitogenic interphotoreceptor retinoid-binding protein (IRBP) peptide-pulsed DCs. On the other hand, Th17 cells are essential to the induction of classical EAU, which is induced by the immunization with IRBP in the presence of strong adjuvants such as complete Freund's adjuvant and *B. pertusis* [23].

3. Th17 cells and cytokines in Behcet's disease and VKH syndrome

Th17 cells, characterized by their production of IL-17, have been reported be associated with the pathogenesis of many autoimmune diseases, including multiple sclerosis, rheumatoid arthritis and systemic lupus erythematosus (SLE). Th17 cells preferentially produce IL-17A, IL 17F, IL 21, and IL 22 [24]. IL 17A, also commonly called IL-17, plays a critical role in the development of allergy and autoimmune responses. IL-17F is mainly involved in mucosal host defense mechanisms, while not required for the induction of experimental autoimmune encephalomyelitis (EAE) and Collagen-induced arthritis (CIA) [25]. As yet no reports have appeared on the role of IL-17F in the pathogenesis of uveitis, thus, whether IL-17F is involved in human uveitis and EAU needs further investigation. This section aims to review studies regarding Th17 cells and related cytokines in the development of BD and VKH syndrome.

Various studies have shown that Th17 cells contribute to the pathogenesis of BD and VKH syndrome. The previous reports from ours and others have shown that the level of IL-17 by polyclonally stimulated peripheral blood mononuclear cells (PBMCs) and $CD4^{+}T$ cells, and the frequency of IL-17–producing $CD4^{+}T$ cells in PBMCs was higher in patients with active BD or VKH syndrome than the controls [11-12, 26]. Geri et al reported an increase of Th17 cells in peripheral blood and in CSF from active BD patients [27]. Animal studies showed that IL-17 may play a major role in the pathogenesis of EAU. The neutralization of IL-17 by monoclonal antibodies prevented or reversed the intraocular inflammation in the EAU model [28-30]. Adoptive transfer of Th17 cells could induce EAU in the absence of INF-γ [29]. These results indicate that IL-17 plays a proinflammatory and pathogenic role in autoimmune uveitis, and the blockade of IL-17 signaling may represent a therapeutic target in BD and VKH syndrome as well as in other Th17 cell-mediated autoimmune diseases.

IL-21, a member of the IL-2 family of cytokines, can drive Th17 differentiation in an autocrine manner [31-32]. We recently reported a higher level of serum IL-21 and IL-21 mRNA in PBMCs from patients having chronic or recurrent active VKH syndrome as compared with patients having inactive VKH syndrome or healthy controls. Moreover, in vitro experiments showed that IL-21 significantly increased IL-17 production, but had no influence on IFN-γ production by PBMCs or $CD4^{+}T$ cells obtained from either patients or healthy controls [33]. Geri et al observed higher levels of serum IL-21 and IL-21-producing $CD4^{+}T$ cells in BD patients. IL-21 was found to be able to drive Th1 and Th17 differentiation and suppressed the frequency of Treg cells. More importantly, they demonstrated the presence of IL-21-producing T cells in the CSF, choroid plexus, brain parenchyma inflammatory infiltrates and intracerebral blood vessels in active BD with CNS involvement [27]. These results suggest that IL-21 may be involved in the pathogenesis of BD and VKH syndrome and may represent a novel therapeutic target for these diseases. The pathogenic role of IL-21 in autoimmune uveitis is supported by animal models. IL-21R-deficient mice are resistant to EAU, and adoptive transfer of IL-$21R^{-/-}$T cells reduced the EAU severity. Increased IL-21 in lymph nodes and spleens has been reported during the development of EAU [34-35]. All these findings provide evidence for a role of IL-21 in the pathogenesis of uveitis by promoting Th1 and Th17 cell responses and inhibiting Treg cell development.

IL-22, a member of the IL-10 cytokine family, has recently been reported to be involved in a number of human diseases, including mucosal-associated infections and inflammatory disorders of the intestine, skin and joints. In view of the biological function, controversial effects of IL-22 have been observed in different animal models and human disease. IL-22 seems to play a pathogenic role in experimental arthritis and dermatitis, whereas a protective effect was found in inflammatory bowel disease, experimental hepatitis and collagen-induced arthritis [36-37]. Sugita et al showed that the frequency of IL-22-producing T cell clones from aqueous humor of Behcet's uveitis was higher than that from normal controls. Furthermore, they demonstrated that CD4⁺T cells from PBMCs secrete increased amounts of IL-22 in BD patients with active uveitis. Higher IL-22 levels in the supernatants of stimulated PBMCs and CD4⁺T cells and an increased frequency of IL-22-producing CD4⁺T cells in BD patients with active uveitis were also reported by our group. In addition, increased IL-22 mRNA expression was found in erythema nodosum (EN) skin lesions, and positively correlated with the presence of EN [38]. The group of Nussenblatt reported an upregulated expression of IL-22 in PBMCs of clinical uveitis patients. IL-22 was shown to damage the physiological integrity of primary fetal retinal epithelium cells and induced their apoptosis [39]. These results suggest that an increased IL-22 may also be involved in the pathogenesis of BD. However, studies in a mouse model of uveitis showed that IL-22 can protect mice from the development of uveitis by inducing the generation of regulatory CD11b⁺antigen-presenting cells, which were able to convert pathogenic T cells into regulatory T cells [40]. As mentioned, the role of IL-22 in human clinical uveitis and animal models remains controversial and needs further investigation.

4. Molecules modulating Th1 or Th17 cells in Behcet's disease and VKH syndrome

The induction and maintenance of Th1 and Th17 cells requires a large set of molecules. The differentiation of Th17 cells from naïve CD4⁺T cells is regulated by cytokines [41]. Transforming growth factor-β (TGF-β) and IL-6, broadly expressed by many cell types in the body, including dendritic and epithelial cells, are dominant in the initiation of Th17 cell differentiation [42-45]; IL-23, IL-1β and IL-21, which are products of activated DCs, macrophages, activated T cell or inflamed epithelial cells, possibly expand and maintain the differentiated Th17 cells in the presence of IL-6 and TGF-β1 [31-32, 43, 46-47]. Furthermore, signal transducer and activator of transcription 3 (STAT3) has been found to mediate the initiation of Th17 cell differentiation by these inducing cytokines [48]. IL-12 is an important cytokine responsible for Th1 cell differentiation. IL-27 can induce Tr1 cell differentiation while inhibiting Th17 cell differentiation.

IL-6 has been shown to be a critical mediator of the autoimmune response and inflammation. Various studies have demonstrated that IL-6 was associated with disease activity in BD [49-50]. Studies by Norose et al showed that the level of IL-6 was significantly increased and correlated with the number of lymphocytes in aqueous humor from VKH patients [51]. The infiltrated T cells in the aqueous humor or PBMCs obtained from VKH patients showed an enhanced capability to secrete IL-6 as compared to normal controls [51-52]. Ozdamar et al found that serum levels of IL-6 were higher in BD patients with active uveitis than in those without uveitis [53]. A higher level of IL-6 was also reported in the CSF of patients with active BD with nervous system involvement [54-55]. A case report by Hirano et al showed that tocilizumab, a humanized anti-interleukin 6 receptor antibody, could suppress the clinical manifestations in a patient with refractory BD [56]. Consistent with observations in clinical uveitis, IL-6-deficient mice were not able to generate Th17 cells and were resistant to EAU. Systemic administration of anti-IL-6 receptor antibody ameliorated EAU by suppressing both systemic and regional Th17 responses [57-58]. Taken together, these findings suggest that IL-6 is involved in the pathogenesis of BD and VKH syndrome, and IL-6 blockade may provide a therapeutic efficacy in treating ocular inflammation in patients with BD or VKH syndrome.

IL-23, which is composed of a unique p19 subunit and a shared p40 subunit of IL-12, is essential in the survival and maintenance of pathogenic Th17 cells. Our earlier studies provided evidence for the involvement of IL-23 in the occurrence of uveitis in BD and VKH syndrome. Active uveitis in both diseases showed a higher level of IL-23 in the serum and supernatants of PBMCs as compared to inactive patients and normal controls [11-12]. IL-23p19 mRNA expression was increased in the EN-like skin lesions from BD patients [59]. Studies by Habibagahi et al showed that the IL-23 expression was strongly associated with the disease activity of uveitis with BD [60]. These results suggest that IL-23 may be a biomarker in the course of BD and VKH syndrome. Animal studies have shown that IL-23 is necessary for the induction of EAU due to its capacity to promote a Th17 effector response. It has been shown that IL-23KO mice are resistant to EAU and specific anti-IL-23 antibody prevented EAU induction [29]. These findings support the hypothesis that the IL-23/IL-17 pathway is involved in the pathogenesis of intraocular inflammation in BD and VKH syndrome.

IL-1β is a key proinflammatory cytokine that promotes Th17 cell differentiation. We recently observed a higher IL-1β production by peptidoglycan (PGN)/lipopolysaccharide (LPS)–induced monocyte-derived macrophages from active ocular BD patients [61]. Pay et al showed a significantly increased level of IL-1β in synovial fluid from BD patients as compared to that from osteoarthritis patients [62]. These results suggest that IL-1β may play a critical role in the pathogenesis of BD. The pathogenic role of IL-1β in uveitis was also proven directly by the observation that IL-1 receptor deficient mice were completely resistant to EAU [63].

IL-12, a heterodimeric cytokine composed of the subunits p40 andp35, is known to induce the differentiation of naïve $CD4^{+}T$ cells into Th1 cells. Studies on the role of IL-12 in clinical uveitis have shown that IL-12 levels in plasma and PBMC culture supernatants were higher in BD with active uveitis [64-65]. Actual measurements of IL-12 in VKH syndrome have not yet been reported. Many studies have shown that Th1 cells are involved in VKH syndrome [13-14], which makes it likely that IL-12 is involved in the pathogenesis.

IL-27, a member of the IL-12 family of cytokines, has been shown to be able to inhibit Th17 cells and that it can induce regulatory Tr1 cells. IL-27 is composed of a unique p28 subunit and a shared EBI3 subunit with IL-35. Our studies on VKH found a decreased IL-27P28 mRNA expression by PBMCs and the lower IL-27 levels in the serum and supernatants of PBMCs in active VKH patients as compared to the inactive patients and normal controls, while the shared EBI3 mRNA expression was not different between the three groups. Furthermore, IL-27 was shown to inhibit the Th17 cell response in a direct manner on $CD4^{+}T$ cells as well as by modulating DCs. Treatment with corticosteroids has been shown to upregulate IL-27 production in vivo and in vitro [66]. An increased levels of IL-27 have been reported in the serum of uveitis patients with BD [67]. Various animal models have been used to examine the role of IL-27 in autoimmune disease and found that the presence of IL-27 could protect mice from

EAE and CIA [68-69]. In the EAU model, an increased expression of IL-27 was observed at the peak of EAU, and further experiments showed that IL-27 could suppress the expansion of Th17 cells in the retina [70]. These observations suggest that an upregulated IL-27 response may contribute to the self-limited inflammation seen in the EAU model. Further clinical studies are needed in clinical uveitis and EAU to obtain further support whether IL-27 may be a potential therapeutic target for BD and VKH syndrome.

Tumor necrosis factor-alpha (TNF-α) is a proinflammatory cytokine that plays a significant role in the pathogenesis of many inflammatory and autoimmune diseases. It has been reported that the level of TNF-α was increased in the ocular fluids, serum and in the supernatants of stimulated $CD4^+$T cells from active uveitis patients with BD. Furthermore, TNF-α could induce the polarization of Th17 cells in BD patients [71-72]. A similar result was seen in the aqueous humor of VKH patients concerning the expression of TNF-α [18]. In the animal models of EAU it was shown that TNFR1-deficient mice were resistant to EAU through a TNFR1-dependent deficit in macrophage migration to the inflammatory site [73]. Treatment with systemic or local TNF-α inhibition with etanercept in the induction phase of EAU could effectively alleviate the severity of uveitis [74]. The pathogenic role of TNF-α in uveitis was also supported by experiments that showed that TNF-α could disrupt morphologic and functional barrier properties of polarized retinal pigment epithelium cells [75]. Thus, these results also indicate that TNF-α plays an important role in the pathogenesis of uveitis and has provided the basis as a major target for treating inflammatory and autoimmune eye diseases. In clinical trials, a number of reports have shown encouraging results in treating BD and VKH syndrome with anti-TNF-α antibody, such as infliximab [76-77].

A number of other immune-related molecules were also found to be associated with the pathogenesis of BD or VKH syndrome. Our most recent studies have revealed that other proinflammatory mediators, such as osteopontin (OPN), IL-7 and leptin, were also involved in the pathogenesis of BD and/or VKH syndrome. We observed the increased serum levels of OPN, IL-7 and leptin in patients with active BD and/or VKH syndrome, which may promote both Th1 and/or Th17 polarization [78-81]. Consistent with our findings, it has been shown that OPN aggravated the severity of EAU, and blockade of OPN with siRNA prevented the uveitis development [82-83]. IL-7 and leptin have been reported to be involved in the induction and progress of EAE, a model that shares many immunopathogenic mechanisms with EAU [84-85].

Other regulatory molecules may also play a critical role in controlling autoimmunity. 1,25-Dihydroxyvitamin D, miRNA155, IFN-α and IFN-β have all been shown to have an anti-inflammatory role in autoimmune disease. Levels of 1,25-Dihydroxyvitamin D3 and miRNA155 have been shown to be decreased in BD and VKH syndrome. Furthermore, 1,25-Dihydroxyvitamin D3 and miRNA155 were shown to inhibit Th17 cell responses [86-87], supporting its protective role in both BD and VKH syndrome. IFN-α has been effective in treating uveitis in patients with BD and our studies on the possible mechanisms showed that it could inhibit the Th17 cell response and was able to induce the expression of the regulatory cytokine IL-10 [88]. Studies in the animal model of uveitis showed that IFN-β exerted its inhibitory effect on EAU by inhibiting the Th1 and Th17 cell response [89], suggesting a protective role in uveitis.

5. Treg cells in Behcet's disease and VKH syndrome

Treg cells maintain the immune balance between effector and tolerogenic immune responses. It is well documented that a deficiency in Treg cells can result in the development of autoimmune disease and adoptive transfer of Treg cells effectively prevented and suppressed the severity of inflammation and/or autoimmune disease. Up to now, several subsets of Treg cells have been identified, such as the TGF-β-secreting Th3 regulatory cells [90], $CD8^+CD28^-$T cells [91] and NKT regulatory cells [92]. However, the best characterized subsets of $CD4^+$regulatory T cells are $CD4^+CD25^+FoxP3^+$Tregs and Tr1 cells that secrete IL-10 and lack FoxP3 expression. The important protective role played by these T-regulatory cells in the control of inflammatory and autoimmune disease has generated considerable interest in patients with noninfectious uveitis including BD and VKH syndrome.

$CD4^+CD25^+FoxP3^+$Tregs can be divided into two subpopulations: natural Treg cells (nTreg), which are develop as a distinct lineage of cells in the thymus, and the induced Treg cells (iTreg), which are generated in the periphery from naïve $CD4^+$T cells. They can also be induced in vitro. The difference and relative contributions in immune response of nTreg and iTreg cells are difficult to distinguish. A recent study found that a cell surface molecule neuropilin-1 was expressed on thymus-derived nTreg cells, but not on mucosa-generated $Foxp3^+$iTreg cells [93-94]. This marker can now be used to distinguish the subsets of $CD4^+CD25^+$Tregs. Our studies showed a decreased frequency of $CD4^+CD25^+$Treg cells and $CD4^+CD25^+Foxp3^+$Treg cells in the peripheral blood from active VKH patients. $CD4^+CD25^+$Treg cells from active VKH patients showed a diminished function in suppressing the proliferation of $CD4^+CD25^-$T cells and were less potent in inhibiting the production of IFN-γ and IL-13 by $CD4^+CD25^-$Tcells [95]. These results suggest that a decreased frequency and diminished function of $CD4^+CD25^+$Treg cells are associated with the active uveitis seen in VKH patients. However, Commodaro et al found no significant differences in the frequency of $CD4^+Foxp3^+$and $CD25^+Foxp3^+$T cells as well as no reduction in FOXP3 mRNA expression in mononuclear cells from VKH patients with active or inactive uveitis as compared with healthy controls [96]. The discrepancy may be due to the difference in Tregs subtypes investigated in the two studies (iTreg or nTreg). Patients with BD showed a significantly decreased frequency of Treg cells [27, 97], suggesting that the low level of Treg cells may contribute to the pathogenesis of ocular attacks in BD patients.

Tr1 cells are defined by their high expression of IL-10 and their ability to suppress antigen-specific effector T cell. Unlike $CD4^+CD25^+$Treg cells, which are present from birth, Tr1 cells are inducible cells and can be generated both in vitro and in vivo. It has been reported that IL-27 or CD46 activation in the presence of IL-2 can induce the differentiation of Tr1 cells [98-99]. A defect of CD46-mediated Tr1 cells has been reported in multiple sclerosis [98]. A study by our group revealed a decreased IL-10 production by naïve $CD4^+$T cells under Tr1 cell polarizing conditions in active VKH patients as compared with inactive VKH patients and healthy controls [66], suggesting that a defect of Tr1 cells might contribute to the pathogenesis of VKH syndrome.

Animal studies showed that Treg cells are involved in the remission of ocular inflammation. nTreg cells and iTreg cells induced by LPS-activated bone marrow dendritic cells inhibited the development of EAU. An increased frequency of $CD4^{+}CD25^{+}$Treg cells was associated with the EAU activity, and these Treg cells from EAU mice have a stronger ability to inhibit the proliferation of $CD4^{+}CD25^{-}$T cells and decreased IFN-γ production by $CD4^{+}CD25^{-}$T cells compared with those obtained from normal control mice. Moreover, transfer of $CD4^{+}CD25^{+}$Treg cells obtained from EAU mice on day 14 or 28 inhibited EAU induction [100]. These results suggest that the increased frequency and inhibitory effect of $CD4^{+}CD25^{+}$Treg cells in EAU mice may contribute to the monophasic nature and rapid resolution of EAU. Shao and his colleagues found that the suppressive function of Treg cells from animals with recurrent EAU was weaker than those from animals with the monophasic form, indicating that the dysregulation and malfunction of Treg cells in the eye contributed to disease recurrence [101]. Taken together, these results offer an explanation why the uveitis in the BD and VKH syndrome is recurrent while the uveitis in the EAU model is monophasic. The observations demonstrate the important role of $Foxp3^{+}$Treg cells in maintaining immune tolerance and preventing autoimmunity. Thus, it could be hypothesized that Treg cells in vitro expansion and adoptive transfer back to the patient might be a potential treatment for BD and VKH syndrome.

6. Genetic factors in Behcet's disease and VKH syndrome

The majority of BD is sporadic, but its familial aggregation has been reported [102-103]. BD can be found all over the world, however, its prevalence is particularly high in a peculiar region along the Silk Road extending from the Mediterranean basin to China [2, 104]. BD has been shown to be strongly associated with HLA-B51, which has been confirmed in different ethnic groups [105-106]. Previous studies showed that VKH syndrome is more prevalent in particular ethnic groups, particularly in pigmented groups [7] including Latin-American and Asian populations and displays a familial aggregation pattern [107]. Several HLA genes such as HLA-DR4 and HLA-DRw53, were strongly associated with VKH in a variety of ethnic groups [10, 108-109]. The aforementioned evidence as provided a strong genetic basis for BD and VKH confirmed by familial aggregation, geographical ethnic distribution, and strong association with especially Human leukocyte antigen (*HLA*) antigens. The genes associated with Behcet's disease and VKH syndrome are summarized in Tables 1 and 2, respectively.

6.1. Risk genes in Th1 cell pathway associated with Behcet's disease and VKH syndrome

STAT4, a transcription factor belonging to the Signal Transducer and Activator of Transcription protein family, is required for Th1 development of naive $CD4^{+}$T cells. Our study has identified an associated locus at STAT4 for BD in a Chinese Han population, and indicated that the risk SNP rs897200 in the STAT4 gene played a pathogenic role through an effect on

STAT4 transcription and IL-17 production [110]. The association of STAT4 with BD was confirmed in a Turkish population [111], suggesting that STAT4 is a common risk gene for BD in different ethnic cohorts.

C-C chemokine receptor type 1 (CCR1) and CCR3 play important roles in the accumulation and activation of inflammatory cells such as the Th1 cell. Recent studies showed that a locus at CCR1/CCR3 was associated with BD in Chinese Han and Turkish populations [111-112]. Functional studies showed a higher expression of CCR1 and migration of monocytes was found in individuals with the risk genotype [111], suggesting that impaired clearance of pathogens may contribute to the development of BD.

IL-18 is a proinflammatory cytokine that stimulates the production of IFN-γ in collaboration with IL-12 by Th1 cells. Studies from Turkish and Korean populations have shown the consistent association with BD in spite of inconsistent result in Korean cohorts [113].

TNF-α has been implicated in the pathogenesis of BD and anti-TNF-α represents an important treatment modality for BD patients [114]. A meta analysis showed an association of TNF-α gene polymorphisms with BD in various ethnic populations [115-117].

6.2. Risk genes in the Th17 cell pathway associated with Behcet's disease and VKH syndrome

Accumulative evidence supports the important role of the IL-23/Th17/IL-17 pathway in mediating chronic inflammatory or immune diseases such as BD and VKH syndrome [11, 95] and suggests the involvement of genes related to this pathway such as IL23R-IL12RB2, JAK1, STAT3, IL-1β, IL-6, IL17 and OPN in BD and VKH syndrome. We investigated the association of IL23R genes with BD in the Chinese Han population [118]. The results showed that two SNPs in IL23R were associated with the susceptibility to BD. Genome-wide association studies also confirmed the association of IL23R-IL12RB2 with BD in Japanese, Turkish and Iranian patients [8-9, 119]. Additionally, we identified the association of STAT3, JAK1, MCP-1 genes with BD in a Chinese Han population [120-122]. Other genes in the Th17 pathway such as IL-6 and IL-1β also showed an association with BD [123-124].

OPN, also known as bone sialoprotein I or early T-lymphocyte activation, may enhance T cell survival and proliferation, and promotes the responses of Th1 and Th17 cells during chronic inflammatory or immune mediated diseases. We examined the OPN serum level in VKH syndrome and the association of OPN polymorphisms and its receptors with this disease [80]. The results showed that the OPN level was significantly increased in the serum of active VKH patients and identified an association of this gene with VKH syndrome in a Chinese Han population. Furthermore, we found the association of JAK1, IL17F with VKH syndrome [125-126]. These studies suggest that genetic variants of cytokines associated to the Th17 pathway may play an important role in the development of BD and VKH syndrome.

6.3. Risk genes in the Treg cell pathway associated with Behcet's disease and VKH syndrome

Mir-146a, one of the miRNAs prevalently expressed in Treg cells, is known as a negative regulator of innate immunity in a variety of immune diseases [127]. We examined the association of polymorphisms in mir-146a with BD and VKH syndrome in a Chinese Han population and found that a polymorphism in this gene was associated with BD but not with VKH syndrome [128].

7. Innate immunity in Behcet's disease and VKH syndrome

It has been reported that infection may be involved in the pathogenesis of BD and VKH syndrome. Most of the uveitis patients with BD or VKH syndrome have manifestations of a bacterial or viral infection before the prodromal stage [129-130], suggesting that infectious agents may be a triggering factor to the onset of these diseases. DCs serve as professional antigen-presenting cells and provide the first line of defense against pathologic infections. Toll-like receptors (TLRs) expressed on DCs play a critical role in innate immunity against these pathologic infections. Interaction of DCs with TLR ligands results in the secretion of a number of proinflammatory cytokines that can induce the differentiation of naïve $CD4^{+}T$ cells into different $CD4^{+}T$ cells, including Th1, Th17 and Treg cells. Kirino and his colleagues reported that an increased expression of TLR4 is associated with heme oxygenase-1 reduction in PBMCs from patients with BD, leading to augmented inflammatory responses [131]. The study by Do et al showed a higher level of TLR2 and TLR4 in monocytes from active BD patients [132]. Our recent study showed a higher expression of TLR2, TLR3, TLR4 and TLR8 by either PBMCs, $CD4^{+}T$ cells or monocytes obtained from BD patients as compared with controls. Furthermore, significantly higher levels of IL-1β were produced by monocytes from active BD patients stimulated with known TLR ligands such as LPS and PGN [133]. These results suggest that a higher expression of TLR is associated with ocular Behcet's disease and may partly explain the mechanism by which infection was involved in the pathogenesis. It has been reported that DC deregulation was implicated in the pathogenesis of BD [134]. DCs play a critical role in determining the immune balance between self and non-self and this area is becoming a hotspot for researchers to develop tolerogenic DCs for treating autoimmune disease [135].

8. Summary

With the recent progress in immunology and genetics, environmental triggering factors such as viruses, bacteria or other molecular mimicry are thought to be participated in the outbreak of BD and VKH through interacting with TLRs. The imbalance of pathogenic Th1/Th17 and regulatory T cells and abnormalities in the associated immunoregulatory molecules with the abovementioned T cells are now supposed to be involved in the pathogenesis of these two diseases. The understanding of novel pathogenic mechanisms of both diseases may provide a foundation for developing new strategies to better treat the uveitis.

Genes	Odd Ratio	95% Confidence Interval	Ethnic	References
CCR1/CCR3	0.28	0.2–0.4	Chinese	[112]
CCR5	2.37	1.1- 5.1	Italian	[136]
CD40	1.98	1.38-2.83	Chinese	[137]
CPVL	2.26	1.47–3.45	Turkish	[138]
eNOS	1.88	1.27-2.49	Turkish	[139]
	3.2	1.4-7.3	Korean	[140]
	1.26	2.13-3.62	Tunisian	[141]
ERAP1	4.56	2.88-7.22	Turkish	[111]
FCRL3	0.7	0.5–0.9	Chinese	[142]
ICAM1	1.26	2.13-3.62	Tunisian	[143]
	4.2	1.9-9.3	Italian	[144]
IL1β	3.63	1.23–12.97	Turkish	[123]
IL4	3.40	1.72–7.12	Turkish	[145]
IL6	3.5	1.2-10.0	Korean	[124]
IL10	1.20	1.02-1.40	Iran	[119]
	1.45	1.34-1.58	Turkish, Arab, Greek, UK, Korean, Japanese	[9]
	1.45	1.32–1.60	Japanese, Turkish, Korean	[8]
IL12B	1.8	1.0–3.3	Japanese	[146]
IL18	1.48	1.10–1.97	Turkish	[147]
IL23R-IL12RB2	1.51	1.27–1.78	Iran	[119]
	1.28	1.18-1.39	Turkish	[9]
	1.35	0.95–1.91	Japanese,Turkish, Korean	[8]
	1.86	1.39 -2.49	Chinese	[118]
IRF-1	3.71	1.778-7.770	Korean	[148]
KIAA1529	2.04	1.45–2.88	Turkish	[138]
LOC100129342	1.84	1.32–2.58	Turkish	[138]
m.709G >A	1.40	1.0-1.97	Iranian	[149]
MCP1	1.51	1.05–2.17	Chinese	[122]

Genes	Odd Ratio	95% Confidence Interval	Ethnic	References
MDR1	3.03	1.41-6.54	Turkish	[150]
MIF	1.46	1.19–1.79	Chinese	[151]
miR-146a	1.33	1.17-1.52	Chinese	[128]
MMP2	0.6	0.44-0.87	Korean	[152]
MMP9	0.371	0.152-0.905	Korean	[153]
MTHFR	1.70	1.23–2.35	Turkish	[154]
NRAMP1	1.88	1.21-2.93	Turkish	[155]
PDGFRL	0.59	0.49–0.72	Chinese	[156]
Protein Z	6.8	2.6-17.9	Turkish	[157]
PTPN22	2.4	1.2 to 4.7	UK, Middle East	[158]
SLC11A1	0.60	0.37-0.95	Korean	[159]
STAT3	1.712	1.238–2.369	Chinese	[121]
STAT4	1.45	1.3-1.6	Chinese	[110, 160]
	1.27	1.17–1.37	Turkish	[111]
SUMO4	23.40	2.33-235.54	Korean	[161]
	1.41	1.01-1.97	Tunisian	[162]
	1.7	1.3–2.2	Chinese	[106]
TGFBR3	0.617	0.441-0.863	Chinese	[163]
TLR4	1.96	1.26-3.26	Korean	[164]
	1.67	1.08-2.60	Japanese	[165]
TNF-α	1.68	1.10-2.56	Moroccan	[116]
	3.08	1.73-5.47	Iranian Azeri Turk	[117]
TNFAIP3	2.03	1.65-2.49	Chinese	[166]
TREM-1	2.723	1.285-5.770	Korean	[167]
UBAC2	1.5	1.2-1.7	Chinese	[168]
UBASH3B	1.71	1.23–2.38	Turkish	[138]
VDR	1.89	1.32-2.71	Tunisians	[169]
VEGF	0.10	0.011-0.875	Korean	[170]

Table 1. Summary of the associated genes with Behcet's disease

Author details

Peizeng Yang[1*], Chaokui Wang[1], Shengping Hou[1], Bo Lei[1], Aize Kijlstra[2] and De-Quan Li[3*]

*Address all correspondence to: peizengycmu@126.com; dequanl@bcm.tmc.edu

1 The First Affiliated Hospital of Chongqing Medical University, Chongqing Key Lab of Ophthalmology, Chongqing Eye Institute, Chongqing, P. R. China

2 University Eye Clinic Maastricht, Maastricht, Netherlands

3 Ocular Surface Center, Cullen Eye Institute, Department of Ophthalmology, Baylor College of Medicine, Houston, Texas, USA

References

[1] Wakefield D.,J.H. Chang. Epidemiology of uveitis. Int Ophthalmol Clin 2005; 45(2): 1-13.

[2] Sakane T., M. Takeno, N. Suzuki,G. Inaba. Behcet's disease. N Engl J Med 1999; 341(17):1284-91.

[3] Evereklioglu C. Current concepts in the etiology and treatment of Behcet disease. Surv Ophthalmol 2005; 50(4):297-350.

[4] Yang P., W. Fang, Q. Meng, Y. Ren, L. Xing,A. Kijlstra. Clinical features of chinese patients with Behcet's disease. Ophthalmology 2008; 115(2):312-318 e4.

[5] Moorthy R.S., H. Inomata,N.A. Rao. Vogt-Koyanagi-Harada syndrome. Surv Ophthalmol 1995; 39(4):265-92.

[6] Murakami S., Y. Inaba, M. Mochizuki, A. Nakajima,A. Urayama. [A nation-wide survey on the occurrence of Vogt-Koyanagi-Harada disease in Japan]. Nihon Ganka Gakkai Zasshi 1994; 98(4):389-92.

[7] Yang P., Y. Ren, B. Li, W. Fang, Q. Meng,A. Kijlstra. Clinical characteristics of Vogt-Koyanagi-Harada syndrome in Chinese patients. Ophthalmology 2007; 114(3):606-14.

[8] Mizuki N., A. Meguro, M. Ota, S. Ohno, T. Shiota, T. Kawagoe, N. Ito, J. Kera, E. Okada, K. Yatsu, Y.W. Song, E.B. Lee, N. Kitaichi, K. Namba, Y. Horie, M. Takeno, S. Sugita, M. Mochizuki, S. Bahram, Y. Ishigatsubo,H. Inoko. Genome-wide association studies identify IL23R-IL12RB2 and IL10 as Behcet's disease susceptibility loci. Nat Genet 2010; 42(8):703-6.

[9] Remmers E.F., F. Cosan, Y. Kirino, M.J. Ombrello, N. Abaci, C. Satorius, J.M. Le, B. Yang, B.D. Korman, A. Cakiris, O. Aglar, Z. Emrence, H. Azakli, D. Ustek, I. Tugal-Tutkun, G. Akman-Demir, W. Chen, C.I. Amos, M.B. Dizon, A.A. Kose, G. Azizlerli,

B. Erer, O.J. Brand, V.G. Kaklamani, P. Kaklamanis, E. Ben-Chetrit, M. Stanford, F. Fortune, M. Ghabra, W.E. Ollier, Y.H. Cho, D. Bang, J. O'Shea, G.R. Wallace, M. Gadina, D.L. Kastner,A. Gul. Genome-wide association study identifies variants in the MHC class I, IL10, and IL23R-IL12RB2 regions associated with Behcet's disease. Nat Genet 2010; 42(8):698-702.

[10] Islam S.M., J. Numaga, Y. Fujino, R. Hirata, K. Matsuki, H. Maeda,K. Masuda. HLA class II genes in Vogt-Koyanagi-Harada disease. Invest Ophthalmol Vis Sci 1994; 35(11):3890-6.

[11] Chi W., P. Yang, B. Li, C. Wu, H. Jin, X. Zhu, L. Chen, H. Zhou, X. Huang,A. Kijlstra. IL-23 promotes CD4+T cells to produce IL-17 in Vogt-Koyanagi-Harada disease. J Allergy Clin Immunol 2007; 119(5):1218-24.

[12] Chi W., X. Zhu, P. Yang, X. Liu, X. Lin, H. Zhou, X. Huang,A. Kijlstra. Upregulated IL-23 and IL-17 in Behcet patients with active uveitis. Invest Ophthalmol Vis Sci 2008; 49(7):3058-64.

[13] Li B., P. Yang, H. Zhou, X. Huang, H. Jin, L. Chu, Y. Gao, L. Zhu,A. Kijlstra. Upregulation of T-bet expression in peripheral blood mononuclear cells during Vogt-Koyanagi-Harada disease. Br J Ophthalmol 2005; 89(11):1410-2.

[14] Liu X., P. Yang, X. Lin, X. Ren, H. Zhou, X. Huang, W. Chi, A. Kijlstra,L. Chen. Inhibitory effect of Cyclosporin A and corticosteroids on the production of IFN-gamma and IL-17 by T cells in Vogt-Koyanagi-Harada syndrome. Clin Immunol 2009; 131(2): 333-42.

[15] Zhao C., P. Yang, H. He, X. Lin, L. Du, H. Zhou,A. Kijlstra. Retinal S-antigen Th1 cell epitope mapping in patients with Behcet's disease. Graefes Arch Clin Exp Ophthalmol 2009; 247(4):555-60.

[16] Ben Ahmed M., H. Houman, M. Miled, K. Dellagi,H. Louzir. Involvement of chemokines and Th1 cytokines in the pathogenesis of mucocutaneous lesions of Behcet's disease. Arthritis Rheum 2004; 50(7):2291-5.

[17] Miyazawa I., T. Abe, K. Narikawa, J. Feng, T. Misu, I. Nakashima, J. Fujimori, M. Tamai, K. Fujihara,Y. Itoyama. Chemokine profile in the cerebrospinal fluid and serum of Vogt-Koyanagi-Harada disease. J Neuroimmunol 2005; 158(1-2):240-4.

[18] El-Asrar A.M., S. Struyf, D. Kangave, S.S. Al-Obeidan, G. Opdenakker, K. Geboes,J. Van Damme. Cytokine profiles in aqueous humor of patients with different clinical entities of endogenous uveitis. Clin Immunol 2011; 139(2):177-84.

[19] Yokoi H., K. Kato, T. Kezuka, J. Sakai, M. Usui, H. Yagita,K. Okumura. Prevention of experimental autoimmune uveoretinitis by monoclonal antibody to interleukin-12. Eur J Immunol 1997; 27(3):641-6.

[20] Egwuagu C.E., J. Sztein, R.M. Mahdi, W. Li, C. Chao-Chan, J.A. Smith, P. Charukamnoetkanok,A.B. Chepelinsky. IFN-gamma increases the severity and accelerates the

onset of experimental autoimmune uveitis in transgenic rats. J Immunol 1999; 162(1): 510-7.

[21] Caspi R.R., C.C. Chan, B.G. Grubbs, P.B. Silver, B. Wiggert, C.F. Parsa, S. Bahmanyar, A. Billiau,H. Heremans. Endogenous systemic IFN-gamma has a protective role against ocular autoimmunity in mice. J Immunol 1994; 152(2):890-9.

[22] Fukushima A., T. Yamaguchi, W. Ishida, K. Fukata, K. Udaka,H. Ueno. Mice lacking the IFN-gamma receptor or fyn develop severe experimental autoimmune uveoretinitis characterized by different immune responses. Immunogenetics 2005; 57(5): 337-43.

[23] Damsker J.M., A.M. Hansen,R.R. Caspi. Th1 and Th17 cells: adversaries and collaborators. Ann N Y Acad Sci 2010; 1183:211-21.

[24] Korn T., E. Bettelli, M. Oukka,V.K. Kuchroo. IL-17 and Th17 Cells. Annu Rev Immunol 2009; 27:485-517.

[25] Iwakura Y., H. Ishigame, S. Saijo,S. Nakae. Functional specialization of interleukin-17 family members. Immunity 2011; 34(2):149-62.

[26] Hamzaoui K., E. Bouali, I. Ghorbel, M. Khanfir, H. Houman,A. Hamzaoui. Expression of Th-17 and RORgammat mRNA in Behcet's Disease. Med Sci Monit 2011; 17(4):CR227-34.

[27] Geri G., B. Terrier, M. Rosenzwajg, B. Wechsler, M. Touzot, D. Seilhean, T.A. Tran, B. Bodaghi, L. Musset, V. Soumelis, D. Klatzmann, P. Cacoub,D. Saadoun. Critical role of IL-21 in modulating TH17 and regulatory T cells in Behcet disease. J Allergy Clin Immunol 2011; 128(3):655-64.

[28] Peng Y., G. Han, H. Shao, Y. Wang, H.J. Kaplan,D. Sun. Characterization of IL-17+interphotoreceptor retinoid-binding protein-specific T cells in experimental autoimmune uveitis. Invest Ophthalmol Vis Sci 2007; 48(9):4153-61.

[29] Luger D., P.B. Silver, J. Tang, D. Cua, Z. Chen, Y. Iwakura, E.P. Bowman, N.M. Sgambellone, C.C. Chan,R.R. Caspi. Either a Th17 or a Th1 effector response can drive autoimmunity: conditions of disease induction affect dominant effector category. J Exp Med 2008; 205(4):799-810.

[30] Zhang R., J. Qian, J. Guo, Y.F. Yuan,K. Xue. Suppression of experimental autoimmune uveoretinitis by Anti-IL-17 antibody. Curr Eye Res 2009; 34(4):297-303.

[31] Nurieva R., X.O. Yang, G. Martinez, Y. Zhang, A.D. Panopoulos, L. Ma, K. Schluns, Q. Tian, S.S. Watowich, A.M. Jetten,C. Dong. Essential autocrine regulation by IL-21 in the generation of inflammatory T cells. Nature 2007; 448(7152):480-3.

[32] Korn T., E. Bettelli, W. Gao, A. Awasthi, A. Jager, T.B. Strom, M. Oukka,V.K. Kuchroo. IL-21 initiates an alternative pathway to induce proinflammatory T(H)17 cells. Nature 2007; 448(7152):484-7.

[33] Li F., P. Yang, X. Liu, C. Wang, S. Hou,A. Kijlstra. Upregulation of interleukin 21 and promotion of interleukin 17 production in chronic or recurrent Vogt-Koyanagi-Harada disease. Arch Ophthalmol 2010; 128(11):1449-54.

[34] Wang L., C.R. Yu, H.P. Kim, W. Liao, W.G. Telford, C.E. Egwuagu,W.J. Leonard. Key role for IL-21 in experimental autoimmune uveitis. Proc Natl Acad Sci U S A 2011; 108(23):9542-7.

[35] Liu L., Y. Xu, J. Wang,H. Li. Upregulated IL-21 and IL-21 receptor expression is involved in experimental autoimmune uveitis (EAU). Mol Vis 2009; 15:2938-44.

[36] Sarkar S., X. Zhou, S. Justa,S.R. Bommireddy. Interleukin-22 reduces the severity of collagen-induced arthritis in association with increased levels of interleukin-10. Arthritis Rheum 2013; 65(4):960-71.

[37] Sanjabi S., L.A. Zenewicz, M. Kamanaka,R.A. Flavell. Anti-inflammatory and pro-inflammatory roles of TGF-beta, IL-10, and IL-22 in immunity and autoimmunity. Curr Opin Pharmacol 2009; 9(4):447-53.

[38] Cai T., Q. Wang, Q. Zhou, C. Wang, S. Hou, J. Qi, A. Kijlstra,P. Yang. Increased expression of IL-22 is associated with disease activity in Behcet's disease. PLoS One 2013; 8(3):e59009.

[39] Li Z., B. Liu, A. Maminishkis, S.P. Mahesh, S. Yeh, J. Lew, W.K. Lim, H.N. Sen, G. Clarke, R. Buggage, S.S. Miller,R.B. Nussenblatt. Gene expression profiling in autoimmune noninfectious uveitis disease. J Immunol 2008; 181(7):5147-57.

[40] Ke Y., D. Sun, G. Jiang, H.J. Kaplan,H. Shao. IL-22-induced regulatory CD11b+APCs suppress experimental autoimmune uveitis. J Immunol 2011; 187(5):2130-9.

[41] Zheng X., F. Bian, P. Ma, C.S. De Paiva, M. Stern, S.C. Pflugfelder,D.Q. Li. Induction of Th17 differentiation by corneal epithelial-derived cytokines. J Cell Physiol 2010; 222(1):95-102.

[42] Zhou L., Ivanov, II, R. Spolski, R. Min, K. Shenderov, T. Egawa, D.E. Levy, W.J. Leonard,D.R. Littman. IL-6 programs T(H)-17 cell differentiation by promoting sequential engagement of the IL-21 and IL-23 pathways. Nat Immunol 2007; 8(9):967-74.

[43] Veldhoen M., R.J. Hocking, C.J. Atkins, R.M. Locksley,B. Stockinger. TGFbeta in the context of an inflammatory cytokine milieu supports de novo differentiation of IL-17-producing T cells. Immunity 2006; 24(2):179-89.

[44] Mangan P.R., L.E. Harrington, D.B. O'Quinn, W.S. Helms, D.C. Bullard, C.O. Elson, R.D. Hatton, S.M. Wahl, T.R. Schoeb,C.T. Weaver. Transforming growth factor-beta induces development of the T(H)17 lineage. Nature 2006; 441(7090):231-4.

[45] Bettelli E., Y. Carrier, W. Gao, T. Korn, T.B. Strom, M. Oukka, H.L. Weiner,V.K. Kuchroo. Reciprocal developmental pathways for the generation of pathogenic effector TH17 and regulatory T cells. Nature 2006; 441(7090):235-8.

[46] Manel N., D. Unutmaz,D.R. Littman. The differentiation of human T(H)-17 cells requires transforming growth factor-beta and induction of the nuclear receptor RORgammat. Nat Immunol 2008; 9(6):641-9.

[47] Hunter C.A. New IL-12-family members: IL-23 and IL-27, cytokines with divergent functions. Nat Rev Immunol 2005; 5(7):521-31.

[48] Yang X.O., A.D. Panopoulos, R. Nurieva, S.H. Chang, D. Wang, S.S. Watowich,C. Dong. STAT3 regulates cytokine-mediated generation of inflammatory helper T cells. J Biol Chem 2007; 282(13):9358-63.

[49] Adam B.,E. Calikoglu. Serum interleukin-6, procalcitonin and C-reactive protein levels in subjects with active Behcet's disease. J Eur Acad Dermatol Venereol 2004; 18(3): 318-20.

[50] Nalbant S., B. Sahan, M. Durna, D. Ersanli, M. Kaplan, O. Karabudak,M. Unal. Cytokine profile in Behcet uveitis. Bratisl Lek Listy 2008; 109(12):551-4.

[51] Norose K., A. Yano, X.C. Wang, T. Tokushima, J. Umihira, A. Seki, M. Nohara,K. Segawa. Dominance of activated T cells and interleukin-6 in aqueous humor in Vogt-Koyanagi-Harada disease. Invest Ophthalmol Vis Sci 1994; 35(1):33-9.

[52] Norose K.,A. Yano. Melanoma specific Th1 cytotoxic T lymphocyte lines in Vogt-Koyanagi-Harada disease. Br J Ophthalmol 1996; 80(11):1002-8.

[53] Ozdamar Y., N. Berker, G. Bahar, E. Soykan, T. Bicer, S.S. Ozkan,J. Karakaya. Inflammatory mediators and posterior segment involvement in ocular Behcet disease. Eur J Ophthalmol 2009; 19(6):998-1003.

[54] Akman-Demir G., E. Tuzun, S. Icoz, N. Yesilot, S.P. Yentur, M. Kurtuncu, M. Mutlu,G. Saruhan-Direskeneli. Interleukin-6 in neuro-Behcet's disease: association with disease subsets and long-term outcome. Cytokine 2008; 44(3):373-6.

[55] Wang C.R., C.Y. Chuang,C.Y. Chen. Anticardiolipin antibodies and interleukin-6 in cerebrospinal fluid and blood of Chinese patients with neuro-Behcet's syndrome. Clin Exp Rheumatol 1992; 10(6):599-602.

[56] Hirano T., N. Ohguro, S. Hohki, K. Hagihara, Y. Shima, M. Narazaki, A. Ogata, K. Yoshizaki, A. Kumanogoh, T. Kishimoto,T. Tanaka. A case of Behcet's disease treated with a humanized anti-interleukin-6 receptor antibody, tocilizumab. Mod Rheumatol 2012; 22(2):298-302.

[57] Hohki S., N. Ohguro, H. Haruta, K. Nakai, F. Terabe, S. Serada, M. Fujimoto, S. Nomura, H. Kawahata, T. Kishimoto,T. Naka. Blockade of interleukin-6 signaling suppresses experimental autoimmune uveoretinitis by the inhibition of inflammatory Th17 responses. Exp Eye Res 2010; 91(2):162-70.

[58] Yoshimura T., K.H. Sonoda, N. Ohguro, Y. Ohsugi, T. Ishibashi, D.J. Cua, T. Kobayashi, H. Yoshida,A. Yoshimura. Involvement of Th17 cells and the effect of anti-IL-6 therapy in autoimmune uveitis. Rheumatology (Oxford) 2009; 48(4):347-54.

[59] Lew W., J.Y. Chang, J.Y. Jung,D. Bang. Increased expression of interleukin-23 p19 mRNA in erythema nodosum-like lesions of Behcet's disease. Br J Dermatol 2008; 158(3):505-11.

[60] Habibagahi Z., M. Habibagahi,M. Heidari. Raised concentration of soluble form of vascular endothelial cadherin and IL-23 in sera of patients with Behcet's disease. Mod Rheumatol 2010; 20(2):154-9.

[61] Liang L., X. Tan, Q. Zhou, Y. Zhu, Y. Tian, H. Yu, A. Kijlstra,P. Yang. IL-1beta triggered by peptidoglycan and lipopolysaccharide through TLR2/4 and ROS-NLRP3 inflammasome-dependent pathways is involved in ocular Behcet's disease. Invest Ophthalmol Vis Sci 2013; 54(1):402-14.

[62] Pay S., H. Erdem, A. Pekel, I. Simsek, U. Musabak, A. Sengul,A. Dinc. Synovial proinflammatory cytokines and their correlation with matrix metalloproteinase-3 expression in Behcet's disease. Does interleukin-1beta play a major role in Behcet's synovitis? Rheumatol Int 2006; 26(7):608-13.

[63] Su S.B., P.B. Silver, R.S. Grajewski, R.K. Agarwal, J. Tang, C.C. Chan,R.R. Caspi. Essential role of the MyD88 pathway, but nonessential roles of TLRs 2, 4, and 9, in the adjuvant effect promoting Th1-mediated autoimmunity. J Immunol 2005; 175(10): 6303-10.

[64] Guenane H., D. Hartani, L. Chachoua, O.S. Lahlou-Boukoffa, F. Mazari,C. Touil-Boukoffa. [Production of Th1/Th2 cytokines and nitric oxide in Behcet's uveitis and idiopathic uveitis]. J Fr Ophtalmol 2006; 29(2):146-52.

[65] Belguendouz H., D. Messaoudene, D. Hartani, L. Chachoua, M.L. Ahmedi, K. Lahmar-Belguendouz, O. Lahlou-Boukoffa,C. Touil-Boukoffa. [Effect of corticotherapy on interleukin-8 and-12 and nitric oxide production during Behcet and idiopathic uveitis]. J Fr Ophtalmol 2008; 31(4):387-95.

[66] Wang C., Y. Tian, B. Lei, X. Xiao, Z. Ye, F. Li, A. Kijlstra,P. Yang. Decreased IL-27 expression in association with an increased Th17 response in Vogt-Koyanagi-Harada disease. Invest Ophthalmol Vis Sci 2012; 53(8):4668-75.

[67] Shen H., L.P. Xia,J. Lu. Elevated levels of interleukin-27 and effect on production of interferon-gamma and interleukin-17 in patients with Behcet's disease. Scand J Rheumatol 2013; 42(1):48-51.

[68] Fitzgerald D.C., B. Ciric, T. Touil, H. Harle, J. Grammatikopolou, J. Das Sarma, B. Gran, G.X. Zhang,A. Rostami. Suppressive effect of IL-27 on encephalitogenic Th17 cells and the effector phase of experimental autoimmune encephalomyelitis. J Immunol 2007; 179(5):3268-75.

[69] Pickens S.R., N.D. Chamberlain, M.V. Volin, A.M. Mandelin, 2nd, H. Agrawal, M. Matsui, T. Yoshimoto,S. Shahrara. Local expression of interleukin-27 ameliorates collagen-induced arthritis. Arthritis Rheum 2011; 63(8):2289-98.

[70] Amadi-Obi A., C.R. Yu, X. Liu, R.M. Mahdi, G.L. Clarke, R.B. Nussenblatt, I. Gery, Y.S. Lee,C.E. Egwuagu. TH17 cells contribute to uveitis and scleritis and are expanded by IL-2 and inhibited by IL-27/STAT1. Nat Med 2007; 13(6):711-8.

[71] Sugita S., Y. Kawazoe, A. Imai, Y. Yamada, S. Horie,M. Mochizuki. Inhibition of Th17 differentiation by anti-TNF-alpha therapy in uveitis patients with Behcet's disease. Arthritis Res Ther 2012; 14(3):R99.

[72] Evereklioglu C., H. Er, Y. Turkoz,M. Cekmen. Serum levels of TNF-alpha, sIL-2R, IL-6, and IL-8 are increased and associated with elevated lipid peroxidation in patients with Behcet's disease. Mediators Inflamm 2002; 11(2):87-93.

[73] Raveney B.J., D.A. Copland, A.D. Dick,L.B. Nicholson. TNFR1-dependent regulation of myeloid cell function in experimental autoimmune uveoretinitis. J Immunol 2009; 183(4):2321-9.

[74] Busch M., D. Bauer, M. Hennig, S. Wasmuth, S. Thanos,A. Heiligenhaus. Effects of systemic and intravitreal TNF-alpha inhibition in experimental autoimmune uveoretinitis. Invest Ophthalmol Vis Sci 2013; 54(1):39-46.

[75] Shirasawa M., S. Sonoda, H. Terasaki, N. Arimura, H. Otsuka, T. Yamashita, E. Uchino, T. Hisatomi, T. Ishibashi,T. Sakamoto. TNF-alpha disrupts morphologic and functional barrier properties of polarized retinal pigment epithelium. Exp Eye Res 2013; 110:59-69.

[76] Khalifa Y.M., M.R. Bailony,N.R. Acharya. Treatment of pediatric vogt-koyanagi-harada syndrome with infliximab. Ocul Immunol Inflamm 2010; 18(3):218-22.

[77] Cantini F., L. Niccoli, C. Nannini, O. Kaloudi, E. Cassara, M. Susini,I. Lenzetti. Efficacy of infliximab in refractory Behcet's disease-associated and idiopathic posterior segment uveitis: a prospective, follow-up study of 50 patients. Biologics 2012; 6:5-12.

[78] Liu L., P. Yang, H. He, X. Lin, L. Jiang, W. Chi, C. Zhao,H. Zhou. Leptin increases in Vogt-Koyanagi-Harada (VKH) disease and promotes cell proliferation and inflammatory cytokine secretion. Br J Ophthalmol 2008; 92(4):557-61.

[79] Chu M., P. Yang, S. Hou, F. Li, Y. Chen,A. Kijlstra. Behcet's disease exhibits an increased osteopontin serum level in active stage but no association with osteopontin and its receptor gene polymorphisms. Hum Immunol 2011; 72(6):525-9.

[80] Chu M., P. Yang, R. Hu, S. Hou, F. Li, Y. Chen,A. Kijlstra. Elevated serum osteopontin levels and genetic polymorphisms of osteopontin are associated with Vogt-Koyanagi-Harada disease. Invest Ophthalmol Vis Sci 2011; 52(10):7084-9.

[81] Yang Y., X. Xiao, F. Li, L. Du, A. Kijlstra,P. Yang. Increased IL-7 expression in Vogt-Koyanagi-Harada disease. Invest Ophthalmol Vis Sci 2012; 53(2):1012-7.

[82] Iwata D., M. Kitamura, N. Kitaichi, Y. Saito, S. Kon, K. Namba, J. Morimoto, A. Ebihara, H. Kitamei, K. Yoshida, S. Ishida, S. Ohno, T. Uede, K. Onoe,K. Iwabuchi. Prevention of experimental autoimmune uveoretinitis by blockade of osteopontin with small interfering RNA. Exp Eye Res 2010; 90(1):41-8.

[83] Kitamura M., K. Iwabuchi, N. Kitaichi, S. Kon, H. Kitamei, K. Namba, K. Yoshida, D.T. Denhardt, S.R. Rittling, S. Ohno, T. Uede,K. Onoe. Osteopontin aggravates experimental autoimmune uveoretinitis in mice. J Immunol 2007; 178(10):6567-72.

[84] Liu X., S. Leung, C. Wang, Z. Tan, J. Wang, T.B. Guo, L. Fang, Y. Zhao, B. Wan, X. Qin, L. Lu, R. Li, H. Pan, M. Song, A. Liu, J. Hong, H. Lu,J.Z. Zhang. Crucial role of interleukin-7 in T helper type 17 survival and expansion in autoimmune disease. Nat Med 2010; 16(2):191-7.

[85] Matarese G., A. Di Giacomo, V. Sanna, G.M. Lord, J.K. Howard, A. Di Tuoro, S.R. Bloom, R.I. Lechler, S. Zappacosta,S. Fontana. Requirement for leptin in the induction and progression of autoimmune encephalomyelitis. J Immunol 2001; 166(10): 5909-16.

[86] Tian Y., C. Wang, Z. Ye, X. Xiao, A. Kijlstra,P. Yang. Effect of 1,25-dihydroxyvitamin D3 on Th17 and Th1 response in patients with Behcet's disease. Invest Ophthalmol Vis Sci 2012; 53(10):6434-41.

[87] Zhou Q., X. Xiao, C. Wang, X. Zhang, F. Li, Y. Zhou, A. Kijlstra,P. Yang. Decreased microRNA-155 expression in ocular Behcet's disease but not in Vogt Koyanagi Harada syndrome. Invest Ophthalmol Vis Sci 2012; 53(9):5665-74.

[88] Liu X., P. Yang, C. Wang, F. Li,A. Kijlstra. IFN-alpha blocks IL-17 production by peripheral blood mononuclear cells in Behcet's disease. Rheumatology (Oxford) 2011; 50(2):293-8.

[89] Sun M., Y. Yang, P. Yang, B. Lei, L. Du,A. Kijlstra. Regulatory effects of IFN-beta on the development of experimental autoimmune uveoretinitis in B10RIII mice. PLoS One 2011; 6(5):e19870.

[90] Weiner H.L. Induction and mechanism of action of transforming growth factor-beta-secreting Th3 regulatory cells. Immunol Rev 2001; 182:207-14.

[91] Najafian N., T. Chitnis, A.D. Salama, B. Zhu, C. Benou, X. Yuan, M.R. Clarkson, M.H. Sayegh,S.J. Khoury. Regulatory functions of CD8+CD28-T cells in an autoimmune disease model. J Clin Invest 2003; 112(7):1037-48.

[92] Taniguchi M., M. Harada, S. Kojo, T. Nakayama,H. Wakao. The regulatory role of Valpha14 NKT cells in innate and acquired immune response. Annu Rev Immunol 2003; 21:483-513.

[93] Weiss J.M., A.M. Bilate, M. Gobert, Y. Ding, M.A. Curotto de Lafaille, C.N. Parkhurst, H. Xiong, J. Dolpady, A.B. Frey, M.G. Ruocco, Y. Yang, S. Floess, J. Huehn, S. Oh, M.O. Li, R.E. Niec, A.Y. Rudensky, M.L. Dustin, D.R. Littman,J.J. Lafaille. Neuropilin 1 is expressed on thymus-derived natural regulatory T cells, but not mucosa-generated induced Foxp3+T reg cells. J Exp Med 2012; 209(10):1723-42, S1.

[94] Yadav M., C. Louvet, D. Davini, J.M. Gardner, M. Martinez-Llordella, S. Bailey-Bucktrout, B.A. Anthony, F.M. Sverdrup, R. Head, D.J. Kuster, P. Ruminski, D. Weiss, D. Von Schack,J.A. Bluestone. Neuropilin-1 distinguishes natural and inducible regulatory T cells among regulatory T cell subsets in vivo. J Exp Med 2012; 209(10):1713-22, S1-19.

[95] Chen L., P. Yang, H. Zhou, H. He, X. Ren, W. Chi, L. Wang,A. Kijlstra. Diminished frequency and function of CD4+CD25high regulatory T cells associated with active uveitis in Vogt-Koyanagi-Harada syndrome. Invest Ophthalmol Vis Sci 2008; 49(8): 3475-82.

[96] Commodaro A.G., J.P. Peron, J. Genre, C. Arslanian, L. Sanches, C. Muccioli, L.V. Rizzo,R. Belfort, Jr. IL-10 and TGF-beta immunoregulatory cytokines rather than natural regulatory T cells are associated with the resolution phase of Vogt-Koyanagi-Harada (VKH) syndrome. Scand J Immunol 2010; 72(1):31-7.

[97] Nanke Y., S. Kotake, M. Goto, H. Ujihara, M. Matsubara,N. Kamatani. Decreased percentages of regulatory T cells in peripheral blood of patients with Behcet's disease before ocular attack: a possible predictive marker of ocular attack. Mod Rheumatol 2008; 18(4):354-8.

[98] Astier A.L., G. Meiffren, S. Freeman,D.A. Hafler. Alterations in CD46-mediated Tr1 regulatory T cells in patients with multiple sclerosis. J Clin Invest 2006; 116(12): 3252-7.

[99] Murugaiyan G., A. Mittal, R. Lopez-Diego, L.M. Maier, D.E. Anderson,H.L. Weiner. IL-27 is a key regulator of IL-10 and IL-17 production by human CD4+T cells. J Immunol 2009; 183(4):2435-43.

[100] Sun M., P. Yang, L. Du, H. Zhou, X. Ren,A. Kijlstra. Contribution of CD4+CD25+T cells to the regression phase of experimental autoimmune uveoretinitis. Invest Ophthalmol Vis Sci 2010; 51(1):383-9.

[101] Ke Y., G. Jiang, D. Sun, H.J. Kaplan,H. Shao. Ocular regulatory T cells distinguish monophasic from recurrent autoimmune uveitis. Invest Ophthalmol Vis Sci 2008; 49(9):3999-4007.

[102] Berman L., B. Trappler,T. Jenkins. Behcet's syndrome: a family study and the elucidation of a genetic role. Ann Rheum Dis 1979; 38(2):118-21.

[103] Gul A., M. Inanc, L. Ocal, O. Aral,M. Konice. Familial aggregation of Behcet's disease in Turkey. Ann Rheum Dis 2000; 59(8):622-5.

[104] Verity D.H., J.E. Marr, S. Ohno, G.R. Wallace,M.R. Stanford. Behcet's disease, the Silk Road and HLA-B51: historical and geographical perspectives. Tissue Antigens 1999; 54(3):213-20.

[105] de Menthon M., M.P. Lavalley, C. Maldini, L. Guillevin,A. Mahr. HLA-B51/B5 and the risk of Behcet's disease: a systematic review and meta-analysis of case-control genetic association studies. Arthritis Rheum 2009; 61(10):1287-96.

[106] Hou S., P. Yang, L. Du, H. Zhou, X. Lin, X. Liu,A. Kijlstra. SUMO4 gene polymorphisms in Chinese Han patients with Behcet's disease. Clin Immunol 2008; 129(1): 170-5.

[107] Rutzen A.R., G. Ortega-Larrocea, I.R. Schwab,N.A. Rao. Simultaneous onset of Vogt-Koyanagi-Harada syndrome in monozygotic twins. Am J Ophthalmol 1995; 119(2): 239-40.

[108] Zhao M., Y. Jiang,I.W. Abrahams. Association of HLA antigens with Vogt-Koyanagi-Harada syndrome in a Han Chinese population. Arch Ophthalmol 1991; 109(3): 368-70.

[109] Zhang X.Y., X.M. Wang,T.S. Hu. Profiling human leukocyte antigens in Vogt-Koyanagi-Harada syndrome. Am J Ophthalmol 1992; 113(5):567-72.

[110] Hou S., Z. Yang, L. Du, Z. Jiang, Q. Shu, Y. Chen, F. Li, Q. Zhou, S. Ohno, R. Chen, A. Kijlstra, J.T. Rosenbaum,P. Yang. Identification of a susceptibility locus in STAT4 for Behcet's disease in Han Chinese in a genome-wide association study. Arthritis Rheum 2012; 64(12):4104-13.

[111] Kirino Y., G. Bertsias, Y. Ishigatsubo, N. Mizuki, I. Tugal-Tutkun, E. Seyahi, Y. Ozyazgan, F.S. Sacli, B. Erer, H. Inoko, Z. Emrence, A. Cakar, N. Abaci, D. Ustek, C. Satorius, A. Ueda, M. Takeno, Y. Kim, G.M. Wood, M.J. Ombrello, A. Meguro, A. Gul, E.F. Remmers,D.L. Kastner. Genome-wide association analysis identifies new susceptibility loci for Behcet's disease and epistasis between HLA-B*51 and ERAP1. Nat Genet 2013; 45(2):202-7.

[112] Hou S., X. Xiao, F. Li, Z. Jiang, A. Kijlstra,P. Yang. Two-stage association study in Chinese Han identifies two independent associations in CCR1/CCR3 locus as candidate for Behcet's disease susceptibility. Hum Genet 2012; 131(12):1841-50.

[113] Jang W.C., S.B. Park, Y.H. Nam, S.S. Lee, J.W. Kim, I.S. Chang, K.T. Kim,H.K. Chang. Interleukin-18 gene polymorphisms in Korean patients with Behcet's disease. Clin Exp Rheumatol 2005; 23(4 Suppl 38):S59-63.

[114] Arida A., K. Fragiadaki, E. Giavri,P.P. Sfikakis. Anti-TNF agents for Behcet's disease: analysis of published data on 369 patients. Semin Arthritis Rheum 2011; 41(1):61-70.

[115] Touma Z., C. Farra, A. Hamdan, W. Shamseddeen, I. Uthman, H. Hourani,T. Arayssi. TNF polymorphisms in patients with Behcet disease: a meta-analysis. Arch Med Res 2010; 41(2):142-6.

[116] Radouane A., M. Oudghiri, A. Chakib, S. Bennani, I. Touitou,M. Barat-Houari. SNPs in the TNF-alpha gene promoter associated with Behcet's disease in Moroccan patients. Rheumatology (Oxford) 2012; 51(9):1595-9.

[117] Bonyadi M., Z. Jahanafrooz, M. Esmaeili, S. Kolahi, A. Khabazi, A.A. Ebrahimi, M. Hajialilo,S. Dastgiri. TNF-alpha gene polymorphisms in Iranian Azeri Turkish patients with Behcet's Disease. Rheumatol Int 2009; 30(2):285-9.

[118] Jiang Z., P. Yang, S. Hou, L. Du, L. Xie, H. Zhou,A. Kijlstra. IL-23R gene confers susceptibility to Behcet's disease in a Chinese Han population. Ann Rheum Dis 2010; 69(7):1325-8.

[119] Xavier J.M., F. Shahram, F. Davatchi, A. Rosa, J. Crespo, B.S. Abdollahi, A. Nadji, G. Jesus, F. Barcelos, J.V. Patto, N.M. Shafiee, F. Ghaderibarim,S.A. Oliveira. Association study of IL10 and IL23R-IL12RB2 in Iranian patients with Behcet's disease. Arthritis Rheum 2012; 64(8):2761-72.

[120] Hou S., J. Qi, Q. Zhang, D. Liao, Q. Li, K. Hu, Y. Zhou, A. Kijlstra,P. Yang. Genetic variants in the JAK1 gene confer higher risk of Behcet's disease with ocular involvement in Han Chinese. Hum Genet 2013.

[121] Hu K., S. Hou, Z. Jiang, A. Kijlstra,P. Yang. JAK2 and STAT3 polymorphisms in a Han Chinese population with Behcet's disease. Invest Ophthalmol Vis Sci 2012; 53(1): 538-41.

[122] Hou S., P. Yang, L. Du, Z. Jiang, L. Mao, Q. Shu, H. Zhou,A. Kijlstra. Monocyte chemoattractant protein-1-2518 A/G single nucleotide polymorphism in Chinese Han patients with ocular Behcet's disease. Hum Immunol 2010; 71(1):79-82.

[123] Ozcimen A.A., K. Dilek, U. Bingol, H. Saricaoglu, A. Sarandol, O. Taskapilioglu, M. Yurtkuran, M.A. Yurtkuran,H.B. Oral. IL-1 cluster gene polymorphisms in Turkish patients with Behcet's disease. Int J Immunogenet 2011; 38(4):295-301.

[124] Chang H.K., W.C. Jang, S.B. Park, S.M. Han, Y.H. Nam, S.S. Lee, J.U. Kim,H.S. Lee. Association between interleukin 6 gene polymorphisms and Behcet's disease in Korean people. Ann Rheum Dis 2005; 64(2):339-40.

[125] .Hu K., S. Hou, F. Li, Q. Xiang, A. Kijlstra,P. Yang. JAK1, but not JAK2 and STAT3, confers susceptibility to Vogt-Koyanagi-Harada (VKH) syndrome in a Han Chinese population. Invest Ophthalmol Vis Sci 2013; 54(5):3360-5.

[126] Shu Q., P. Yang, S. Hou, F. Li, Y. Chen, L. Du,Z. Jiang. Interleukin-17 gene polymorphism is associated with Vogt-Koyanagi-Harada syndrome but not with Behcet's disease in a Chinese Han population. Hum Immunol 2010; 71(10):988-91.

[127] Tang Y., X. Luo, H. Cui, X. Ni, M. Yuan, Y. Guo, X. Huang, H. Zhou, N. de Vries, P.P. Tak, S. Chen,N. Shen. MicroRNA-146A contributes to abnormal activation of the type I interferon pathway in human lupus by targeting the key signaling proteins. Arthritis Rheum 2009; 60(4):1065-75.

[128] Zhou Q., S. Hou, L. Liang, X. Li, X. Tan, L. Wei, B. Lei, A. Kijlstra,P. Yang. MicroRNA-146a and Ets-1 gene polymorphisms in ocular Behcet's disease and Vogt-Koyanagi-Harada syndrome. Ann Rheum Dis 2012.

[129] Sugita S., H. Takase, T. Kawaguchi, C. Taguchi,M. Mochizuki. Cross-reaction between tyrosinase peptides and cytomegalovirus antigen by T cells from patients with Vogt-Koyanagi-Harada disease. Int Ophthalmol 2007; 27(2-3):87-95.

[130] Narikawa S., Y. Suzuki, M. Takahashi, A. Furukawa, T. Sakane,Y. Mizushima. Streptococcus oralis previously identified as uncommon 'Streptococcus sanguis' in Behcet's disease. Arch Oral Biol 1995; 40(8):685-90.

[131] Kirino Y., M. Takeno, R. Watanabe, S. Murakami, M. Kobayashi, H. Ideguchi, A. Ihata, S. Ohno, A. Ueda, N. Mizuki,Y. Ishigatsubo. Association of reduced heme oxygenase-1 with excessive Toll-like receptor 4 expression in peripheral blood mononuclear cells in Behcet's disease. Arthritis Res Ther 2008; 10(1):R16.

[132] Do J.E., S.Y. Kwon, S. Park,E.S. Lee. Effects of vitamin D on expression of Toll-like receptors of monocytes from patients with Behcet's disease. Rheumatology (Oxford) 2008; 47(6):840-8.

[133] Liu X., C. Wang, Z. Ye, A. Kijlstra,P. Yang. Higher expression of Toll-like receptors 2, 3, 4 and 8 in ocular Behcet's disease. Invest Ophthalmol Vis Sci 2013.

[134] Pay S., I. Simsek, H. Erdem,A. Dinc. Immunopathogenesis of Behcet's disease with special emphasize on the possible role of antigen presenting cells. Rheumatol Int 2007; 27(5):417-24.

[135] Harry R.A., A.E. Anderson, J.D. Isaacs,C.M. Hilkens. Generation and characterisation of therapeutic tolerogenic dendritic cells for rheumatoid arthritis. Ann Rheum Dis 2010; 69(11):2042-50.

[136] Atzeni F., L. Boiardi, B. Casali, E. Farnetti, D. Nicoli, P. Sarzi-Puttini, N. Pipitone, I. Olivieri, F. Cantini, F. Salvi, R. La Corte, G. Triolo, D. Filippini, G. Paolazzi,C. Salvarani. CC chemokine receptor 5 polymorphism in Italian patients with Behcet's disease. Rheumatology (Oxford) 2012; 51(12):2141-5.

[137] Chen F., S. Hou, Z. Jiang, Y. Chen, A. Kijlstra, J.T. Rosenbaum,P. Yang. CD40 gene polymorphisms confer risk of Behcet's disease but not of Vogt-Koyanagi-Harada syndrome in a Han Chinese population. Rheumatology (Oxford) 2012; 51(1):47-51.

[138] Fei Y., R. Webb, B.L. Cobb, H. Direskeneli, G. Saruhan-Direskeneli,A.H. Sawalha. Identification of novel genetic susceptibility loci for Behcet's disease using a genome-wide association study. Arthritis Res Ther 2009; 11(3):R66.

[139] Oksel F., G. Keser, M. Ozmen, K. Aksu, G. Kitapcioglu, A. Berdeli,E. Doganavsargil. Endothelial nitric oxide synthase gene Glu298Asp polymorphism is associated with Behcet's disease. Clin Exp Rheumatol 2006; 24(5 Suppl 42):S79-82.

[140] Kim J.U., H.K. Chang, S.S. Lee, J.W. Kim, K.T. Kim, S.W. Lee,W.T. Chung. Endothelial nitric oxide synthase gene polymorphisms in Behcet's disease and rheumatic diseases with vasculitis. Ann Rheum Dis 2003; 62(11):1083-7.

[141] Ben Dhifallah I., H. Houman, M. Khanfir,K. Hamzaoui. Endothelial nitric oxide synthase gene polymorphism is associated with Behcet's disease in Tunisian population. Hum Immunol 2008; 69(10):661-5.

[142] Li K., M. Zhao, S. Hou, L. Du, A. Kijlstra,P. Yang. Association between polymorphisms of FCRL3, a non-HLA gene, and Behcet's disease in a Chinese population with ophthalmic manifestations. Mol Vis 2008; 14:2136-42.

[143] Ben Dhifallah I., E.F. Karray, F. Sassi,K. Hamzaoui. Intercellular adhesion molecule 1 K469E gene polymorphism is associated with presence of skin lesions in Tunisian Behcet's disease patients. Tissue Antigens 2010; 75(1):74-8.

[144] Boiardi L., C. Salvarani, B. Casali, I. Olivieri, G. Ciancio, F. Cantini, F. Salvi, R. Malatesta, M. Govoni, F. Trotta, D. Filippini, G. Paolazzi, D. Nicoli, E. Farnetti,L. Macchioni. Intercellular adhesion molecule-1 gene polymorphisms in Behcet's Disease. J Rheumatol 2001; 28(6):1283-7.

[145] Oral H.B., K. Dilek, A.A. Ozcimen, O. Taskapilioglu, U. Bingol, A. Sarandol, H. Saricaoglu, M. Yurtkuran,M.A. Yurtkuran. Interleukin-4 gene polymorphisms confer Behcet's disease in Turkish population. Scand J Immunol 2011; 73(6):594-601.

[146] Yanagihori H., N. Oyama, K. Nakamura, N. Mizuki, K. Oguma,F. Kaneko. Role of IL-12B promoter polymorphism in Adamantiades-Behcet's disease susceptibility: An involvement of Th1 immunoreactivity against Streptococcus Sanguinis antigen. J Invest Dermatol 2006; 126(7):1534-40.

[147] Htoon J., A. Nadig, T. Hughes, S. Yavuz, H. Direskeneli, G. Saruhan-Direskeneli,A.H. Sawalha. IL18 polymorphism is associated with Behcet's disease but not lupus in patients from Turkey. J Rheumatol 2011; 38(5):962-3.

[148] Lee Y.J., S.W. Kang, J.K. Song, H.J. Baek, H.J. Choi, Y.D. Bae, H.J. Ryu, E.Y. Lee, E.B. Lee,Y.W. Song. Associations between interferon regulatory factor-1 polymorphisms and Behcet's disease. Hum Immunol 2007; 68(9):770-8.

[149] Xavier J.M., N.M. Shafiee, F. Ghaderi, A. Rosa, B.S. Abdollahi, A. Nadji, F. Shahram, F. Davatchi,S.A. Oliveira. Association of mitochondrial polymorphism m.709G>A with Behcet's disease. Ann Rheum Dis 2010; 70(8):1514-6.

[150] Rustemoglu A., U. Gul, G. Gumus-Akay, M. Gonul, S. Yigit, N. Bozkurt, A. Karadag, E. Piskin, A. Sunguroglu,A. Kadikiran. MDR1 gene polymorphisms may be associated with Behcet's disease and its colchicum treatment response. Gene 2012; 505(2): 333-9.

[151] Zheng X., D. Wang, S. Hou, C. Zhang, B. Lei, X. Xiao, A. Kijlstra,P. Yang. Association of macrophage migration inhibitory factor gene polymorphisms with Behcet's disease in a Han Chinese population. Ophthalmology 2012; 119(12):2514-8.

[152] Park K.S., Y. Min, S.R. Park, E.H. Kim, D.J. Lee, D. Bang,E.S. Lee. Matrix metalloproteinase 2, 9, 12, and tissue inhibitor of metalloproteinase 2 gene polymorphisms and cutaneous expressions in patients with Behcet's disease. Tissue Antigens 2012; 79(5): 333-9.

[153] Lee Y.J., S.W. Kang, H.J. Baek, H.J. Choi, Y.D. Bae, E.H. Kang, E.Y. Lee, E.B. Lee,Y.W. Song. Association between matrix metalloproteinase 9 promoter polymorphisms and Behcet's disease. Hum Immunol 2010; 71(7):717-22.

[154] Karakus N., S. Yigit, G. Kalkan, A. Rustemoglu, A. Inanir, U. Gul, G.S. Pancar, S. Akkanet,O. Ates. Association between the methylene tetrahydrofolate reductase gene C677T mutation and colchicine unresponsiveness in Behcet's disease. Mol Vis 2012; 18:1696-700.

[155] Ates O., L. Dalyan, G. Hatemi, V. Hamuryudan,A. Topal-Sarikaya. Genetic susceptibility to Behcet's syndrome is associated with NRAMP1 (SLC11A1) polymorphism in Turkish patients. Rheumatol Int 2009; 29(7):787-91.

[156] Hou S., X. Xiao, Y. Zhou, X. Zhu, F. Li, A. Kijlstra,P. Yang. Genetic variant on PDGFRL associated with Behcet disease in Chinese Han populations. Hum Mutat 2013; 34(1):74-8.

[157] Demir H.D., F.N. Yalcindag, A. Ozturk,N. Akar. Intron F G79A polymorphism of the protein Z gene in Turkish Behcet patients. Curr Eye Res 2012; 37(7):630-2.

[158] Baranathan V., M.R. Stanford, R.W. Vaughan, E. Kondeatis, E. Graham, F. Fortune, W. Madanat, C. Kanawati, M. Ghabra, P.I. Murray,G.R. Wallace. The association of the PTPN22 620W polymorphism with Behcet's disease. Ann Rheum Dis 2007; 66(11): 1531-3.

[159] Kim S.K., W.C. Jang, S.B. Park, D.Y. Park, K.T. Bang, S.S. Lee, J.B. Jun, D.H. Yoo,H.K. Chang. SLC11A1 gene polymorphisms in Korean patients with Behcet's disease. Scand J Rheumatol 2006; 35(5):398-401.

[160] Hou S., A. Kijlstra,P. Yang. The genetics of Behcet's disease in a Chinese population. Front Med 2012; 6(4):354-9.

[161] Park G., H.S. Kim, J.Y. Choe,S.K. Kim. SUMO4 C438T polymorphism is associated with papulopustular skin lesion in Korean patients with Behcet's disease. Rheumatol Int 2012; 32(10):3031-7.

[162] Kamoun M., I. Ben Dhifallah, E. Karray, L. Zakraoui,K. Hamzaoui. Association of small ubiquitin-like modifier 4 (SUMO4) polymorphisms in a Tunisian population with Behcet's disease. Clin Exp Rheumatol 2010; 28(4 Suppl 60):S45-9.

[163] Chen Y., P. Yang, F. Li, S. Hou, Z. Jiang, Q. Shu,A. Kijlstra. Association analysis of TGFBR3 gene with Vogt-Koyanagi-Harada disease and Behcet's disease in the Chinese Han population. Curr Eye Res 2012; 37(4):312-7.

[164] Horie Y., A. Meguro, M. Ota, N. Kitaichi, Y. Katsuyama, Y. Takemoto, K. Namba, K. Yoshida, Y.W. Song, K.S. Park, E.B. Lee, H. Inoko, N. Mizuki,S. Ohno. Association of TLR4 polymorphisms with Behcet's disease in a Korean population. Rheumatology (Oxford) 2009; 48(6):638-42.

[165] Meguro A., M. Ota, Y. Katsuyama, A. Oka, S. Ohno, H. Inoko,N. Mizuki. Association of the toll-like receptor 4 gene polymorphisms with Behcet's disease. Ann Rheum Dis 2008; 67(5):725-7.

[166] Li H., Q. Liu, S. Hou, L. Du, Q. Zhou, Y. Zhou, A. Kijlstra, Z. Li,P. Yang. TNFAIP3 gene polymorphisms confer risk for Behcet's disease in a Chinese Han population. Hum Genet 2013; 132(3):293-300.

[167] Jung E.S., S.W. Kim, C.M. Moon, D.J. Shin, N.H. Son, E.S. Kim, H.J. Lee, S.P. Hong, T.I. Kim, W.H. Kim,J.H. Cheon. Relationships between genetic polymorphisms of triggering receptor expressed on myeloid cells-1 and inflammatory bowel diseases in the Korean population. Life Sci 2011; 89(9-10):289-94.

[168] Hou S., Q. Shu, Z. Jiang, Y. Chen, F. Li, F. Chen, A. Kijlstra,P. Yang. Replication study confirms the association between UBAC2 and Behcet's disease in two independent Chinese sets of patients and controls. Arthritis Res Ther 2012; 14(2):R70.

[169] Karray E.F., I. Ben Dhifallah, K. Ben Abdelghani, I. Ben Ghorbel, M. Khanfir, H. Houman, K. Hamzaoui,L. Zakraoui. Associations of vitamin D receptor gene polymorphisms FokI and BsmI with susceptibility to rheumatoid arthritis and Behcet's disease in Tunisians. Joint Bone Spine 2012; 79(2):144-8.

[170] Nam E.J., S.W. Han, S.U. Kim, J.H. Cho, K.H. Sa, W.K. Lee, J.Y. Park,Y.M. Kang. Association of vascular endothelial growth factor gene polymorphisms with behcet disease in a Korean population. Hum Immunol 2005; 66(10):1068-73.

[171] Du L., P. Yang, S. Hou, X. Lin, H. Zhou, X. Huang, L. Wang,A. Kijlstra. Association of the CTLA-4 gene with Vogt-Koyanagi-Harada syndrome. Clin Immunol 2008; 127(1):43-8.

[172] Hu K., P. Yang, Z. Jiang, S. Hou, L. Du,F. Li. STAT4 polymorphism in a Chinese Han population with Vogt-Koyanagi-Harada syndrome and Behcet's disease. Hum Immunol 2010; 71(7):723-6.

[173] Li H., Q. Liu, S. Hou, L. Du, Q. Zhou, Y. Zhou, A. Kijlstra,P. Yang. TNFAIP3 gene polymorphisms in a Chinese Han population with Vogt-Koyanagi-Harada syndrome. PLoS One 2013; 8(3):e59515.

8

Paranasal Sinus Mucoceles – Opthalmic Manifestations, Radiological Imaging, Endoscopic Endonasal Marsupialization and Outcome

Balwant Singh Gendeh

1. Introduction

Langeback first described paranasal sinus mucoceles in 1820. It was only in the early 1900s that mucoceles were given their name by Rollet and popularized by Gerber, who published 178 cases. In 1995, Lambert attributed frontal or ethmoid mucoceles as the most common nasal condition to produce proptosis [1]

A mucocele is an epithelial-lined mucus containing sac that fills a paranasal sinus and is able to expand by alternative bone resorption and bone formation. A mucocele occurs when a sinus ostium or a compartment of a septated sinus becomes obstructed, thus causing the sinus cavity to become filled with mucus or to become airless. Paranasal sinus mucoceles may result from inflammation, tumor, trauma or surgical manipulation [2].Because of the anatomic proximity of the orbit, the pathologic process of paranasal sinus mucocele will easily affect the orbit [3,4]. Anatomically, the frontal, ethmoid, sphenoid and maxillary sinuses all interface with the orbit. The maxillary sinus shares the floor of the orbit, the frontal sinus is part of the orbital roof, the ethmoid extends along most of the medial wall of orbit and the sphenoid almost completely surrounds the orbital apex [3, 4]. Thus, mucoceles of the paranasal sinuses can easily affect the orbit and cause ophthalmic symptoms such as proptosis, blurred vision and displacement of globe [4,5]. Patients with paranasal mucoceles with orbital symptoms are often seen by the ophthalmologist first and then referred to otorhinolaryngologist [5].Occasionally they can present with intracranial complications.

It is essential to differentiate a mucocele from a mucus retention cyst. A mucus retention cyst is just a fluid filled sac along the sinus lining which does not expand and push into the eye socket, nose or brain and does not cause problems in the vast majority of cases. Notably, mucus retention cysts in the sinuses are more common than expected. Infact, about 30-40% of the population with absolutely no complaints of sinus problems will have cysts of the paranasal sinuses when they have CT scans performed. Most retention cysts of sinuses spontaneously shrink or do not change in size over the long term [6]. In the absence of associated complaints "wait and see" may be the appropriate management strategy for these retention cysts.

2. Material and methods

From 2005 to 2012, 13 patients with paranasal sinus mucoceles were treated with wide endoscopic endonasal marsupilization at the UKM Medical Center in Kuala Lumpur, Malaysia. Review of the patients' complete medical records, including out-patient clinical records, operative notes and reports of imaging and histopathology were performed. The radiological imaging (CT/MRI) on preoperative coronal and axial views were reviewed.

3. Results

The demographic data on the 13 patients includes the age, sex, race, clinical presentation, type of radiological imaging performed, the surgical details and the post-operative follow-up are listed in Table 1. The most common sinus involved was the frontal, followed by the ethmoid, maxillary and sphenoid (Table 2). The most common clinical presentation was headache followed by eye and nasal symptoms (Table 3). Figure 1 shows a radiological image of a right ethmoidal mucocele in an adult patient with diplopia and headache. Figure 2 shows a radiological image of a gross right frontal mucocele in an adult patient with headache, reduced vision and proptosis. Figure 3 shows a radiological image of a sphenoid mucocele in a child with headache and vomiting. Figure 4 shows a radiological image of left maxillary mucocele in an adult patient with nasal blockage and foul smelling discharge.

Patient / Age/sex/ race	**Presentation**	**Sinus involvement on endoscopy**	**Imaging**	**Surgery**	**Follow-up**
1. 40/M/C	supra orbital swelling, no diplopia or nasal symptoms	Left frontal and ethmoid sinuses involvement	CT: Expansile cystic mass Lt fronto ethmoid region	Endoscopic marsupialization of fronto-ethmoidal mucocele	Symptom free at 1 year follow up with no sign of recurrence
2. 59/M/C	Right frontal swelling with diplopia	Right frontal sinus involvement	CT: Expansile cystic lesion pushing interfrontal sinus septum with	Bicoronal flap cranialization with endoscopic endonasal frontal sinusotomy and marsupilization	Symptom free at 1 year follow up with no evidence of recurrence

Patient / Age/sex/ race	Presentation	Sinus involvement on endoscopy	Imaging	Surgery	Follow-up
			orbital roof involvement		
3. 40/M/M	Nasal block, rhinorrhoea with anosmia	Right frontal sinus involvement with bilateral nasal polyposis	CR & MRI: Right frontal expansile cystic mass with intracranial extension, no evidence of mass effect or ring enhancement	Endoscopic right frontal sinusotomy and bilateral ethmoidectomy with marsupilization	Symptoms improvement with no evidence of recurrence of nasal polyps at 6 month follow-up
4. 55/F/M	Headaches with, right diplopia	Right ethmoid sinuses involvement	CT & MRI: Expansile right ethmoidal mass with thinning of lamina papyracea	Endoscopic anterior and posterior ethmoidectomy with marsupilization	Symptom free at 6 month follow up with no evidence of recurrence
5. 59/M/Bengali	Headaches, proptosis with reduced left eye movement	Bilateral frontal sinus involvement	CT: Expansile mass involving bilateral frontal sinuses	Endoscopic drainage of bilateral frontal mucopyocele with marsupilization	Symptom free at 6 month follow up with no evidence of recurrence
6. 73/M/C	Reduced vision, eye pain, headaches with nasal blockage	Sphenoid sinus involvement	CT: Expansile mass within sphenoid sinus compressing on optic nerves	Endoscopic sphenoethmoidectomy and marsupialization	Symptom free at 1 year follow up with no evidence of recurrence
7. 75/F/C	Left epiphora with swelling at medial cantus	Left Fronto-Ethmoid sinuses involvement	CT: Opacification of left frontal and ethmoidal sinuses	Endoscopic left frontal sinustomy with anterior and posterior ethmoidectomy with marsupialization	Symptom free at 1 year follow up with no evidence of recurrence
8. 71/F/C	Right nasal blockage, rhinorrhea, sneezing with epiphora	Right maxillary sinus involvement	CT: Hypodense mass in right maxillary sinus with remodeling of maxillary wall and hard plate	Endoscopic right MMA with Marsupialization	Symptom free at 6 months follow up with no evidence of recurrence

Patient / Age/sex/ race	Presentation	Sinus involvement on endoscopy	Imaging	Surgery	Follow-up
9. 63/F/C	Pain left eye with reduced vision and headaches	Left spheno-Ethmmoid sinuses involvement	CT & MRI: Bilateral opacity of ethmoid and sphenoid sinuses with evidence of compression of optic nerve and cavernous sinus	Endoscopic ethmosphenoidectomy with marsupialization	Symptom free at 1 year follow up with no evidence of recurrence
10. 39/M/I	Headaches with right protosis, and diplopia	Right frontal sinus involvement	MRI: Opacity within right frontal sinus with mass effect on right superior and medial wall	Endoscopic right frontal sinusotomy with marsupialization	Symptoms improvement with no evidence of recurrence at 1 year follow up
11. 8/M/I	Headaches with vomitting	Sphenoid sinus involvement	MRI: Expansile mass within sphenoid sinus involving the sphenoethmoidal recess	Endoscopic sphenoethmoidectomy with marsupialization	Symptoms improved with no recurrence at 3 months
12. 62/M/C	Lt nasal blockage with foul smelling nasal discharge	Left maxillary sinus involvement	CT: Expansile left maxillary mass	Endoscopic wide left MMA with marsupilization	Post DXT NPC with no recurrence at 3 months
13. 58/M/M	Rt nasal blockage with foul smelling nasal discharge	Right maxillary sinus involvement	CT: Expansile right maxillary mass	Endoscopic wide right MMA with marsupilization	Symptoms improved with no recurrence at 6 months

M – Male

F – Female

Race-M (Malay), C (Chinese), I (Indian)

Rt– Right

Lt – Left

MMA – Middle meatal antrostomy

Table 1. Dermographic presentation of 13 patients with paranasal sinus mucocele

	Frontal	Ethmoid	Maxillary	Sphenoid
Number of cases	6	4	3	3

Table 2. Sites of involvement of paranasal sinuses

	Headache	Diplopia	Proptosis	Reduced vision	Reduced eye movement	Nasal symptoms	Vomiting
Number of cases	7	2	5	3	2	5	1

Table 3. Clinical presentation of head and eye symptoms

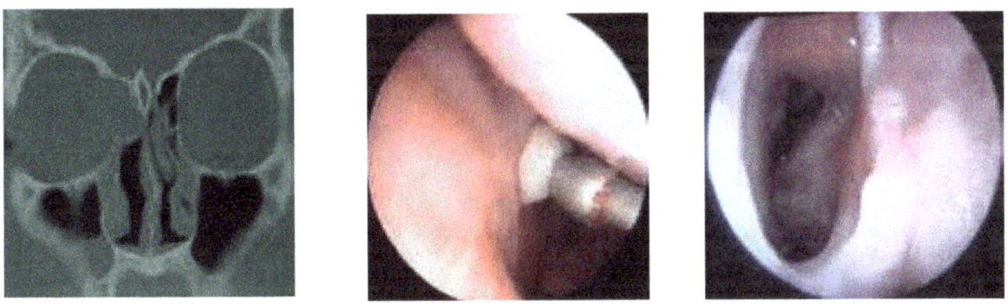

Figure 1. Coronal CT imaging of patient number 4 showing a right iatrogenic frontoethmoid mucocele with intraoperative endoscopic drainage and follow up at 3 months post surgery showing a patent frontal sinustomy

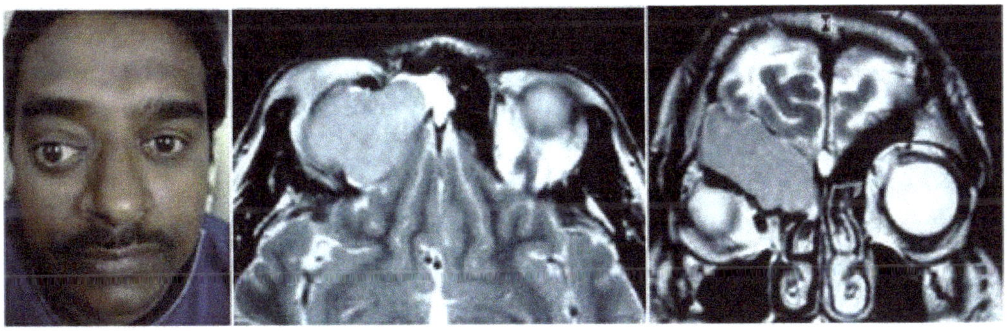

Figure 2. Picture of patient number 10 showing gross right protosis and the respective axial and coronal MRI sections revealing expansile frontal sinus lesion with loss of scalloping suggestive of a mucocele

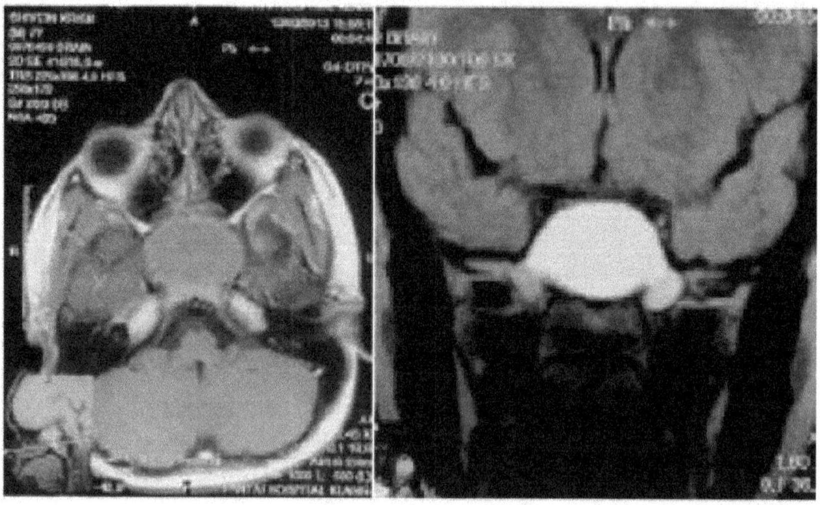

Figure 3. Axial views and coronal sections of T1 and T2 weighted MRI images of patient number 11 showing an expansile sphenoid lesion suggestive of mucocele in a 8-year Indian male.

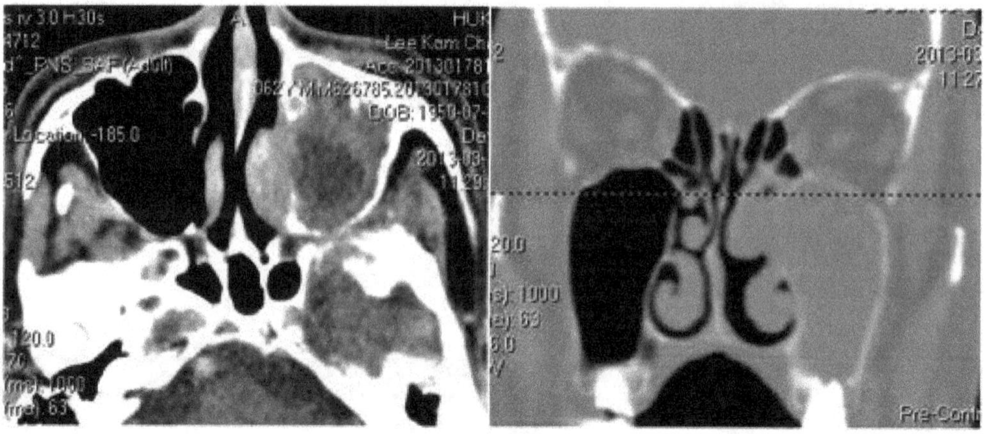

Figure 4. Axial views and coronal sections of CT images of patient number 12 showing a left expansile mass in the maxillary sinus suggestive of a mucocele in a 62 year male Chinese.

3.1. Surgical technique

All patients were operated under general aneasthesia. The patient is placed in supine position with head slightly elevated. Packing that has been soaked in a 4% cocaine solution is placed in the nasal cavity to initiate mucosal vasoconstriction. Both eyes are exposed in the surgical field. Under endoscopic visualization, submucosal injections of 1% lidocaine with epinephrine are administred along the lateral nasal wall and middle turbinate. Briefly the endoscopic endonasal marsupilization is as follows: wide middle meatal antrostomy and marsupilization for maxillary mucocele; initially complete ethmoidectomy followed by removal of antero-inferior wall of the sphenoid mucocele and marsupilizing the cavity for ethmoid and sphenoid mucocele;uncinectomy, anterior ethmoidectomy and widening of the frontal recess (Draf type 2 procedure) and marsupilization for fronto-ethmoid mucocele.Patients' are observed at weekly follow-up with secretion aspirated and sinonasal washing with saline solution upto one month post-surgery. Patients are checked upon at follow-ups every three months for first year than once a year.

4. Discussion

Paranasal sinus mucoceles are rare in children but relatively common in adults. In the literature, the etiologies of pediatric mucoceles have focused on impaired secretion process such as cystic fibrosis, pathological pneumatization processus, atopy and trauma, [7,8].

Mucoceles are commonly caused by post-operative ostial obstruction or secondary to trauma but can also present as primary disease. Paranasal sinus mucoceles predorminently occur in the fronto-ethmoid region (64%), followed by the maxillary sinus (18.6%), the sphenoid sinus (8.4%) and the posterior ethmoid sinus (6.7%) [9] which was similar to that in our study. Another common site for occurrence of mucocele is within the supraorbital ethmoid region. Primary sphenoid mucoceles can be found in association with chronic ethmoid sinusitis and/ or nasal polyposis and are uncommon in isolation [10].

In the literature review, proptosis, periorbital pain and impairment of ocular mobility were the most common manifestations of mucoceles in the anterior paranasal sinuses while blurred vision and impairment of ocular mobility [11] were frequently seen in mucoceles in the posterior sinuses. Mucoceles of the anterior paranasal sinuses may expand the anterior and medial sinus walls, pushing the globe outward and downward and restrict movement of the extraocular muscles, thus causing proptosis and impairment of ocular mobility [4, 12, 13].

The natural development of sinus mucoceles consists of gradual expansion. This slow growing expansion can result in bone remodeling, bulging and erosion and reaches adjacent structures such as other sinuses, orbit, clivus, skull base or brain. In case of an intracranial complication, infection may even lead to conditions such as meningitis, subdural or brain abcess [14]. By extension into adjacent structures, the mucocele gives rise to a variety of clinical manifestations. The most common symptoms reported are headaches, facial pain, anosmia, ocular displacement, ocular palsy and visual failure. Visual symptoms in patients with sphenoid mucocele include diplopia, ocular muscle paresis, exopthalmus and complete visual loss [15, 16, 17, 18]. One should also be aware of unusual presentation including hypopituitarism [19, 20, 21].

The anatomical proximity and fragility of the orbital structures explains the high occurrence of ocular complications in sinusopathy. As the optic nerve enters the orbital apex from the intracranial portion, the nerve is encompassed by the narrow bony canal and is in close proximity to the posterior ethmoid and/or sphenoid sinus. In majority of cases the bony wall between the nerve and the sinuses is as thin as 40-60um [22, 23]. Intracranially the optic nerve is covered by the pia mater, arachnoid and CSF. As the nerve enters the canal, it is surrounded by two layers of nerve sheath, the outer which is continuous with the periorbita and the inner which en sheaths the nerve to the eyeball. The optic nerve canal can be identified as a semi-circular tube when viewed from the inside of the posterior ethmoid or sphenoid sinus. Since the optic nerve canal contains the nerve and two layers of nerve sheath without any soft tissues such as fat, pressure due to expansion of the mucocele may easily impact the nerve if the thin protecting bony wall is resorbed or if it is dehiscent congenitally.

Blurred vision is more often associated with mucoceles in the posterior than anterior paranasal sinuses and can affect the optic or other cranial nerves via two pathways. Firstly, expansion of the paranasal sinus wall may compress the optic nerve or compromise its blood supply with subsequent optic atrophy [12, 24, 25]. Secondly, optic neuritis may result from direct spread of suppuration from adjacent paranasal sinuses via bone loss or bone fissure [12, 26]. Both optic nerve compression and neuritis can cause deterioration of visual acuity [12, 26]. Besides the optic nerve, other cranial nerves (abducent or oculomotor) passing through the orbital apex or superior orbital fissure may be involved, thus resulting in impairment of ocular mobility [12, 25, 26, 27].

In a review of 47 patients suffering from ethmoid or sphenoid mucoceles, Moriyama et al [28] highlighted 70 per cent of patients first sought help from the ophthalmology department. The mucocele may compress the optic canal and cause visual disturbances, leading to loss of eye sight in severe cases. Further to direct pressure, ischemia or venous congestion around the optic nerve subsequently occurs [28]. Besides compression and its local effects, inflammation due to infection of the mucocele can spread to the nerve through zones of bony erosion. Therefore, the visual loss may be due to a local inflammatory response which responds to steroid therapy [29] but further diagnosis and immediate surgical drainage are imperative.

Preoperative diagnosis is usually based on CT and MRI. On CT scan, mucoceles usually fill a sinus structure and bulge against adjacent anatomical structures, but without infiltration and usually the bony margins of the lesion are well defined. MRI of mucoceles in both T1 and T2 weighted images show variable signal intensities as depicted in Fig 3. CT scans are preferable for definitive evaluation, assessment of bony involvement and presurgical planning. MRI scans are helpful in the evaluation of orbital or intracranial extension and in ruling out a neoplasm or fungus disease [30]. Therefore, CT and MRI imaging are complementary for the diagnostic evaluation of an expansile mass around the posterior ethmoid and sphenoid sinus. In the differential diagnosis, one should rule out a mucopyocele, sinus malignancy, hypophyseal tumor, craniopharyngioma, meningioma or optic nerve glioma, intracranial chordoma,cholesteatoma and neoplastic lesions of nasopharynx.

An urgent surgical intervention is advocated in a paranasal sinus mucocele with vision loss. The endoscopic endonasal approach is the most convenient for the treatment of mucocele in view of easy access, lower morbidity and a reduction in potential complications compared to intracranial route [31]. Several recent literatures have reported successful results in the management of mucoceles with endoscopic marsupilization as the main choice of treatment [32]. It has the advantage of magnification of the operative field, is minimally invasive, preserves the sinus architecture and produces good long-term results with adequate post-operative care. Some conditions are not suitable for endoscopic surgery alone including a far laterally placed frontal mucocele, hypertrophic bone occluding the area of the fronto-nasal recess and a mucocele arising secondarily from a malignancy [33]. With respect to patient number 2, the extensive mucocele with intraorbital extension was removed using both an endoscopic and an external approach through bicoronal flap and cranialization [34].

The paranasal sinus mucocele is widely opened and a sufficient part of the wall or outflow pathway is resected for adequate drainage and ventilation. With exposure of the dura or peri-orbital wall, the wall of the mucocele acts as a cover and no attempts are made to remove this mucosal lining to protect the orbit, optic nerve, dura and carotid artery. On adequate marsu-pilization of the mucocele, one should expect a rapid improvement of visual acuity but in cases with complete loss of vision prior to surgery, the prognosis may be much poorer. The micro-debrider is used in endonasal surgery with great easiness and good surgical outcome. The degree of improvement of the visual acuity after mucocele marsupilization depends on the severity of the initial loss prior to surgery, the mode of development and the location of the mucocele and the time from onset of the opthalmological disorder until the surgical marsu-pilization [9]. Prompt surgical treatment is necessary in order to avoid permanent visual impairment and other sequel [3, 18]. If vision is seriously impaired, immediate surgery should be performed, preferably within 24 hours after the onset of visual disturbances [35].

5. Differential diagnosis

5.1. Paranasal sinus tumors

The differential diagnosis of mucocele includes paranasal sinus tumors as shown in Table 4.

Non-neoplastic	Neoplastic
Mucosal cyst	Papillomas
Antrochonal polyp	Mesenchymal tumors (fibroma, lipoma, myxoma)
Fungal disease	Vasiform tumors (hemangioma, aneurysmal bone cyst, hemangiopericytoma)
Cholesterol granuloma	Tumors of muscle origin (leiomyoma, rhabdomyoma)
Hematoma	Odontogenic tumors
Antrolithiasis	Fibroosseous lesions (osteoma, ossifying fibroma, fibrous dysplasia, osteoblastoma)
Eosinophilic angiocentric fibrosis	Neuroectodermal tumors (schwannoma, neurofibroma)

Table 4. Classification of benign lesions of the paranasal sinus tumors

6. Non-neoplastic

6.1. Mucosal cyst

Mucosal cyct of the paranasal sinuses are common with and incidence between 12 and 36% detected on radiography [36, 37, 38]· They are broadly classified into secretory and non-secretary cysts [39]. Obstruction of mucosal gland leads to formation of secretory cysts which are less common. The more common non secretory cysts are presumably caused by an accumulation of exudates in the sinus mucosa lifting the epithelial lining. The aetiologic factors behind cyst formation remain unknown. They are mostly unilateral but can be bilateral in 10 to 20% cases [40], [41]. They are usually seen as homogenous, dome-shaped opacities on CT scanning and are usually a chance diagnosis on sinus radiography.

6.2. Antrochoanalpolyp (ACP)

ACP is a benign lesion that originates from the mucosa of the maxillary sinus and grows into the nasal cavity to reach the choana (Fig 5). ACPs account for 4 to 6% of all nasal polyps with increased incidence of 33% in children [42], [43]. ACPs are usually unilateral with only a small number of reported cases with bilateral polyps [16]. It has been suggested that most ACPs originate from the posterior-medial wall [44]. Mean age of presentation is 17 years and it is reported to be twice as common in males than females [44].

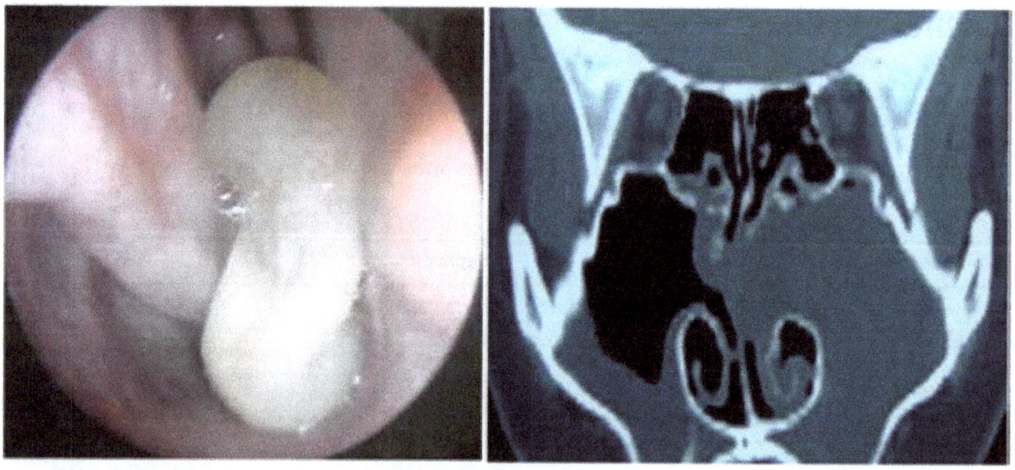

Figure 5. (A) A zero degree endoscope view of a left antrochoanal polyp in an adult male and (B) a coronal CT section of same patient showing a homogenous opaque mass in the maxillary sinus with opasification of the middle meatus and extension into choana.

Clinical manifestations usually start with unilateral nasal obstruction but other symptoms have been reported such as epistaxis, purulent rhinorrhea, post-nasal drip, snoring, obstructive sleep apnea, dysphonia and dysphagia [42, 44].

6.3. Fungal disease

Most sinus fungal infections are caused by Aspergillus species. Aspergilus flavus is the most common cause of sinus fungal ball. Infections by dematiaceous fungi such as Bipolaris, Curvularia or Alternaria are commonly seen in patients with allergic fungal sinusitis. Zygomycetes, such as Mucorales or Rhizopus are well-described aggressive organisms implicated in many cases of invasive fungal sinusitis [45, 46, 47].Fungal rhinosinusitis can be classified as invasive or non-invasive (Table 5). The prognosis of the fungal sinus infections is more dependent on the manifestation of the disease than on the specific causative species.

Noninvasive	Invasive
Saprophytic	Acute invasive fungal sinusitis
Allergic fungal sinusitis	Chronic granulomatous invasive sinusitis
Fungal ball	Chronic invasive fungal sinusitis

Table 5. Classification of fungal sinusitis

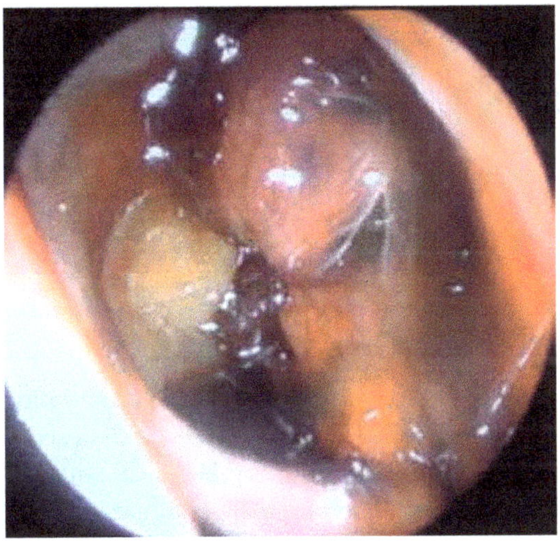

Figure 6. A zero degree endoscopic view of right nasal cavity showing evidence of allergic mucin in an adult male presenting with chronic rhinosinusitis

Associated nasal polyposis is seen in up to 10% due to the chronic inflammatory response. Maxillary sinus fungal ball often presents with unilateral sinus disease and unrelenting symptoms of rhinosinusitis. Allergic fungal sinusitis is characterized by the presence of allergic mucin in patients with symptoms of chronic rhinosinusitis, polyposis and an IgE-mediated hypersensitivity reaction to fungal elements resulting in a self-perpetuating inflammatory cascade (Fig 6). A high index of suspicion for invasive fungal sinusitis is necessary in patients with immunodeficiency, fever and symptoms referable to the paranasal sinuses. CT of paranasal sinuses is often ordered to evaluate refractory symptoms. Complete or subtotal opacification of the involved sinus is not uncommon. Up to 41% demonstrated heterogenous opacification with calcifications (Fig 7). Bony erosion or sclerosis from mass effect can be identified in 17 to 36% [48, 49, 50].

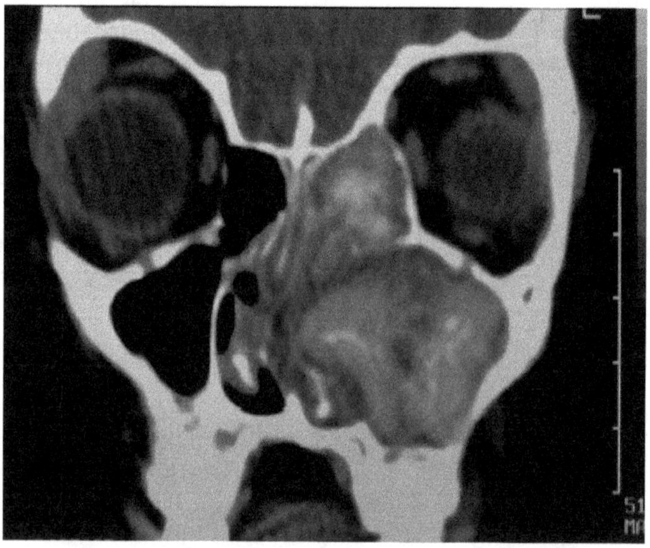

Figure 7. A CT scan coronal section showing heterogenous opacification of the left nasal cavity with calcification in an adult female with fungal sinusitis

6.4. Cholesterol granuloma (CG)

CG is a histologic term used to describe the coexistence of granulation tissue with cholesterol crystals and foreign body giant cells [51].The condition is well described in the temporal bone but is rarely encountered in the paranasal sinuses [52]. The maxillary sinus is most commonly involved [52, 53]. Only one case of bilateral maxillary sinus involvement has been reported [53]. CG has been observed more in men with 3:1 male to female ratio and an average age of 41 years.Only a small number of patients had a history of previous trauma or surgery [52, 53].

The factors contributing to the formation of CG includes disturbed ventilation in a bony cavity, impaired drainage and hemorrhage [52, 53, 54, 55]. Impaired drainage would result in obstruction to venous and lymphatic circulation thus predisposing to mucosal hemorrhage. The insufficient lymphatic drainage would fail to eliminate lipid components in red blood cells and contribute to accumulation of cholesterol crystals. These act as foreign material that stimulates the granulomatous reaction in the sinus cavity [52, 53, 56].

Patients with CG present with symptoms and signs resembling chronic sinusitis [52, 53]. Most of the patients present with nasal obstruction, post-nasal drip, rhinorrhea, facial pain or headaches (Fig 8 A). CT shows a cyst-like opacity which does not enhance with contrast (Fig 8B). Bony erosion or expansion has been reported in a small number of cases [53, 56].

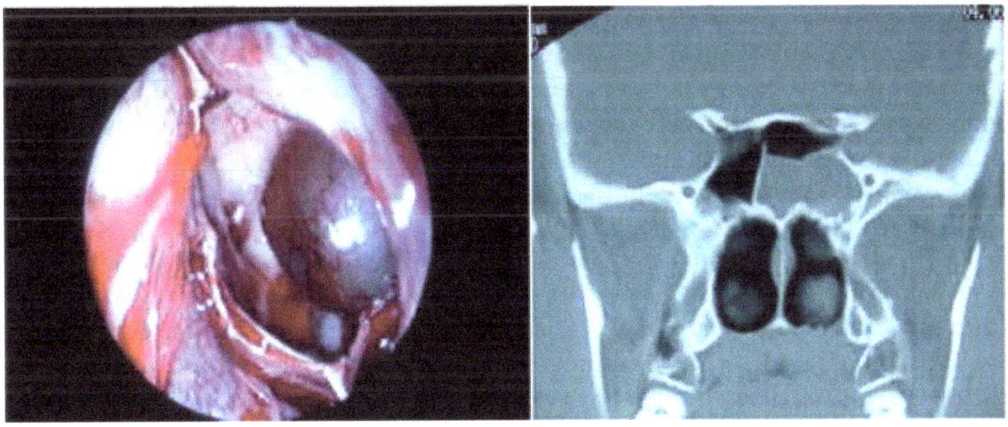

Figure 8. (A) Intraoperative view with 45 degree endoscope showing a polypoid left sphenoid sinus cholesterol granuloma in a young adult female presenting with persistent vertax headaches and (B) a CT scan coronal section showing a homogenous partial opacification of the affected sphenoid sinus

6.5. Hematoma

Hematoma of the maxillary sinus is also known as organized hematoma or hemorrhagic pseudotumor [57, 58, 59]. It is an uncommon cause of maxillary sinus mass with only a small number of reported cases from Korea and Japan [58]. Some of the hematoma have been reported in patients with bleeding diathesis such as Von Willebrand disease but there are several patients who present with what appears to be a spontaneous etiology [58, 59, 60]. Initially, a blood clot accumulates in the maxillary sinus secondary to facial trauma, operative bleeding, recurrent epistaxis or bleeding diathesis. Subsequently the hematoma develops and due to poor ventilation and obstruction of drainage it transforms into an organized hematoma by means of neovascularization and fibrosis [58, 59]. Encapsulation of the blood clot by fibrous tissue prevents reabsorption of the hematoma. Further bleeding causes increasing pressure and progressive expansion which leads to erosion of adjacent structures [59], [60].

The most common symptom at presentation is epistaxis followed by unilateral obstruction and facial swelling [57, 58]. Symptoms due to pressure on adjacent structures such as proptosis and infraorbital hypoaesthesia have been reported [61, 62]. CT scanning shows the hematoma as a nonenhancing soft tissue mass which can be heterogeneous or homogenous. Histologically the hematoma has a peripheral wall that consists of dense fibrous tissue with a spindle-shaped myofibroblast cells. The center of the hematoma consist of loose fibrous tissue which is relatively acellular and contains some intact erythrocytes [57, 58, 62].

6.6. Antrolithiasis

Antrolithiasis are calcified bodies that are formed from mineral salt deposition around a nucleus within the maxillary sinus cavity [63]. These are synonymous with rhinoliths which are reported within the nasal cavity. Anthroliths result from either endogenous (blood clot, mucus or pus) or exogenous factors (teeth and roots or other foreign material. The majority of cases reported had tooth extraction prior to presentation. The patients can be asymptomatic and may present with symptoms of unilateral chronic maxillary sinusitis. CT scan shows antroliths as radiopaque masses of varying sizes and shapes with irregular borders.

6.7. Eosinophilic Angiocentric Fibrosis (EAF)

EAF is an uncommon inflammatory fibrotic lesion that affects the submucosa of the nose, larynx and orbit [64, 65]. The pathologic process is manifested by predorminently eosinophilic perivascular inflammation and gradual replacement with progressive fibrosis [64, 67]. EAF is found with slightly higher incidence in young to middle-aged women than men [64]. The etiology of EAF is unknown but it has been closely linked to granuloma faciale [64, 68]. Majority of the lesions involve the nasal septum and lateral nasal wall with only few cases involving the maxillary sinus.

EAF is slow growing and can take many years to manifest [64, 65]. Symptoms are non specific and can initially include nasal obstruction, rhinorrhea,epistaxis and facial pain [64, 67, 68]. Due to mass expansion the patients will present later with facial swelling [64, 65]. Involvement of the orbit can lead to periorbital edema and proptosis [64]. Nasal endoscopy reveals thickening of the nasal septum with an intranasal mass [64, 65].

7. Neoplastic

7.1. Papillomas

Papillomas are the most common benign epithelial tumor found in the sinonasal area accounting for 10% of all neoplasms in this region [66].Histologically they are divided into inverted,cylindrical and everted [67]. Everted papilloma more often arises on the nasal septum whereas both inverted and cylindrical papillomas mostly arise on the lateral nasal wall within the middle meatus (Fig 9). The age of presentation is from 35 to 60 years with a male preponderance of 3.5: 1 [66, 68]. It is more common in Caucasions compared with other racial groups. A viral aetiology has been suggested with a link to papilloma viral subtypes 6, 11,16 and 18 [68].

Patients generally present with obstructive nasal symptoms, rhinorrhea and chronic rhinosinusitis [66, 68]. CT scans shows a mass in lateral nasal wall with areas of apparent calcification and there may be sclerosis of the walls of the sinus [81] (Fig 10). Both a high recurrence rate and malignant transformation have been documented. A recent review of the literature of over 200 cases calculated 7.1% synchronous carcinoma and 3.6% metachronous carcinoma [70].

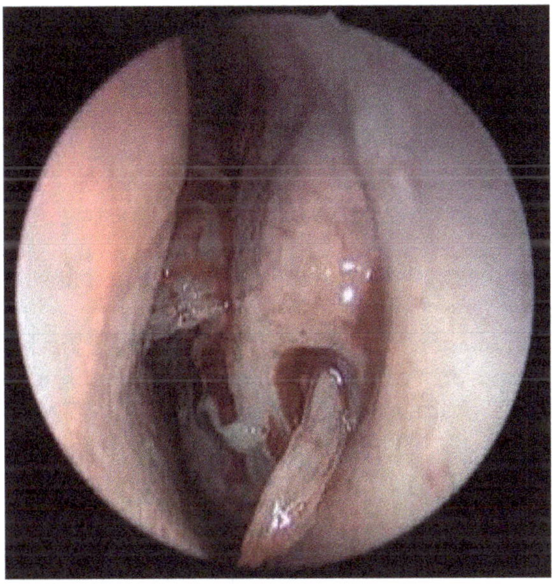

Figure 9. A zero degree endoscopic view of a left inverted papilloma arising from the lateral nasal wall in an elderly male

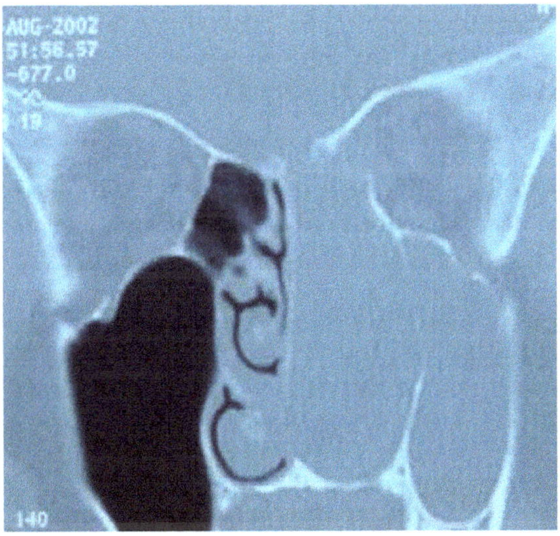

Figure 10. A coronal CT scan section showing an aggressive inverted papilloma (hybrid tumor) arising from the left nasal cavity with evidence of anterior skull base erosion in an elderly Chinese male presenting with CSF rhinorrhea

7.2. Mesenchymal tumors: Fibroma, lipoma and myxoma

These rare tumors may be encountered in the nose and sinuses and generally present prior to adulthood. Isolated tumors within maxillary sinus are very rare.

7.2.1. Fibromas

Fibromas result from progressive inflammation or fibroblastic proliferation of the nasal mucosa [71]. They present as slow-growing, grey-white, smooth surfaced masses producing obstructive nasal symptoms.

7.2.2. Lipoma

Lipoma is the most common soft tissue tumor in adulthood in contrast to intraosseouslipoma which is a rare condition.The etiology of intraosseous lipoma is unknown but infaction, ischaemia, trauma and irradiation may be contributing factors [72]. Cases have been reported within the nasal cavity and very rarely in the maxillary sinus. The presentation is of nasal swelling and possible nasal obstruction.

7.2.3. Myxoma

Myxoma of the maxillary sinus is very rare but more frequent than fibromas and lipomas [73]. The age of presentation is between 2 and 15 years and may be related to dental malformations or missing teeth.

7.3. Vasiform Tumors: Hemangioma, Aneurysmal Bone Cyst and Hemangiopericytoma

These benign lesions arise from vascular tissue within the mucosa or bone of the nose and sinuses.

7.3.1. Hemangiomas

Hemangiomas represent about 20% of benign non-epithelial tumors of nasal cavity and paranasal sinuses [74]. Mean age of diagnosis is 40 years and the most frequent presenting symptoms are nasal obstruction and epistaxis. Invovement of maxillary sinus have been reported less frequently [91]. Both cavernous and capillary hemangiomas have been reported.

7.3.2. Aneurysmal bone cyst (ABCs)

ABCs are expansile lesions of unknown etiology that involves long bones and vertebrae of patients younger than 20 years. About 2% of ABCs are encountered in the head and neck region with jaw being the most frequently involved site. The present with facial swelling and obstructive nasal symptoms in the age group between 5 and 23 years. ABCs consist of multiple cavities filled with blood and serous fluids which are separated by septa and surrounded by rim of bone [75]. ABCs have a "honeycomb"appearance on gadolinium-enhanced MRI studies [75].

7.3.3. Hemangiopericytoma (HPC)

HPC is a rare benign vascular tumor derived from extracapillary cells (pericytes). Less than one-third of HPC occur in the head and neck and 5% are located in the nasal cavity and paranasal sinuses [76, 77]. Sphenoid and ethmoid sinuses are involved more frequently than the maxillary sinus. Both sexes are equally affected and can occur at any age but often develop after the second decade. The patients usually present with epistaxis and nasal obstruction with reddish submucosal nasal mass (Fig 11).

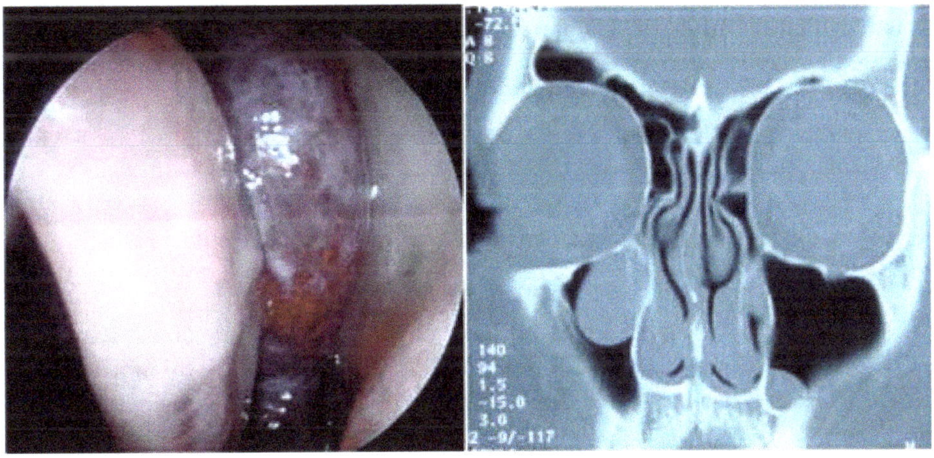

Figure 11. (A) View with 30 degree endoscope in an adult Chinese female presenting with right nasal obstruction and maxillary sinus discomfort and (B) CT scan coronal section showing a polypoidal mass arising from the right maxillary sinus and histopathology report consistent with hemangiopericytoma

7.4. Tumors of muscle origin: Leiomyoma and rhabdomyoma

7.4.1. Leiomyoma

Leiomyoma is a smooth muscle tumor that originates in areas of abundance of muscle like the uterus.

It is extremely rare for these tumors to present in the sinonasal tract because of the paucity of smooth muscle. And only a handful of cases have been reported in the maxillary sinus [78]. The tumor seem to be slow-growing and non-aggressive and presenting with obstructive nasal symptoms.

7.4.2. Rhabdomyoma

Rhabdomyomais a skeletal muscle tumor and is extremely rare in the paranasal sinus.,which has a benign behavior and low recurrence rate [79, 80].

7.5. Odontogenic tumors

Odontogenic tumors originate either within the maxillofacial skeleton (intraosseous) or within the gingival or alveolar mucosa overlying the tooth bearing areas (extraosseous). They are usually slow growing and have been associated with non-eruption of the teeth. Patients usually present with swelling of alveolar process along with nasal obstruction and epistaxis. Superior displacement of globe has been reported with large odontogenic tumors.

7.5.1. Ameloblastoma

Ameloblastomais the most common odontogenic tumor. It is slow growing, locally invasive and has a high rate of recurrence if not treated effectively. Patients between the ages of 16 and 60 years are generally affected with the region of canine tooth and maxilla being the most common sites. They are often asymptomatic but can present with a painless swelling of the cheek, gingival and palate that may reach a large size. Ameloblastoma presents as a unilocular or multilocular radiolucency that may be associated with an impacted tooth.

7.6. Fibro-osseous lesions: Osteoma, ossifying fibroma, fibrous dysplasia and osteoblastoma

Fibro-osseous lesions represent a class of bony abnormalities: osteoma, ossifying fibroma, fibrous dysplasia and osteoblastoma. They are distinct but lie along a continuum from the most to the least content. They have some similarities in appearance but their clinical implications differ.

7.6.1. Osteomas

Osteomas are frequent incidental finding in up to 3% of CT scans of the paranasal sinuses [81] (Fig 12). Eighty percent occur in the frontal sinuses followed by the ethmoids and least in the maxillary sinuses. The etiology is either embryologic or secondary to trauma or an infective process. There is an association with Gardner syndrome which is an autosomal dominant condition characterized by intestinal polyposis and pigmented skin lesions in addition to osteomas [82]. Maxillary sinus osteomas are slow growing and usually asymptomatic but they may become symptomatic depending on the location and onset [83].

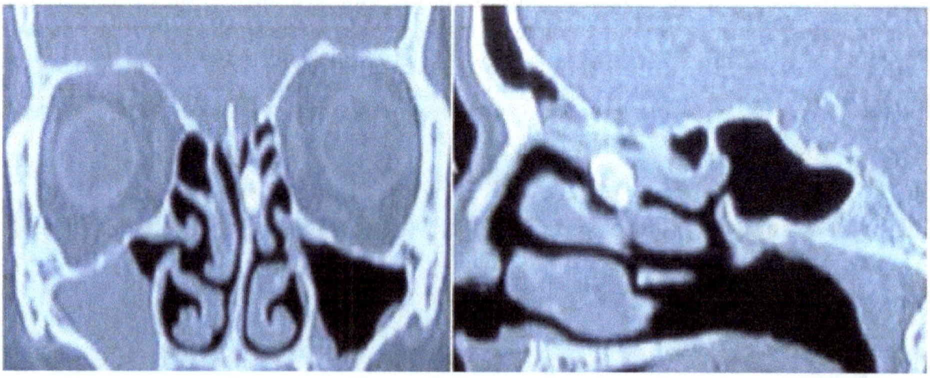

Figure 12. (A) A CT scan coronal and (B) sagittal section showing osteoma arising from the anterior ethmoid sinuses in an adult female presenting with frequent headaches

7.6.2. Ossifying fibroma (OF)

OF is a well-circumscribed lesion that continues to grow after sexual maturity and can attain dramatic proportions [81, 84]. The vast majority is located in the posterior region of the mandible; those involving the maxillary sinus are uncommon [85]. Patient usually present between the third and forth decades and the lesion is more common in women [85]. The most common presentation is of painless cheek swelling but involvement of the orbit or nasal cavity may be signified by proptosis, loss of visual acuity, epiphora, nasal obstruction and epistaxis [81, 85]. Radiologically, the lesion is sharply circumscribed with an egg shell rim and central radiolucency which differentiates it from fibrous dysplasia with its indistinguishable borders.

7.6.3. Fibrous dysplasia (FD)

FD is a slow, progressive disorder where normal bone is replaced by fibrous tissue and immature woven bone [81, 84]. There are two main forms of FD: monostatic (70-85%) that involves only one bone and polystatic (15-30%) where multiple bones can be involved (Fig 13). The maxilla and mandible are the most commonly involved bones generally in the monostatic form. FD is a disease of the young where patients present in their first or second decade and is assumed to be "burnt out" as the patients reach skeletal maturity. The usual symptom is of painless facial deformity although other complaints such as loosening of teeth, nasal obstruction or epistaxis have been encountered [86]. CT scans shows lesions with indistinct borders and a homogenous "ground glass" appearance.

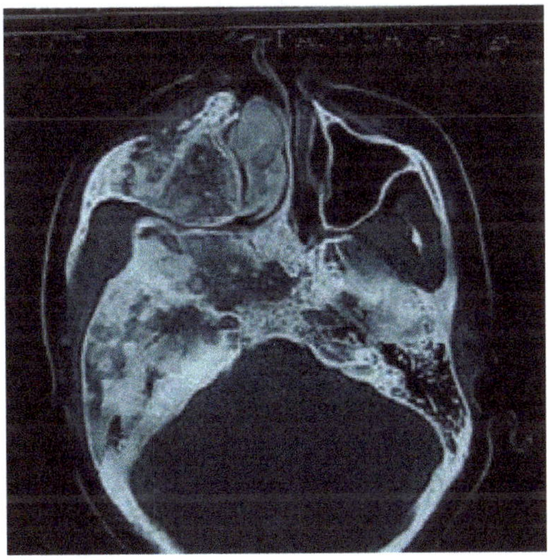

Figure 13. An axial CT section showing a polystatic fibrous dysplasia in an adult female

7.6.4. Osteoblastoma

Osteoblastoma is an uncommon neoplasm characterized by proliferation of osteoblasts forming bone trabeculae set in a vascularized fibrous connective tissue stroma [87]. The tumor occur predorminantly in vertebrae and long bones and can affect craniofacial bones with the mandible being the most commonly involved. It is reported less in the maxillary bone and rarely in the maxillary sinus [88]. The majority of the patients are under 30 years and present with a facial swelling and is often painful [87]. CT scan features range from radiolucent to radiopaque lesions and are often mistaken for other fibro-osseous lesions.

7.7. Neuroectodermal tumors: Schwannoma and neurofibroma

7.7.1. Schwannomas

Schwannomas are benign nerve sheath tumors of which 50% occur in the head and neck region. They are very uncommon in the paranasal sinuses (only 4%) and a very small number involve the maxillary sinus [84]. The lesion slowly expands in the sinus cavity resulting in swelling, pressure symptoms and bony necrosis. The patients mostly present with nasal obstruction but other symptoms such as proptosis, epiphora, headaches, facial anesthesia and epistaxis have been reported [90]. CT scan shows a homogenous radio-opaque mass with evidence of bone remodeling (Fig 14).

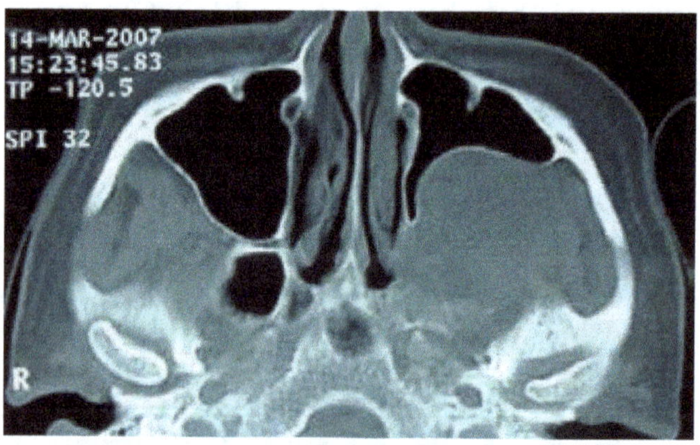

Figure 14. An axial CT section showing a left homogenous radio-opaque mass involving the maxillary sinus and infra-temporal region in an adult female

7.7.2. Neurofibromas

Neurofibromas are heterogenous peripheral nerve tumors that arise from the connective tissue of the nerves especially the endoneurium [91]. They may occur as sporadic lesions but are much more common in association with neurofibromatosis type 1 (NF 1). Neurofibromas of the maxillary sinus are exceedingly rare.As with schwannomas, they slowly grow and expand within the sinus cavity causing swelling, pressure symptoms and bone necrosis. Presentation is similar to other expanding masses in the maxillary sinus. CT scan shows a well-circumscribed mass with some bony erosion.

8. Conclusion

Mucocele of the paranasal sinuses are well described complication of chronic sinusitis in adults but they rarely occur in the pediatric population. Mucocele can be associated with ophthalmic complications or intracranial complications. Radiological imaging includes CT-scan and sometimes MRI when intracranial complications are suspected. The differential diagnosis of mucocele includes paranasal sinus tumors. Usually a wide endoscopic endonasal marsupilization of paranasal sinus mucocele is a safe and less invasive than external approaches. Thus, a good understanding of paranasal sinus mucoceles by ophthalmologists and otorhinolaryngologists is essential for early diagnosis and rapid surgical intervention.

Author details

Balwant Singh Gendeh*

Address all correspondence to: bsgendeh@gmail.com

Department of Otorhinolaryngology-Head Neck Surgery, UKM Medical Center, Jalan Yaacob Latif, Bandar Tun Razak, Kuala Lumpur, Malaysia

References

[1] Alberti PW, Marshall HF, Black JI. 1968. Fronto-ethmoidalmucocele as a cause of unilateral proptosis. Br J Ophthalmol52: 833-838

[2] Johnson JT, Ferguson BJ. 1998. Infection in: Cummings CW, Fredrickson JM, Harker LA, Krause CJ, Schuller DE, Rhicharson MA, eds Otolaryngology Head Neck Surgery, 3rd edition. St Louis: Mosby1115-1116

[3] Maniglia AJ, Kronberg FG, Culbertson W. 1984. Visual loss associated with orbital and sinus disease. Laryngoscope 94(8): 1050-1059

[4] Curtin HD, Rabinov JD. 1998. Extension to the orbit from paraorbital disease. Radiol Clin North Am 36: 1201-1213

[5] Moriyama H, Hesaka H, Tachibana T, Honda Y. 1992. Mucoceles of ethmoid and sphenoid sinus with visual disturbance. Arch Otolaryngol Head Neck Surg 118: 141-146

[6] Wang JW, JangYT, Lee BJ. 2007. Natural course of retention cysts of the maxillary sinus: long term follow-up results. Laryngoscope 117(2):341-344

[7] Olze H, Matthias C, Degenhardt P. 2006. Pediatr ic paranasal sinus mucoceles. Eur J Pediatr ic Surg 16: 192-196

[8] Timon CL, O'Dwyer TP. 1989. Ethmoidal mucoceles in children. J Laryngol Otol 103: 284-246

[9] Rombaux Ph, Bertrand B, Eloy Ph, Collet S, Daela J, Bachert C, Claes J. 2000. Endoscopic endonasal surgery for paranasal sinus mucoceles. Acta Oto-Rhinol-Laryngologica Belg 54:115-122

[10] Daniilidis J, Nikolaou A, Kondopoulos V. 1992. An unusual case of sphenoid sinus mucocele with severe intracranial extension. Rhinology 31:135-137

[11] Tseng CC, Ho CY, Kao SC. 2005. Ophthalmic manifestation of paranasal sinus mucocele. J Chin Med Ass 68(6): 260-264

[12] Shimo-Oku M, Miyazaki S, Shiraki K, Sugimoto T, Sotani H. 1989. Optic nerve involvement in posterior paranasal sinus diseases. Neuroophthalmology 9:145-155

[13] Lund VJ, Rolfe ME. 1989. Ophthalmic considerations in fronto-ethmoid mucoceles. J Laryngol Otol 103:667-669

[14] Nugert GR, Sprinkle P, Bloor BM. 1970. Sphenoid sinus mucocele. J Neurosurg 32:443-451

[15] McCarthy WL, Frenkel M. 1972. Visual loss as the only symptom of sphenoid sinus mucocele. Am J Ophthalmol 74: 1140-1143

[16] Casteels F, De Loof E, Brock P, Jorissen M, Dralands L, Missotten L, Wilms G. 1992. Sudden blindness in a child: Presenting symptoms of sphenoid sinus mucocele. Br J Opthalmol 76: 502-504

[17] Hao SP. 1994. Mucocele of sphenoid sinus with acute blindness: report of a case. J Formosan Med Ass 93: 519-521

[18] Munee A, Jones NS. 1997. Unilateral abducens nerve palsy: a presenting sign of sphenoid mucoceles. J Laryngol Otol 111: 644-646

[19] Valvassoori G, Putterman AM. 1973. Ophthalmological and radiological findings in sphenoid mucoceles. Arch Ophthal 90:416-419

[20] Rosselet PO. Gomez F, Mange B, Savery M, Grigorin D. 1984. Sphenoid sinusitis and panhypopituitarism. Schweiz Med Wonchenschr 114: 1340-1342

[21] Pitkaranta A, Atula T, Lindokl P, Saxen H, Malmberg H. 2000. Unilateral blindness in a child with acute sinusitis. Rhinology 38:43-44

[22] Slavin ML, Glacer JS. 1987. Acute severe irreversible visual loss with sphenoethmoiditis – "Posterior" orbital cellulitis. Arch Ophthal 105: 345-348

[23] Kainz J, Stammberger H. 1992. Danger areas of the posterior rhinobasis. Acta Otolaryngol 112:852-861

[24] McCrary JA. 1997. Spheno-ethmoidal mucocele, chondrosarcoma and unilateral visual loss. In: Smith JL, ed. Neuroophthalmology Update. New York: Masson Publishing, 105-109

[25] Weille FL, Vang RR. 1953. Sinusitis as focus of infection in uveitis, keratitis and retrobulbar neuritis. Arch Ophthalmol, 58:154-165

[26] Rothstein J, Maisel RH, berlinger NT, Writschaffer JD. 1984. Relationship of optic neuritis to disease of the paranasal sinuses. Laryngoscope 94:1501-1508

[27] Lundgren A, Olin T. 1961. Mucopyocele of sphenoidal sinus or posterior ethmoidal cells with special reference to apex orbital syndrome. Acta Otolaryngol 53:61-79

[28] Moriyama H, Nakajima T, Honda Y. 1992. Studies on mucoceles of the ethmoid and sphenoid sinuses. Analysis of 47 cases. J Laryngol Otol 106:23-27

[29] Fujitani T, Takahashi T, Asai T. 1984. Optic nerve disturbance caused by frontal and fronto-ethmoidal mucopyoceles. Arch otolaryngol 110:257-269

[30] Kennedy DW, Josephson JS, Zinreich SJ, Mattox DE, Goldsmith MW. 1989. Endoscopic sinus surgery for mucoceles: A viable alternative. Laryngoscope 99:885-895

[31] Bheasley NTP, Jones NS. 1995. Paranasal sinus mucoceles: modern management. Am J Rhinol 9: 251-256

[32] Kennedy DW, Keogh B, Senior B, Lanza DC. 1996. Endoscopic approach to tumors of anterior skull base and orbit. Oper Tech Otolaryngol Head Neck Surg 7:257-263

[33] Conboy PJ, Jones NS. 2003. The place of endoscopic sinus surgery in the treatment of paranasal sinus mucoceles. Clin Otolaryngol Allied Sci 28;207-210

[34] Namavar E, loh JCN, Gendeh BS. 2012. Paranasal sinus mucocele:Endoscopicmarsupilization and surgical outcome, Egyptian J Otolaryngol 28(2): 95-97

[35] Yomoto E, Hyodo M, Kawatika S, Aibara R. 1997. Effect of sinus surgery on visual disturbances caused by Sphenoethmoidal mucoceles. Am j Rhinol 11: 337-343

[36] Bhattacharyya N. 2000. Do maxillary sinus retention cysts reflect obstructive sinus phenomena? Arch Otolaryngol Head Neck Surg 126(11):1369-1371

[37] Harar RPS, Chadha NK, Rogers G. 2007. Are maxillary sinus mucosal cysts a manifestation of inflammatory sinus disease? J Laryngol Otol 121(8):751-754

[38] Kanagalingham J, Bhatia K, Georgalas C, Fokkens W, Miszkiel K, Lund VJ. 2009. Maxillary mucosal cyst is not a manifestation of rhinosinusitis: results of prospective three-dimentional CT study of ophthalmic patients. Laryngoscope 119(1):8-12

[39] Gardner DG. Pseudocysts and retention cysts of the maxillary sinus. 1984. Oral Surg Oral Med Oral Pathol 58(5):561-567

[40] Casamassimo PS, lilly GE. 1980. Mucosal cysts of the maxillary sinus: a clinical and radiographic study. Oral Surg Oral Med Oral Pathol 50(3):282-286

[41] Fisher EW, Whittet HB, Croft CB. 1989. Symptomatic mucosal cysts of the maxillary sinus:antroscopic treatment. J Laryngol Otol 103(12):1184-1186

[42] Maldonado M, Martinez A, Alobid I, Mullol J. 2004. The antrochoanal polyp. Rhinology 42(4):178-182

[43] Mahfouz ME, Elsheikh MN, Ghoname NF. 2006. Molecular profile of the antrochoanalpolyp:up-regulation of basic fibroblast growth factor and transforming growth factor beta in maxillary sinusmucosa. Am J Rhinol 20(4):178-182

[44] Aydin O, Keskin G, Ustundag E, Iseri M, Ozkarakas H. 2007. Choanal polyps:an evaluation of 53cases. Am j Rhinol 21(2):164-168

[45] Deshazo RD, 2009. Syndromes of invasive fungal sinusitis. Med Mycol 47(Suppl 1):S309-S314

[46] Michael RC, Michael JS, Ashbee RH, Matthews MS. 2008. Mucological profile of fungal sinusitis:an audit of specimens over a 7-year period in a tertiary care hospital in Tamil Nadu. Indian J PatholMicrobiol 51(4): 493-496 Abstract

[47] Plszewski J, Milonski J. 2008. The analysis of the bacterial and fungal flora in maxillary sinuses in patients operated due to FESS method. Otolaryngol Pol 62(4):458-461

[48] Ferguson BJ. 2000. Fungal balls of the paranasal sinuses. Otolaryngol Clin North Am 33(2):389-398

[49] Ferreiro JA, Carlson BA, Cody DT. 1997. Paranasal sinus fungal balls. Head Neck 19(6):481-486

[50] Klossek JM, Serrano E, Peloquin L, Percodi J, Fontanel JP, Pessey JJ. 1997. Functional endoscopic sinus surgery and 109 mycetomas of paranasal sinuses. Laryngoscope 107(1):112-117

[51] Friedmann I, Osborn DA. 1982. Pathology of granulomas and neoplasms of the nose and paranasal sinuses. In: WStCSymmers, ed. Systemic Pathology. Edinburgh/London/New York:Churchill Livingston:1920235

[52] Astarci HM, Sungu N, Samim EE, Ustun H. 2008. Presence of cholesterol granuloma in the maxillary and ethmoid sinuses. Oral Maxillofac Surg 12(2):101-103

[53] Chao TK. 2006. Cholesterol granuloma of the maxillary sinus. Eur Arch Otorhinolaryngol 263(6):592-597

[54] Graham J, Michaels L. 1978. Cholesterol, granuloma of the maxillary antrum. Clin Otolaryngol Allied Sci 3(@):155-160

[55] Niho M. 1986. Cholesterol crystals in the temporal bone and the paranasal sinuses. Int J Pediatr Otorhinolaryngol 11(1):79-95

[56] Kunt T, Ozturkan S, Egilmez R. 1998. Cholesterol granuloma of the maxillary sinus: six cases from the same region. J Laryngol Otol 112(1):65-68

[57] Lim M, Lew-Ghor S, Beale T, Ramsay A, Lund VJ. 2008. Maxillary sinus haematoma. J Laryngol Otol 122(2): 210-212

[58] Song HM, Jang YJ, Chung YS, Lee BJ. 2007. Organizing hematoma of the maxillary sinus. Otolaryngol Head Neck Surg 136(4):616-620

[59] LeePK, Wu JK, Ludemann JP. 2004. Hemorrhagic pseudotumor of the maxillary sinus. J Otolaryngol 33(3):206-208

[60] Ozhan S, Arac M, Isik S, Oznur 11, Atilla S, Kemaloglu Y. 1996. Pseudotumor of the maxillary sinus in a patient with von Willebrand's disease. Am J Roentgenol 166(4): 950-951

[61] Lee BJ, Park HJ, Hoe SC. 2003. Organized hematoma of the maxillary sinus, Acta Otolaryngol 123(7): 869-872

[62] Tabaee A, Kacker A. 2002. Hematoma of the maxillary sinus presenting as a mass- a case report and review of literature. Int J Pediatr Otorhinolaryngol 65(2):153-157

[63] Guneri P, Kaya A, Caliskan MK. 2005. Antroliths:survey of the literature and report of a case. Oral Surg Oral Med Oral Pathol Oral Radiol Endod 99(4):517-521

[64] Kosarac O, Luna MA, RoJ Y, Ayala AG. 2008. Eosinophilic angiocentric fibrosis of the sinonasal tract. Ann Diagn Pathol 12(4):267-270

[65] Paun S, Lund VJ, Gallimore A. 2005. Nasal fibrosis:long-term follow-up of four cases of Eosinophilic angiocentric fibrosis. J Laryngol Otol 119(2):119-124

[66] Lund VJ. 2000. Optimum management of inverted papilloma. J Laryngol Otol 114(3): 194-197

[67] Michaels L. 1996. Benign mucosal tumors of the nose and paranasal sinuses. Semi-n Diagn Pathol 13(2):113-117

[68] Minovi A, Kollert M, Draf W, Bockmuhl U. 2006. Inverted papilloma: feasibility of endonasal surgery and long-term results of 87 cases. Rhinology 44(3):205-210

[69] Savy L, Lloyd G, Lund VJ, Howard D. Optimum imaging for inverted papilloma. J Laryngol Otol 114(11):891-893

[70] Mirza S, Bradley PJ, Acharya A, Stacey M, Jones NS. 2007. Sinonasal inverted papillomas:recurrence and synchoronous and metachronous malignancy. J Laryngol Otol 121(9):857-864

[71] Lin HL, Huang CC, Lee TJ. 2004. Endoscopic sinus surgery treatment for a huge sinonasal fibroma. Chang Gung Med J 27(3):233-237

[72] Uysal A, Kayiran O, Cuzdan SS, Bektas CI, Aslan G, Caydere M. 2007. Maxillary sinus lipoma:an unanticipated diagnosis. J Craniofac Surg 18(5):1153-1155

[73] Gregor RT, Loftus-Coll B. 1994. Myxoma of the paranasal sinuses. J Laryngol Otol 108(8):679-681

[74] Rabaso E, Rosell A, Plaza G, Martinez-Vidal A. Haemangioma of the maxillary sinus. J Laryngol Otol 111(7):638-640

[75] Fyrmpas G, Constantinidis J, Televantou D, Konstantinidis I, Daniilidis J. 2006. Primary aneurismal bone cyst of the maxillary sinus in a child: case report and review of the literature. Eur Arch Otorhinolaryngol 263(7):695-698

[76] Herve S, AbdAlsamad I, Beautru R, et al. 1993. Management of sinonasal hemangiopericytomas. Rhinology 37(4):153-158

[77] Stomeo F, Fois V, Cossu A, Meloni F, Pastore A, Bozzo C. 2004. Sinonasal hemangiopericytoma: a case report. Eur Arch Otorhinolaryngol 261(10): 555-557

[78] LaBruna A, Reagan B, Papageorge A, 1995. Leiomyoma of the maxillary sinus; a diagnostic dilemma. Otolaryngol Head Neck Surg 112(4): 595-598

[79] Fu YS, Perkin KH. 1976. Nonepithelial tumors of the nasal cavity, paranasal sinuses and nasopharynx: a clinicopathologic study of skeletal muscle tumors(rhabdomyoma and rhabdosarcoma). Cancer 37(1):364-376

[80] Reitter GS. 1921. Rhabdomyosarcoma of the nose: report of case. JAMA 76:22-23

[81] Eller R, Sillers M. 2006. Common fibro-osseous lesions of the paranasal sinuses. Otolaryngol Clin North Am 39(3): 585-600

[82] Alexander AA, Patel AA, Odland R. 2007. Paranasal sinus osteomas and Gardner's syndrome. Ann OtolRhinolLaryngol 116(6):658-662

[83] Park W, Kim HS. 2006. Osteoma of maxillary sinus: a case report. Oral Surg Oral Med Oral Pathol Oral Radiol Endod 102(6):e26-e27

[84] Harrison DF. 1984. Osseous and fibro-osseous conditions affecting the craniofacial bones. Ann OtolRhinolLaryngol 93(3 Pt 1):199-203

[85] Chong VF, Tan LH. 1997. Maxillary sinus ossifying fibroma. Am J Otolaryngol 18(6): 419-424

[86] Muraoka H, Ishihara A, Kumagai J. 2001. Fibrous dysplasia with cystic appearance in maxillary sinus. Auris Nasus Larynx 28(1):103-105

[87] Jones AC, Prihoda TJ, Kacher JE, Odingo NA, Freedman PD. 2006. Osteoblastoma of the maxilla and mandible: A report of 24 cases and review of literature and discus-

sion of its relationship to osteodosteoma of the jaw. Oral Surg Oral Med Oral Pathol Oral Radiol Endod 102(5):639-650

[88] Osguthorpe JD, Hungerford GD. 1983. Benign osteoblastoma of the maxillary sinus. Head Neck Surg 6(1): 605-609

[89] Sarioglu S, Ozkal S, Guneri A, et al 2002. Cystic schwannoma of the maxillary sinus. Auris Nasus Larynx 29(3):297-300

[90] Sheikh HY, Chakravathy RP, Slevin NJ, Sykes AJ, Banerjee SS. 208. Benign schwannoma in paranasl sinuses: a clinic-patological study of five cases emphasizing diagnostic difficulties. J Laryngol Otol 122(6):598-602

[91] Boedeker CC, Ridder GJ, Kayser G, Schipper J, Maier W. 2005. Solitary neurofibroma of the maxillary sinus and pterygopalatine fossa. Otolaryngol Head Neck Surg 133(3): 458-459

Permissions

All chapters in this book were first published by InTech Open; hereby published with permission under the Creative Commons Attribution License or equivalent. Every chapter published in this book has been scrutinized by our experts. Their significance has been extensively debated. The topics covered herein carry significant findings which will fuel the growth of the discipline. They may even be implemented as practical applications or may be referred to as a beginning point for another development.

The contributors of this book come from diverse backgrounds, making this book a truly international effort. This book will bring forth new frontiers with its revolutionizing research information and detailed analysis of the nascent developments around the world.

We would like to thank all the contributing authors for lending their expertise to make the book truly unique. They have played a crucial role in the development of this book. Without their invaluable contributions this book wouldn't have been possible. They have made vital efforts to compile up to date information on the varied aspects of this subject to make this book a valuable addition to the collection of many professionals and students.

This book was conceptualized with the vision of imparting up-to-date information and advanced data in this field. To ensure the same, a matchless editorial board was set up. Every individual on the board went through rigorous rounds of assessment to prove their worth. After which they invested a large part of their time researching and compiling the most relevant data for our readers.

The editorial board has been involved in producing this book since its inception. They have spent rigorous hours researching and exploring the diverse topics which have resulted in the successful publishing of this book. They have passed on their knowledge of decades through this book. To expedite this challenging task, the publisher supported the team at every step. A small team of assistant editors was also appointed to further simplify the editing procedure and attain best results for the readers.

Apart from the editorial board, the designing team has also invested a significant amount of their time in understanding the subject and creating the most relevant covers. They scrutinized every image to scout for the most suitable representation of the subject and create an appropriate cover for the book.

The publishing team has been an ardent support to the editorial, designing and production team. Their endless efforts to recruit the best for this project, has resulted in the accomplishment of this book. They are a veteran in the field of academics and their pool of knowledge is as vast as their experience in printing. Their expertise and guidance has proved useful at every step. Their uncompromising quality standards have made this book an exceptional effort. Their encouragement from time to time has been an inspiration for everyone.

The publisher and the editorial board hope that this book will prove to be a valuable piece of knowledge for researchers, students, practitioners and scholars across the globe.

List of Contributors

Pinakin Gunvant Davey
Western University of Health Sciences, College of Optometry, Pomona, CA, USA

Fatih C. Gundogan
GATA Medical School, Ophthalmology, Ankara, Turkey

Umit Yolcu
Siirt Military Hospital, Ophthalmology, Siirt, Turkey

Jie Shen
College of Optometry, Western University of Health Sciences, USA

Vikas Tah
Stoke Mandeville Hospital, UK
Moorfields Eye Hospital, UK

Sonia Mall
Oxford Eye Hospital, UK

James Myerscough
Colchester Hospital University Foundation Trust, UK

Kamran Saha and Daren Hanumunthadu
Moorfields Eye Hospital, UK

Elizabeth Emsley
Imperial College London, UK

Ganeshan Ramsamy and Mandeep Bindra
Stoke Mandeville Hospital, UK

Bennett McAllister
Low Vision, American Academy of Optometry, USA
Primary Care Service, College of Optometry, Western University of Health Sciences, Pomona, California, USA

Andrew Swampillai
Barts and The London School of Medicine and Dentistry, UK

Rebecca Kammer
Low Vision, American Academy of Optometry, USA

Cintia S. de Paiva, De-Quan Li and Stephen C. Pflugfelder
The Ocular Surface Center, Cullen Eye Institute, Department of Ophthalmology, Baylor College of Medicine, USA

Andrew J.W. Huang
Department of Ophthalmology and Visual Sciences, School of Medicine, Washington University, St. Louis, MO, USA

Peizeng Yang, Chaokui Wang, Shengping Hou and Bo Lei
The First Affiliated Hospital of Chongqing Medical University, Chongqing Key Lab of Ophthalmology, Chongqing Eye Institute, Chongqing, P. R. China

Aize Kijlstra
University Eye Clinic Maastricht, Maastricht, Netherlands

Balwant Singh Gendeh
Department of Otorhinolaryngology-Head Neck Surgery, UKM Medical Center, Jalan Yaacob Latif, Bandar Tun Razak, Kuala Lumpur, Malaysia

Index

www.ingramcontent.com/pod-product-compliance
Lightning Source LLC
LaVergne TN
LVHW062234200926
848484LV00006B/1537